# YOGA OF THE GUHYASAMĀJATANTRA

# BUDDHIST TRADITION SERIES

Edited by
ALEX WAYMAN



**VOLUME 17**

# Yoga of the Guhyasamājatantra

*THE ARCANE LORE OF FORTY VERSES*
*A Buddhist Trantra Commentary*

ALEX WAYMAN

MOTILAL BANARSIDASS PUBLISHERS
PRIVATE LIMITED • DELHI

*First Edition: Delhi, 1977*
*Reprint: Delhi, 1980, 1991, 1999*



ISBN: 81-208-0872-x

*Also available at:*

MOTILAL BANARSIDASS

41 U.A. Bungalow Road, Jawahar Nagar, Delhi 110 007
8 Mahalaxmi Chamber, Warden Road, Mumbai 400 026
120 Royapettah High Road, Mylapore, Chennai 600 004
Sanas Plaza, 1302 Baji Rao Road, Pune 411 002
16 St. Mark's Road, Bangalore 560 001
8 Camac Street, Calcutta 700 017
Ashok Rajpath, Patna 800 004
Chowk, Varanasi 221 001

PRINTED IN INDIA
BY JAINENDRA PRAKASH JAIN AT SHRI JAINENDRA PRESS,
A-45 NARAINA, PHASE I, NEW DELHI 110 028
AND PUBLISHED BY NARENDRA PRAKASH JAIN FOR
MOTILAL BANARSIDASS PUBLISHERS PRIVATE LIMITED,
BUNGALOW ROAD, DELHI 110 007

To

Professor Murray B. Emeneau,

Who set the standard

difficult to sustain

# FOREWORD

This work is based on the Sanskrit-Tibetan commentarial tradition. The chief commentary on the *Guhyasamājatantra* in the Tibetan tradition is the *Pradīpoddyotana*; and when the first edition of the present work was prepared, and published in 1977, there was available the photographic manuscript of the *Pradīpoddyotana*, first at the Bihar Research Society and subsequently at the K.P. Jayaswal Research Institute, both in Patna. This manuscript was much utilized in the form supplied by the Jayaswal Institute. In 1984 a Sanskrit version of the *Pradīpoddyotana* was published by the Jayaswal Institute in the form edited by Chintaharan Chakravarti; and which presumably inspired a review of *Yoga of the Guhyasamājatantra* in ABORI, 1988 (Poona, 1989). The work *Yoga of* must have made it easy to notice that this Sanskrit edition has a number of errors. This was necessarily the case for a Sanskrit edition of a Tantra being made from a unique manuscript without consultation of the careful Tibetan translation.

Therefore, a few words are necessary about this *Pradīpoddyotana* commentary. At the year-end 1976 to 1977, the writer was at Darbhanga, staying at the K.S.D. Sanskrit University, whose Vice-Chancellor at that time was Dr. Ram Karan Sharma. Dr. Anantalal Thakur, who had been invited by Dr. Sharma, was there with the draft manuscript of the *Pradīpoddyotana* as edited by Prof. Chakravarti and which Dr. Thakur was trying to get in shape for publishing. Dr. Thakur asked the writer if he thought this is a good commentary. It was clear that he was not much impressed with it. Now, it should be explained that the *Pradīpoddyotana* by the tantric author Candrakīrti was accepted in Tibet as the chief commentary on the *Guhyasamāja* (which enjoys a huge commentarial tradition translated into Tibetan), not because it necessarily presents the best comments throughout on the basic text but because it is based on the six alternative interpretations (*ṣaṭkoṭivyākhyā*) and the four kinds of explanation of a given passage (see herein, pp. 116-7). Accordingly, the *Pradīpoddyotana* is the tradition which claims that the *Guhyasamājatantra* cannot be understood by reading it. It is necessary to have gurus to explain it, and the study of the basic text requires commentaries that allow for varying interpretations. Although such information was in the work herein reprinted, some essays have appeared subsequently where the authors write as though they can understand the verses whether or not they consult commentaries. This tradition holds that such a person first deceives oneself and then others. Now, someone might argue that even without a commentary, one may notice the Sanskrit that is there and understand it by one's knowledge of the Sanskrit language. There are numerous examples which could be cited to clarify this issue; but one will suffice, namely, *Guhyasamāja*, Chap. VII, 2, as B. Bhattacharya edits it (I transcribe): */sarvakāmopabhogais tu sevyamānair yathecchataḥ/svādhidaivatayogena parāṅgaiś ca prapūjayet/*Doubtless, B. Bhattacharya and his copier S. Bagchi are excellent Sanskritists and yet neither noticed that *parāṅgaiś* is a corruption; and Yūkei Matsunaga is doubtless competent and yet repeats the same corruption in both his editions of the text. In the present work, Appendix III, I have discussed this verse, and have cited the *Pradīpoddyotana* manuscript entry *svātmānaṃ parāṃś ca* (now confirmed by the edition of the Sanskrit) as indicating its reading of the basic text, namely, *svaṃ parāṃś ca*, or the equivalent. By consultation of a commentary it was possible to show the two objects of the verb *prapūjayet*, and to correct the basic text. It follows that the three editors above named when they came to this verse saw only words and copied only words. No idea of the verse's meaning could flash upon their minds, even in a literal sense. And if anyone had attempted to translate it on the basis of the editions so presented, their translation would not be of a verse of the *Guhyasamājatantra*, since the original author could rightfully declare: "That is not my verse!" One great value of a commentary is of course to get its testimonial on what were the actual words of the basic text. And this is quite apart from whether it is a "good" commentary. Perhaps the question should be reformulated to: "What is it good for?" The *Pradīpoddyotana* is certainly good for showing what the lineage of gurus would themselves like the reader to understand of the basic text. Another commentary I sometimes utilized, that of Celupā, is good for answering questions that the reader might ask about the verses.

The writer has sometimes been asked: What is the oldest Tantra? A difficulty of response to such a question is that the material now called 'Tantra' may have preexisted in a form not called 'Tantra'. That is to say, probably the oldest Tantra of the Western side of India—and in the South—is the *Mañjuśrī-mūla-tantra*; but in the edition of T. Gaṇapati Sāstrī at Trivandrum, it is called *Ārya-Mañjuśrī-mūlakalpa*; and here probably only the first of the three volume should be accepted as 'old', and probably to be placed in the fourth century, A.D. It may be that the *Guhyasamājatantra* is the first Tantra to be called a 'Tantra'; and in the work herein I have tentatively placed it in the fourth century, A.D. and should add that it first circulated in the Eastern side of India, in the country called Vaṅga, later Bengal. The work whose main title is *Vairocanābhisaṃbodhi*, is called a Tantra in Tibet but a Sūtra in Sino-Japanese Buddhism; and in the work *Enlightenment of Vairocana* which is being published by Motilal Banarsidass I have placed it at mid-sixth century in the area now called Maharashtra. Thus, it appears that the works in the tantric section of the Tibetan canon that arose in the Western side of India—and in the South, were not originally called 'tantra'; but the name 'tantra' was applied to certain works that originated in the Eastern side of India, particularly what is now called Bengal. Accordingly, it appears that the term 'tantra' is due to a movement in North-east India. Later, in the commentarial period (approx. eighth through twelfth centuries) the term 'tantra' was more generally applied; and the resultant large literature of 'tantra' had to be sorted out in different classes; and so arose such classifications as Kriyā-tantra, Caryā-tantra, Yoga-tantra, and Anuttarayoga-tantra. In such classifications, the *Mañjuśrī-mūla-kalpa* is put in the Kriyā-tantra; the *Vairocanābhisaṃbodhi* in the Caryā-tantra; and the *Guhyasamājatantra* in the Anuttarayoga-tantra. It follows that such classifying words as 'Kriyā-tantra' are independent of the historical arising of the included works. It is certain that the entirety of the Buddhist tantric movement is to be placed in the time of Mahāyāna Buddhism. Yet certain practices in the tantric works are much older. For example, the practice of mantras is pre-Upaniṣadic, and the practice of *yoga* may be older in India than the Āryan invaders who brought into India the earliest portion of the *Ṛg-veda*. Deities were assigned to the four cardinal directions and then to the four intermediate directions long before the rise of the earliest Buddhism.

The *Chāndogya-upaniṣad* (III, 13) already had the theory of five doorkeepers of the world of heaven, and they are the five 'breaths'. The palace within the Buddhist *maṇḍala* is a kind of elaboration descended from the old Vedic compound, with an intermediary of the Buddhist Stūpa such as the one at Sanchi. A literature called the Yoga-Upaniṣads with many features of the later tantras was circulating probably in the early centuries, A.D.

Thus, when someone raised in a learned Buddhist family and educated in the Sanskrit language from an early age, and steeped in the esoteric traditions of India, decided to write the book known as the *Guhyasamājatantra*, this person did not have to invent new esoteric theories. The task was to combine this ancient lore with the terminology of Mahāyāna Buddhism. In all likelihood, the unknown author of this Tantra was a lay Buddhist who did not feel obligated to defend the formal statements of Buddhist doctrine. Accordingly, when in Chap. II, the author presents the two kinds of *bodhicitta*—the conventional (*saṃvṛti*) and the absolute (*paramārtha*), this is not done in a manner repeating the standard Bodhisattva treatises. The author had a talent for compressing much in small spaces. So in the century following this composition, an extensive literature of 'explanatory tantras' arose. By the time of the named commentators, the *Guhyasamājatantra* had become a sort of mysterious, abstruse cord of jewel-like ideas.

The present writer somehow found out how to approach this Tantra, and used the forty verses as an organizational means to assemble materials from Sanskrit and Tibetan sources. This enabled me to bring into a Western language a fund of materials not previously found in Western languages and which was disconcertingly pertinent to the announced topic, "Yoga of the Guhyasamājatantra".

December, 1990 ALEX WAYMAN

# PREFACE

The work here presented to the public is an organization of materials from the *Guhyasamājatantra* cycle, stressing the aspect of *yoga*, with sufficient introductory treatments to enable the reader to place this remarkable literature within the general frame of Indian thought and religious practice, which has already made world-wide contributions to the theory of *yoga*.

The set of forty verses was memorized for centuries by followers of the 'Ārya' *Guhyasamāja* tradition, which claims that these verses explain the entire (*Guhyasamāja*) Tantra. I made up a title, the '*Guhyasamāja-nidāna-kārikā*', for those verses (*kārikā*) which go with each syllable of the initial sentence (*nidāna*) of the *Guhyasamājatantra*. The verses stem from the Explanatory Tantra *Vajramālā*, and were extant in the original Sanskrit by reason of being cited in the *Pradīpoddyotana* manuscript.

As the synthetic commentary on the verses became increasingly technical, considerable introductory material was indicated; and this grew to three introductions before I was satisfied with the standard of clarification. Thus the reader has a bridge to the verses, which in turn have been sufficiently annotated to bring out their individual character.

Having long ago become aware of the hazards of speculating on the intricate subject of the Tantra, I have tried at every point to bring forward the authentic and reliable passages, whether in Sanskrit or Tibetan. But I do not deny my own contribution of selecting, translating, and organizing this material; and especially the decision to group the forty verses according to the steps of *yoga*.

Since most of the material in this book has not hitherto appeared in Western sources, certainly as far as English is concerned, I have preferred to give the original passages. However, I have omitted the Tibetan for Tsoṅ-kha-pa's *Mchan ḥgrel* on the forty verses, because the interlinear form of this annotation renders it difficult to cite separately; and there are some other omissions of Tibetan. The reader will soon notice my overwhelming use of Tsoṅ-kha-pa's works. His writing is like the personal message of a guru, for it is always to explain, not to conceal. The Tibetan chronicle called *The Blue Annals* has a most eloquent tribute to Tsoṅ-kha-pa for his authoritative works on the *Guhyasamāja* system.

The concluded research is the outcome of a long-time aspiration. My original delving into the major theories is found in my first major published article, "Notes on the Sanskrit term Jñāna" (1955). Already I knew about the forty verses and that they are quoted in the *Pradipoddyotana* because they are mentioned in an important context in *Mkhas grub rje's Fundamentals of the Buddhist Tantras*; the late Professor F.D. Lessing and myself collaborated on a translation of tnis Tibetan book during the 1950's even though it was not published until 1968. I realized that to do anything scholarly with the forty verses I would have to obtain the original Sanskrit, which was presumably in the *Pradipoddyotana* manuscript of the Bihar Research Society. During my faculty research in India from February 1963 to January 1964, sponsored by the American Institute of Indian Studies, it became part of a wonderful memory of 1963 Divāli days in Patna that the Bihar Research Society in conjunction with the K.P. Jayaswal Institute graciously arranged for me to secure an enlargement of the *Pradipoddyotana* manuscript, for which I am most grateful. On December 24, 1963, the author was granted an interview with the Dalai Lama at Dharamsala (Punjab, India) during which His Holiness expressed delight to learn that the forty 'revelation' verses explaining the initial sentence of the *Guhyasamāja* were extant in that unique manuscript. He mentioned a Tibetan tradition that there had been an Indian commentary on these forty verses not translated into the Tibetan language, and asked to be informed if such a Sanskrit commentary were to turn up. It is a special pleasure of this research that the present modest incursion into the vast *Guhyasamāja* lore leads to the publication in India of this commentary on the nidāna verses, which thus becomes an 'Indian commentary' in a sense. If an old Sanskrit commentary ever turns up, the contents should overlap, but the fact that the data has been sifted through a Western consciousness will have brought many changes of outer form.

Upon returning to my position of those days in Madison, Wisconsin, with the help of the Tibetan version I edited the forty verses in Sanskrit, which along with the Tibetan and English translations, heads the 'Documents'. As time went on, I collected materials for a synthetic commentary, on which account I must pay tribute to the remarkably convenient Japanese photographic edition of the Peking Kanjur-Tanjur and of Tsoṅ-kha-pa's collected works, all of which has contributed so much to this endeavor. The early integrating labor was pursued in part-time research in the Fall of 1965 supported by Ford Area funds of The University of Wisconsin; and I tried out some of the subject matter in my seminars on tantric Buddhism at Madison in Spring 1966 and at Columbia (as a visitor) in Fall 1966. In Summer 1966, I put together a manuscript that had considerable information on the subject. The Department of Indian Studies in Madison kindly afforded me secretarial assistance for typing up these technical materials. During the next academic year I decided to include even more new data while publishing such a book. During the Summer 1967 in a special teaching and research arrangement by my department in Madison, I selected from the photographic edition of the Tibetan canon a great amount of works or portions of works dealing with these and kindred topics. My assistant, Mr. Kio Kanda, duplicated all those pages on the excellent machine of the University-Industry Research Program in Madison by the cooperation of the ladies in that office. This provided me maximum ease of consulting texts as desired. In my new position at Columbia University starting in Fall 1967 I found some leisure from time to time for perusing more of the relevant texts, and for making more use of the *Pradīpoddyotana* manuscript, which however, is only of interest to me for completing this book. The sabbatical year (1969-70) allowed me by Columbia University afforded me some leisure for further improvements and corrections. I am confident that the delays have considerably strengthened the contribution to knowledge of this tantric system, and that any future investigator of this or associated Buddhist tantric literature will find in this a rich reference work.

An important observation of comparing the basic text of the *Guhyasamājatantra* with its commentaries, and in particular, with the kind of ideas found in the forty verses and their annotation, is that the commentarial literature brings forth an array of data that is not at all apparent in the basic Tantra. This observation leads to the surprising conclusion that one cannot evaluate the *Guhyasamājatantra* in its edited Sanskrit form simply by reading it, which is the premise of the modern-day condemnation of the Tantra. Adding to the difficulty is the loss in original Sanskrit of most of the commentarial works; which, fortunately, are almost all available in fine Tibetan translations. But few specialists are prepared to exploit these Tibetan works. For example, the only published paper that I know of as employing Tsoṅ-kha-pa's *Mchan ḥgrel* to any extent is Giuseppe Tucci's "Some glosses upon the *Guhyasamāja*." Tucci also explored the *Guhyasamāja maṇḍala* in his *Indo-Tibetica* and in his work translated into English under the title *The Theory and Practice of the Mandala.* Without any reflection on those previous efforts, it still follows that the subject of the *Guhyasamāja* has an importance deserving its own book. I believe it fair to say that the very effort of integrating materials from the vast sources has brought this system into a focus not hitherto possible with those—other than Professor Tucci—who only brushed against it in the dark and then praised or blamed.

It is a pleasure to recall the helpful conversations with Dr. Rasik Vihari Joshi about some of the Sanskrit verses included in this book.

An explanation is due the readers who expected this work to appear some years ago, since it was submitted to a publisher in South India late in 1969. Through no fault of that publisher but only of troubles in his city, it was finally necessary to resubmit it to the present publisher. I am indeed grateful to Shree N. P. Jain of Motilal Banarsidass to have undertaken this work and given it a speedy processing. However, those who appreciate the appendixes should thank the publishing delay. Also, in the meantime Samuel Weiser, Inc. of New York, published another work of mine on the Buddhist Tantras, with materials mostly different from the content of the present work , just as this one is so different from *Mkhas grub rje's Fundamentals of the Buddhist Tantras.* This should point attention to the almost inexhaustible character of the Buddhist Tantras.

New York City — Alex Wayman
July 1977

## CONTENTS

## TABLES

## Part One

# DOCUMENTS

The purpose of placing the documents first is to expose the *Guhyasamājatantra* on its literal level. This was always the initial step in the traditional understanding of Buddhism, pursuant to the 'three instructions' (*śikṣā-traya*), 'insight consisting of hearing', 'insight consisting of contemplation,' 'insight consisting of cultivation (or putting into practice)'. That is to say, Buddhism always acknowledged a kind of 'insight' (*prajñā*) for the elementary step of exposure to the text when it was accompanied by devotion even if necessitating personal discomfort. The subsequent introductions, annotation of the forty verses, and appendices, all represent the 'pondering' level for this study.

While the documents provide the most elementary level of 'insight', the form in which they are exhibited here has some advantage over their service to the reader of edited Sanskrit texts. In particular, a number of corrections have been made to the Sanskrit text of Chapters Six and Twelve, *Guhyasamājatantra*, prior to their translation. Again, a portion of the *Pradīpoddyotana* commentary on Chapter Twelve is presented from an unedited work, and the same holds for the forty verses themselves, here edited in Sanskrit. Also, the translations of the two chapters and the extract of comment on Chapter Twelve have been slightly expanded by the use of commentarial and subcommentarial materials, mainly available in Tibetan. Of course, the theory of 'insight consisting of hearing' takes for granted that the text itself is correct. Thus considerable care has been taken with the Documents to meet this condition laid down for 'insight'.

I. The Guhyasamāja-nidāna - kārikā (Sanskrit - Tibetan-English). This section of the 'documents' exhibits samples of the languages employed: Sanskrit and Tibetan for research purposes, and English for translation and communication purposes.

The *nidāna* is the formula at the outset of the *Guhyasamājatantra* : Evam mayā śrutam ekasmin samaye bhagavān sarvatathāgatakāyavākcittahṛdaya-vajrayoṣidbhageṣu vijahāra. The word *nidāna* is being employed in the sense of 'primary cause', that is to say, the cause of the entire *Guhyasamājatantra*. The forty syllables of that formula serve mnemonic purpose as initials of forty verses (*kārikā*) : (1) E, (2) vaṃ, (3) ma, (4) yā, (5) śru, (6) tam, (7) e, (8) ka, (9) smin, (10) sa, (11) ma, (12) ye, (13) bha, (14) ga, (15) vān, (16) sa, (17) rva, (18) ta, (19) thā, (20) ga, (21) ta, (22) kā, (23) ya, (24) vāk, (25) cit, (26) ta, (27) hṛ, (28) da, (29) ya, (30) va, (31) jra, (32) yo, (33) ṣid, (34) bha, (35) ge, (36) ṣu, (37) vi, (38) ja, (39) hā, (40) ra.

The original Sanskrit of the forty verses is here edited from the *Pradīpoddyotana* manuscript, the Tibetan translation from the Derge Tanjur edition of the *Pradīpoddyotana* and from the version of the Tantra *Vajramālā* in the Peking Tibetan Tripiṭaka edition. There are relatively few textual problems. The Sanskrit manuscript gives the syllables *ci* and *tta* for nidāna verses 25 and 26, but I followed the Tibetan phonetic transcription, since *cit* and *ta* correspond more closely to the initial words of the Sanskrit verses. Nidāna verse 20 has a defective *pāda* in the manuscript, *gacchaty indriyas tat tat*. But the scribe had erased a syllable, leading to my solution : *gacchann asty indriyas tat tat*. The correction *gacchann asty* is justified by the Tibetan equivalence *ḥgro bar ḥgyur ba*.

The Tibetan text here presented follows the *Vajramālā* except for some obvious corruptions remedied with the *Pradīpoddyotana* version. The translation *snaṅ ba gsal ba* is the old one for nidāna verse 4's *ālokābhāsa*; the standard translation is *snaṅ ba mched pa*.

ए । एकारोपि सती प्रज्ञा विरामादिक्षणात्मिका ।

एतन्मूलं विनिर्दिष्टं परिज्ञानं भवत्रये ॥ [1]

ཨེ། ཨེ་ནི་ཤེས་རབ་དམ་པ་སྟེ། |

འདོད་ཆགས་བྲལ་སོགས་སྐད་ཅིག་བདག |

སྲིད་པ་གསུམ་ན་ཡོངས་ཤེས་པ། |

འདི་ནི་རྩ་བར་རྣམ་པར་བསྟན། |

"E" is the Noble woman (satī) Prajñā, the moments of aversion, and so on. This root is designated as the experience in the three worlds.

वं । वंशस्तद्द भवदाभाति रागादिप्रसवान्विताम् ।

आलोकाभासविज्ञानमुपाय इति संज्ञितम् ॥ [2]

བཾ། འོད་མ་བསྐྱིང་བ་ལྟར་མཛེས་ཤིང་། |

ཆགས་ལ་སོགས་པ་རབ་སྐྱེད་ལྡན། |

སྣང་བ་གསལ་བ་རྣམ་པར་ཤེས། |

མིང་ནི་ཐབས་ཞེས་བྱ་བ་ཡིན། |

That Spread-of-Light *vijñāna* called 'means' (*upāya*), attended with begetting of desire, and so on, appears like an emerging bamboo.

म । महाविद्या स्वयं मूलमविद्याया विलोमतः ।

अविद्यया भवेच्चैतत्तस्मादालोकसंभवः ॥ [3]

མ། རིག་ཆེན་རང་ཉིད་རྩ་བ་སྟེ། །
མ་རིག་པ་ནི་ལྡོག་པ་ཡིན། །
མ་རིག་པ་ལས་འདི་འབྱུང་བས། །
དེ་ལས་སྣང་བ་འབྱུང་བའོ། །

In the reverse order, the great Science (=Wisdom) is itself the root of nescience. And the ('Spread-of-Light') arises from nescience (*avidyā*) while from that ('Spread-of-Light') arises Light.

या । याति विज्ञानमादौ तदालोकाभाससंज्ञितम् ।

तन् महाशून्यतां याति सा च याति प्रभास्वरम् ॥ [4]

ཡཱ། འགྲོ་བ་རྣམ་ཤེས་གསུམ་དང་པོ་ནི། །
དེ་མིང་སྣང་བ་གསལ་བ་སྟེ། །
དེ་ནི་སྟོང་པ་ཆེར་འགྱུར་ལ། །
དེ་ཡང་འོད་གསལ་བར་འགྲོའོ། །

At first, that *vijñāna* (i.e. Light) passes to what is called 'Spread-of-Light'. That passes to the great Void, and the latter passes to the Clear Light.

श्रु। श्रुतं यदिह विज्ञानमाभासत्रयलक्षणम् ।
प्रकृतीनामिदं मूलं सत्त्वधातोरशेषतः ।। [5]

ཤྲུ། སྣང་བ་གསུམ་གྱི་མཚན་ཉིད་ཅན། །
གང་འདི་རྣམ་ཤེས་གསུམ་ཐོས་པ། །
སེམས་ཅན་ཁམས་ནི་མ་ལུས་པའི། །
རང་བཞིན་རྩ་བ་འདི་ཡིན་ནོ། །

The *vijñāna* heard here has the characteristics of the three lights. This is entirely the root of the *prakṛtis* (natures) of the sentient-being realm.

तं। तमेकैकमर्थाभासं वायुस् संगृह्य धारयेत् ।
वायुयुक्तं च विज्ञानं शश्वज्जगति वर्तते ।। [6]

ཏཾ། དེ་ནི་རེ་རེའི་དོན་སྣང་བ། །
རླུང་གིས་བླངས་ན་འཛིན་བྱེད་ལ། །
རླུང་དང་ལྡན་པའི་རྣམ་ཤེས་ནི། །
ཀུན་ཏུ་འགྲོ་ལ་གནས་པར་འགྱུར། །

The wind seizing, takes hold of that entity-light in each case, and *vijñāna* joined with wind continually operates in the world of living beings.

ए। एषो वायुर्महाधातुर्विज्ञानत्रयवाहनः।
तेभ्यः प्रकृतयः शश्वन्निर्गच्छन्ति यथा यथा ॥ [7]

ཨེ། འདི་ནི་རླུང་ཁམས་ཆེན་པོ་སྟེ། །
རྣམ་ཤེས་གསུམ་གྱི་བཞོན་པ་ཡིན། །
དེ་ཡིས་རང་བཞིན་དག་དུ་ནི། །
ཇི་ལྟ་ཇི་ལྟར་འགྲོ་བར་འགྱུར། །

This wind, the great element, is the mount of the three *vijñānas*. By means of it, the *prakṛtis* always proceed accordingly.

क। कः खटीधातुरापश्च तेजो वायुस् तथैव च।
उपादाय तु विज्ञानं जायते त्रिभवालये ॥ [8]

ཀ། སྲ་བའི་ས་ཁམས་ཆུ་ཉིད་དང་། །
དེ་བཞིན་མེ་དང་རླུང་དག་ནི། །
རྣམ་པར་ཤེས་པས་བླངས་ནས་སུ། །
སྲིད་གསུམ་གནས་སུ་སྐྱེ་བར་འགྱུར། །

What be the solid realm and of water : likewise that of fire and wind—using these, *vijñāna* takes birth in the womb of triple gestation.

स्मिन् । अस्मिश्चं पञ्च संभूताः स्कन्धास् संस्कृतिलक्षणः ।

रूपविन्नाम संस्कारा विज्ञानं चैव पञ्चमम् ॥ [9]

སྨིན། འདི་ནི་ཕུང་པོ་ལྔ་རྣམས་སུ། |

འབྱུང་བ་འདུས་བྱས་མཚན་ཉིད་ནི། |

གཟུགས་ཚོར་འདུ་ཤེས་འདུ་བྱེད་དང་། |

རྣམ་ཤེས་ཉིད་ནི་ལྔ་པའོ། |

And when this is present, the five skandhas arise with the characteristic of construction:—possessing 'form' is 'name'—the (three) saṃskāras, as is also perception (*vijñāna*), the fifth.

स । समता प्रत्यवेक्षणा कृत्यानुष्ठानमेव च ।

आदर्शो धर्मधातुश्च अस्मिन् विज्ञानपञ्चकः ॥ [10]

ས། མཉམ་ཉིད་སོ་སོར་རྟོག་པ་དང་། |

བྱ་བ་གྲུབ་པ་ཉིད་དང་ནི། |

མེ་ལོང་དང་ནི་ཆོས་ཀྱི་དབྱིངས། |

འདི་ནི་ཡེ་ཤེས་ལྔ་པོ་ཡིན། |

Just (the knowledges) Equality, Discriminative, Procedure-of-duty: as well as (the knowledges) Mirror-like and Dharmadhātu. In this (knowledge-pentad) is the *vijñāna*-pentad.

म । मनआयतनं चैव लोचने श्रवणे तथा ।

घ्राणजिह्वा ततः कायश्चेत्यायतनसंभवः ॥ [11]

མ། ཡིད་ཀྱི་སྐྱེ་མཆེད་ཉིད་དང་ནི། |

མིག་དང་དེ་བཞིན་རྣ་བ་དང་། |

སྣ་དང་ལྕེ་དང་ལུས་རྣམས་དེ། |

འདི་ནི་སྐྱེ་མཆེད་རྣམས་འབྱུང་བའོ། |

The sense base of mind, that of eyes, so of ears, nose, tongue, then of torso—thus is the origination of the sense bases.

ये । ये वै त्रैधातुके सत्त्वाः प्राणायामसमाश्रिताः ।

मन्त्रराजं जपन्त्यज्ञा ध्यानाध्यापनवर्जिताः ॥ [12]

ཡེ། གང་ཡང་ཁམས་གསུམ་སེམས་ཅན་རྣམས། |

སྲོག་དང་རྩོལ་བ་ལ་བརྟེན་པ། |

གསང་སྔགས་རྒྱལ་པོ་ཟློས་བཞིན་དུ། |

མི་ཤེས་བསམ་གཏན་ཀློག་པ་སྤྲངས། |

The beings in the three worlds taking recourse to *prāṇāyāma* (breathing in and out) who recite the 'king of mantras' with ignorance, miss the 'mental reading'.

भ । भविन्यस्मिन्प्रकृतयो रागारागादिकाः पुनः ।

ताभ्यः शुभाशुभं कर्म ततो जन्मसमुद्भवः ॥ [13]

བྷ། འདི་ལས་རང་བཞིན་ཆགས་པ་དང་། །
ཆགས་མེད་ལ་སོགས་པར་ཡང་འགྱུར། །
དེ་ལས་དགེ་དང་མི་དགེའི་ལས། །
དེ་ལས་སྐྱེ་བ་འབྱུང་བ་ཡིན། །

In this gestation are the *Prakṛtis*, desire, aversion, and so on; as a result of those, auspicious and inauspicious *karma*: therefrom the origination of (re)birth.

ग । गतिः संभवति स्कन्धः पञ्चबुद्धात्मकः पुनः ।

पञ्चाकाराभिसंबोधमिति नाम प्रचोदितः ॥ [14]

ག འགྲོ་བ་འབྱུང་བའི་ཕུང་པོ་རྣམས། །
སངས་རྒྱས་ལྔ་ཡི་བདག་ཉིད་དེ། །
མངོན་པར་བྱང་ཆུབ་རྣམ་ལྔ་ཞེས། །
མིང་གིས་རབ་ཏུ་བསྐུལ་བ་ཡིན། །

A *skandha* occurs as a destiny (*gati*), also as (one of) the five Buddhas, and exhorted as (one of) the *abhisaṃbodhi* of five kinds.

वान् । वायुस् तेजो जलं [भूमि]र्लोचनादिचतुष्टयम् ।

ज्ञानत्रयात्मकज्ञेयं बुद्धबोधिप्रदायकम् ॥ [15]

བཤད། རླུང་དང་ཆུ་དང་མེ་དང་ས། |
སྤྱན་ལ་སོགས་པ་བཞི་པོ་སྟེ། |
ཡེ་ཤེས་བདག་ཉིད་ཅན་གསུམ་དུ། |
ཤེས་བྱ་སངས་རྒྱས་བྱང་ཆུབ་སྟེར། |

Wind, fire, water, earth, are the quaternion Locanā and so on, which is to be known by one with the nature of the three gnoses as conferring the enlightenment of the Buddhas.

स । सर्वतथागतकायश्चतुर्मुद्रया मुद्रितः ।

चक्षुराद्यात्मना तत्र क्षितिगर्भादिजिनौरसाः ॥ [16]

ས། ཐམས་ཅད་དེ་བཞིན་གཤེགས་པའི་སྐུར། |
ཕྱག་རྒྱ་བཞིས་ནི་རྒྱས་བཏབ་ཅིང་། |
མིག་ལ་སོགས་པའི་བདག་ཉིད་དེར། |
ས་སྙིང་ལ་སོགས་རྒྱལ་སྲས་སོ། |

Every Tathāgata body is sealed by four seals. By means of the eye, etc. identifications, in that (body) are the Bodhisattvas Kṣitigarbha, etc.

वं। धावन्ति ये तु तुष्टा वै क्रोधराजमहाबलाः।

तान् दिग्विदिक्स्वभावेषु भुजाद्यङ्गेषु लक्षयेत् ॥ [17]

ཝཾ། རོལ་པས་དགའ་བ་གང་ཡིན་པའི། །
ཁྲོ་བོའི་རྒྱལ་པོ་སྟོབས་ཆེན་རྣམས། །
དེ་ཡི་ཕྱོགས་མཚམས་ངོ་བོ་རུ། །
དཔུང་པ་ཡན་ལག་རྣམས་སུ་བདག །

As for the mighty Fury Kings who run delighted, one should depict them in their natural abodes of the quarters and intermediate directions and in the limbs such as the arms.

त। तत्तत्कुलसमुद्भूता देवा देव्यः पृथग्विधाः।

न ते सन्ति न ताः सन्ति सत्त्वार्थं प्रतिदर्शिताः ॥ [18]

ཏ། དེ་དང་དེ་ཡིས་རིགས་ལས་བྱུང་། །
ལྷ་དང་ལྷ་མོ་ཐ་དད་པ། །
དེ་ནི་ཡོད་མིན་དེ་དག་ཡང་། །
འགྲོ་བའི་དོན་ཕྱིར་སྟོན་པའོ། །

Of the different gods and goddesses generated by him and his family, neither the gods nor goddesses exist, but are displayed for the sake of sentient beings.

थ । स्थातव्यं विषयेष्वस्माद् योगिनाद्वयदर्शिना ।

हीनमध्यप्रणीतेषु ज्ञानत्रयनिदर्शनात् ॥ [19]

ཐ། འདི་ལས་གཉིས་མེད་མཐོང་བ་ཡི། །
རྣལ་འབྱོར་པ་ནི་ཡེ་ཤེས་གསུམ། །
མཐོང་ཕྱིར་དམན་དང་བར་མ་དང་། །
དམ་པའི་ཡུལ་ལ་གནས་པར་བྱ། །

Afterwards the yogin who sees the non-duality should be dwelling upon sense objects 'inferior', 'intermediate', and 'superior' by seeing the triple gnosis.

ग । गच्छन्नस्त्यिन्द्रियस्तत्तत् स्वयं स्वविषयं प्रति ।

आभासमात्रकं तत्तद्यद्यदिन्द्रियगोचरम् ॥ [20]

ག དབང་པོ་རང་ཉིད་རང་ཡུལ་ལ། །
འགྲོ་བར་འགྱུར་བ་དེ་དང་དེ། །
དབང་པོ་གང་དང་གང་སྤྱོད་ཡུལ། །
དེ་དེ་སྣང་བ་ཙམ་ཉིད་དོ། །

While each and every sense organ is going by itself toward its own sense object, whatever be the sense organ and its range, each of them is 'light only' (*ābhāsamātra*).

त । तत्तदिन्द्रियमार्गेण विषयं प्राप्य साधकः ।

तथागतेभ्यस् सकलं प्रीणनाय निवेदयेत् ।। [21]

ཏ། དབང་པོ་དེ་དེའི་ལམ་ནས་ནི། |
སྒྲུབ་པ་པོས་ནི་ཡུལ་ཐོབ་ནི། |
དེ་བཞིན་དེ་རྣམས་མ་ལུས་པར། |
ཚོམ་པར་བྱ་ཕྱིར་དབུལ་བར་བྱ། |

While the *sādhaka* is reaching the sense object by way of this and that sense organ, he should make offering completely satisfying the Tathāgatas.

का। कायत्रयं समुद्दिष्टं पृथग्भावेन तायिना ।

एकाकारं पुनर्याति निष्पन्नक्रमयोगतः ।। [22]

ཀཱ། སྐུ་གསུམ་དག་ནི་ཐ་དད་པར། |
སྐྱོབ་པ་ཡིས་ནི་ཡང་དག་བསྟན། |
རྫོགས་པའི་རིམ་གྱིས་སྦྱོར་བ་ཡིས། |
གཅིག་ཏུ་ཡང་ནི་འགྱུར་བ་ཡིན། |

The protector (i.e. the Buddha) well taught the three Bodies as being different. Moreover, their unity occurs through the *yoga* of *niṣpanna-krama*.

य। यत्सत्यं संवृतिः प्रोक्तं बुद्धानां कायलक्षणम् ।

स एषो निष्पन्नयोगः स्यात् प्रभास्वरविशुद्धेः ॥ [23]

ཡ། གང་ཞིག་སངས་རྒྱས་སྐུ་མཚན་ཉིད། །

ཀུན་རྫོབ་བདེན་པར་གསུངས་པ་དེ། །

དེ་ཉིད་རྫོགས་རིམ་སྦྱོར་བ་ཡིས། །

འོད་གསལ་བར་ནི་རྣམ་དག་འགྱུར། །

Whatever body characteristic of the Buddhas has been stated to be 'conventional truth' (*saṃvṛti-satya*), the *niṣpanna-yoga* would be it through purification in the Clear light.

वाक् । वाक्पथस्यैव विषयः कायो ज्ञानमयः प्रभुः ।

सर्वसत्त्वहिताच्चाप दृश्यते शक्रचापवत् ॥ [24]

བཱཀ྄། ཚིག་གི་ལམ་གྱི་ཡུལ་འདི་ཉིད། །

གཙོ་བོ་ཡེ་ཤེས་སྐུ་རང་བཞིན། །

སེམས་ཅན་ཀུན་ལ་ཕན་པའི་ཕྱིར། །

འཇའ་ཚོན་བཞིན་དུ་སྣང་བ་ཡིན། །

The speech-path's topic, namely the Lord—the body made of knowledge—is seen like a rainbow, as well as apart from the benefit of all sentient beings.

चितं । चित्तं चैतसिकाविद्या प्रज्ञोपायोपलब्धिकम् ।

शून्यातिशून्यमहाशून्यमिति चापि प्रगीयते । [25]

ཅིད། སེམས་དང་སེམས་བྱུང་མ་རིག་པ། །
ཤེས་རབ་ཐབས་དང་ཉེར་ཐོབ་དང་། །
སྟོང་དང་ཤིན་ཏུ་སྟོང་པ་དང་། །
སྟོང་ཆེན་ཞེས་ཀྱང་རབ་ཏུ་བརྗོད། །

Thought (*citta*), thought derivative (*caitasika*), and nescience (*avidyā*) are also called respectively Insight (*prajñā*), Means (*upāya*), Culmination (*upalabdhika*) : as well as Void (*śūnya*), Further Void (*atiśūnya*), and Great Void (*mahāśūnya*).

त । ततश्चर्यां प्रकुर्वीत प्रकृत्याभासभेदवित् ।

कर्मकायं परित्यज्य वज्रदेहत्वमाप्नुयात् ।। [26]

ད། རང་བཞིན་སྣང་བའི་དབྱེ་ཤེས་ནས། །
དེ་ནས་སྤྱོད་པ་རབ་ཏུ་བྱ། །
ལས་ཀྱི་ལུས་ནི་ཡོངས་སྤངས་ནས། །
རྡོ་རྗེ་སྐུ་ཉིད་ཐོབ་པར་འགྱུར། །

Then, knowing the differences of the *prakṛtis* and the Lights, one should engage in the *caryā*, (namely) abandoning the body of works (*karmakāya*), he would obtain the diamond body (*vajradeha*).

हृ। हृदि कृत्वार्थचर्यां वै लौकिकीं स तथागतः।

निर्माय संवृतं कायं कामांश्चरेद् यथायथम् ॥ [27]

ཧྲྀ། ཐུགས་ལ་འཇིག་རྟེན་པ་རྣམས་ཀྱི། |
དོན་སྤྱོད་བཞག་ནས་དེ་བཞིན་གཤེགས། |
ཀུན་རྫོབ་ཏུ་ནི་སྤྲུལ་སྐུར་གནས། |
ཇི་ལྟ་ཇི་ལྟར་འདོད་པ་སྤྱོད། |

The worldling praxis of aim having been formed in the heart, he the Tathāgata, creating a conventional body, practises desires exactly as he cares.

द। ददाति प्रार्थितं सर्वं चिन्तामणिरिवापरम्।

हठश्चाहृत्य कुरुते बुद्धानामपि संपदम् ॥ [28]

ད། ཡིད་བཞིན་ནོར་བུ་མཆོག་བཞིན་དུ། |
འདོད་པ་ཐམས་ཅད་སྟེར་བར་འགྱུར། |
སངས་རྒྱས་རྣམས་ཀྱི་ཕུན་ཚོགས་ཀྱང་། |
སྟོབས་ཀྱིས་བླངས་ནས་སྒྲོད་པར་འགྱུར། |

Like the best wish-granting jewel, *haṭha* grants everything desired, and seizing (by force) enacts even the success of the Buddhas.

य। यद्यदिच्छति योगेन्द्रः तत्तत्कुर्यादनावृतः ।

असमाहितयोगेन नित्यमेव समाहितः ॥ [29]

ཡ། རྣལ་འབྱོར་དབང་པོ་གང་གང་འདོད། |

དེ་ནི་སྒྲིབ་བ་མེད་པར་བྱ། |

མཉམ་པར་ལ་བཞག་རྣལ་འབྱོར་གྱིས། |

རྟག་ཏུ་མཉམ་པར་འཇོག་པར་འགྱུར། |

Whatever the powerful one of yoga wishes, just that he would do without hindrance; and by means of the yoga of 'after'-stability, is continually stabilized.

व। वज्रपद्मसमायोगाज् ज्ञानत्रयविभागवित् ।

लिप्तालिप्तमतिस् तत्र सुखेन विहरेत् सदा ॥ [30]

ཝ། རྡོ་རྗེ་པད་མོ་མཉམ་སྦྱོར་བས། |

ཡེ་ཤེས་གསུམ་གྱི་ཆ་རིག་པ། |

བློ་ལ་གོས་དང་མ་གོས་པ། |

དེར་ནི་བདེ་བས་རྟག་ཏུ་གནས། |

Knowing the portions of the three knowledges, through union of thunderbolt and lotus,—the defiled and the undefiled intelligence would dwell therein with bliss forever.

ज्र । जृम्भते सर्वभावात्मा मायोपमसमाधिना ।
करोति बुद्धकृत्यानि सम्प्रदायपदस्थितः ॥ [31]

ཛྲ། སྒྱུ་མ་ལྟ་བུ་ཡི་ཏིང་ངེ་འཛིན་གྱིས། |
དངོས་དག་ཀུན་ལས་རྣམ་པར་རོལ། |
སངས་རྒྱས་མཛད་པ་བྱེད་བཞིན་དུ། |
གདན་ལ་པར་པའི་གཞི་ལ་གནས། |

The universal self of entities sports by means of the illusory *samādhi*. It performs the deeds of a Buddha while stationed at the traditional post.

यो । योगश्चैवातियोगश्च महायोगः स्वयं भवेत् ।
वज्री च डाकिनी चैव तयोर्योगश्च यः स्वयम् ॥ [32]

ཡོ། རྣལ་འབྱོར་ལྷག་པའི་རྣལ་འབྱོར་དང་། |
རྣལ་འབྱོར་ཆེན་པོ་རང་ཉིད་འགྱུར། |
རྡོ་རྗེ་ཅན་དང་མཁའ་འགྲོ་མ། |
གང་ཡང་རྣལ་འབྱོར་དེ་རང་ཉིད། |

Yoga, atiyoga, and mahāyoga occur by themselves; also vajrin, ḍākinī, as well as any union (*yoga*) of both, by themselves.

षिद् । निषिद्धमपि कृत्वा वै कृत्याकृत्यविवर्जितः ।
न लिप्यते स्वभावज्ञः पद्मपत्रमिवाम्भसा ।। [33]

ཥིད། དགག་པ་དག་ཀྱང་བྱེད་པས་ན། |
བྱ་དང་བྱ་མིན་རྣམ་སྤངས་ཏེ། |
པད་མ་ལ་ནི་འདམ་གྱི་བཞིན། |
ངོ་བོ་ཉིད་ཅེས་གོས་མི་འགྱུར། |

Having done even the prohibited, he renounces both the proper and the improper act. The one knowing the intrinsic nature is not adhered to (by sin), any more than is a lotus leaf by water.

भ । भवत्यष्टगुणैश्चर्यैरुपेतः सर्ववित् स्वयम् ।
विचरेज् ज्ञानदेहेन लोकधातोरशेषतः ।। [34]

བྷ། ཡོན་ཏན་བརྒྱད་དང་ཉེར་ལྡན་པས། |
སེམས་ཅན་ཐམས་ཅད་རིགས་འགྱུར་ཞིང་། |
འཇིག་རྟེན་ཁམས་ནི་མ་ལུས་པར། |
བདག་ཉིད་ཡེ་ཤེས་ལུས་ཀྱིས་སྤྱོད། |

Equipped with the eight *guṇas* to be practised, an omniscient being arises, and by himself wanders all over the worldly realm by means of the knowledge body.

**गे । गेहं तस्याम्बरश्चैव यत्र स चरति प्रभुः ।**

**तत्रैव रमते नित्यं महासुखसमाधिना ॥** [35]

གེ། གཙོ་བོ་གང་དུ་སྤྱོད་པ་ཡི། |
དེ་ཡི་ཁྱིམ་ནི་ནམ་མཁའ་ཉིད། |
བདེ་བ་ཆེན་པོའི་ཏིང་འཛིན་གྱིས། |
དེ་ཉིད་དུ་ནི་རྟག་ཏུ་རོལ། |

His home is the sky wherever he the Lord does roam. By the *samādhi* of great ecstasy he forever rejoices in that very place.

**षु । एष्वेवाभासभेदेषु सन्ध्यारात्रिदिनेषु च ।**

**व्यवहारः कृतो लोके ज्ञानत्रयनिदर्शनात् ॥** [36]

ཥུ། འདི་ལ་སྣང་བ་དབྱེ་བ་ལ། |
ཐུན་མཚམས་ཉིན་མོ་མཚན་མོ་ཡི། |
འཇིག་རྟེན་ཐ་སྙད་བྱས་པ་ཡིས། |
ཡེ་ཤེས་གསུམ་ནི་མཐོང་ཕྱིར་རོ། |

A conventional illustration is made in the world regarding just these distinctions of lights as the twilight, the night, and the day—so as to see three gnoses (*jñāna*).

वि । विचित्रव्यवहाराश्च लौकिकैः परिकल्पिताः ।

पथत्रयविभागेन ज्ञानत्रयसमुद्भवाः ॥ [37]

བི། སྣ་ཚོགས་པ་ཡི་ཐ་སྙད་དག། |
འཇིག་རྟེན་པས་ནི་ཡོངས་བརྟགས་པ། |
ལམ་གསུམ་གྱི་ནི་དབྱེ་བ་ཡིས། |
ཡེ་ཤེས་གསུམ་ལས་བྱུང་བའོ། |

Worldlings imagine the multiform conventions, which divided into three paths, originate the three knowledges.

ज । जन्म च स्थितिभङ्गेन ग्रन्तराभवसंस्थितिः ।

यावन्त्यः कल्पना लोके चित्तवायुविजृम्भिताः ॥ [38]

ཛ། སྐྱེ་དང་གནས་དང་འཇིག་པ་དང་། |
སྲིད་པར་བར་མར་གནས་པ་སྟེ། |
ཇི་སྲིད་འཇིག་རྟེན་གྱིས་བརྟགས་པ། |
སེམས་ཀྱི་རླུང་ནི་རྣམ་འཕྲུལ་ལོ། |

(Namely) birth, and by loss of abode—formation of the intermediate state. To the extent there is discursive thought in the world, so is there phenomenal projection of mind and (its vehicular) winds.

हा । हास्यलास्यक्रियाश्चैव नवनाट्यरसान्विताः ।

मुद्रामन्त्रविकल्पाश्च वज्रसत्त्वविचेष्टितम् ॥ [39]

ཧཱ། བགོད་དང་རྩེད་མོ་བྱེད་པ་དང་།
གར་གྱི་ཉམས་དགུར་ལྡན་པ་དང་།
སྔགས་དང་ཕྱག་རྒྱ་རྣམ་རྟོག་པ།
རྡོ་རྗེ་སེམས་དཔའི་སྤྱོད་པའོ།

Both the acts of laughter and accompanied dance with the nine sentiments of dramatic art, as well as mudrā, mantra, and mental formation, are enacted by Vajrasattva (the tantric hierophant).

र। रत्नमन्यं न चास्तीह स्वाधिष्ठानाद् ऋते महत् ।

प्रभास्वरविशुद्धं चेद् वह्निशुद्धो मणिर्यथा ॥ [40]

ར། བདག་བྱིན་བརླབས་ཆེན་མ་གཏོགས་པ།
རིན་ཆེན་གཞན་དག་འདི་ན་མེད།
མེ་ཡིས་སྦྱངས་པའི་ནོར་བུ་བཞིན།
འོད་གསལ་རྣམ་པར་དག་པའོ།

There is no jewel in this world so great as the Svādhiṣṭhāna, if purified by the Clear Light like a gem cleansed by fire

II. Chapters VI and XII of the *Guhyasamājatantra*, translated into English.

These two chapters are selected for translation because they are the most important in terms of commentarial literature for stating explicitly the steps of yoga underlying the entire *Guhyasamājatantra*.

The portions of the two chapters which especially apply to steps of yoga are repeated with explanations in Part Two (III. Introduction to the Yoga of the Guhyasamāja system). Here we may say by way of introduction that the two stages, Stage of Generation and Stage of Completion, are represented by verse blocks in both chapters, while other blocks may go with both stages. In Chapter Six, verses 3-5 belong to the Stage of Completion, verses 6-14 represent the *prāṇāyāma* of the Stage of Generation, and 15-18 show the advancement to the *prāṇāyāma* of the Stage of Completion. In the case of Chapter Twelve the *Pradīpoddyotana*, inaugurating its commentary on verse 50 in that chapter says : "Having taught the mundane *siddhi* by way of the deeds of the yogin belonging to the 'Stage of Generation', now in order to teach the means of accomplishing the *siddhi* of *mahāmudrā* of those situated in the 'Stage of Completion', there are the words '*vajrasamaya*' and so on (of verse 50). Presumably these 'Stage of Completion' verses continue through 59. Then verses 60-63 show the steps of achieving those *siddhis* of the 'Stage of Generation'; while the verse 64 (on which Candrakīrti has the long commentary which is edited in the next section) is understood to allude to the steps of achieving the *siddhis* of the 'Stage of Completion'. The subsequent verses can be understood to indicate both stages, by use of the four expressions of *sādhana* (elucidated in Part Two) which can be construed as the 'shared' (*sādhāraṇa*) terminology of the two stages.

The translations are made from the Bhattacharyya edition of the Tantra with the verse numbering in Dr. S. Bagchi's edition, and with some minimum expansion based on Candrakīrti's *Pradīpoddyotana* commentary in the Tibetan edition with Tsoṅ-kha-pa's *ṭippaṇī* (*Mchan ḥgrel*) thereon. Since the Sanskrit is readily available in Bagchi's edition and in the reprint of Bhattacharyya's edition, there is no reason to reproduce the entire Sanskrit text for the two chapters.

However, it has been necessary to correct the Sanskrit in certain places with the help of the Tibetan translation in the Kanjur and the *Pradīpoddyotana*. And in Chapter XII, the lines of verses 39-41 have been grouped differently from the edited text. After this manuscript was being printed, I received from Professor Yūkei Matsunaga his work, "The *Guhyasamājatantra* : A New Critical Edition." Upon comparing his readings for Chapters VI and XII, I find confirmation for most of my corrections, in some cases from the readings he accepts, and in the remainder from the variants given in the footnotes. Following are the corrections which are observed in the translation :

## CHAPTER SIX

| *Verse* | *Incorrect reading* | *Correct reading* |
|---|---|---|
| 1 | śuddhaṃ | guhyaṃ |
| 3 | manaḥ santoṣaṇapriyām | manaḥsaṃtoṣaṇāṃ priyām |
| 4 | vācā kāya-<br>niṣpādayanti saṃyogam | vācākāya-<br>niṣpādayet trisaṃyogam |
| 5 | bodhicitte ca bhāvanā | bodhir vinā ca bhāvanām |
| 6 | vidhisaṃyogaṃ | bodhisaṃyogaṃ |
| 9 | jñānadaṃ | jñānapadaṃ |
| 17 | mantra | sarva |
| 25 | para karmakṛt | padakarmakṛt |
| 26 | darśanenaiva<br>lakṣitam | darśane naiva<br>laṅghitam |

## CHAPTER TWELVE

| *Verse* | *Incorrect reading* | *Correct reading* |
|---|---|---|
| 2 | pradeśeṣu | pradeśe ca |
| 4 | siddhātmā | śuddhātmā |
| 5 | mañjuśrī | mañju |
| 12 | cintyadharma | vajradharma |
| 15 | vajra | trivajra |
| 16 | trisāhasraṃ mahāśūro<br>brahma narottamaḥ | trisāhasram ekaśūro<br>guhyadharottamaḥ |
| 25 | cakrāgrasādhanam<br>cakrakāyāgrayogataḥ | jñānāgrasādhanam<br>buddhakāyāgrayogataḥ |
| 40 | parakarmakṛt | padakarmakṛt |
| 41 | sarvasiddhīnāṃ | sarvabuddhānāṃ |
| 45 | sattvaṃ | sarvaṃ |
| 48 | vajrasattvatvam āpnuyāt | trivajratvam avāpnuyāt |
| 50 | siddhyarthaṃ | siddhyagre |
| 51 | siddhyante | siddhyagre |
| 53 | sarvasiddhīnāṃ | sarvabuddhānāṃ |

| | | |
|---|---|---|
| 58 | kāryaiḥ | kāyaiḥ |
| | dṛḍhāgra | ṛddhyagra |
| 59 | vajrapāṇī | vajrapado |
| 64 | sarvamantrārtha | mantratattvārtha |
| 66 | mantreṇa | samena |
| 68 | abdam | ardham |
| 72 | dharmo vai vākpathaḥ | dharmatāvākpathaḥ |

## CHAPTER SIX

Then the Tathāgata Akṣobhya-vajra entered the samādhi called 'Secret Diamond of the Body, Speech, and Mind of all the Tathāgatas' and pronounced this mantra which empowers the mind :

*Oṃ sarvatathāgatacittavajrasvabhāvātmako 'ham/*

"Oṃ. I am the self-existence of the cittavajra of all the Tathāgatas."

Then the Lord, the Tathāgata Vairocana-vajra, entered the samādhi called 'Dustless Diamond Abode' and pronounced this mantra which empowers the body :

*Oṃ sarvatathāgatakāyavajrasvabhāvātmako 'ham/*

"Oṃ. I am the self existence of the kāyavajra of all the Tathāgatas."

Then the Lord, the Tathāgata Amitāyur-vajra, entered the samādhi called 'Nondual Diamond which is the Sameness of all Tathāgatas' and pronounced this mantra which empowers speech:

*Oṃ sarvatathāgatavāgvajrasvabhāvātmako 'ham/*

"Oṃ. I am the self-existence of the vāgvajra of all the Tathāgatas."

(1) One may perfect by these preeminences the triple diamond which has the Tathāgata-secrets and the (absolute) abode which contemplates the (conventional) abode and is symbolized by the characteristic of mantras.

Then the Lord, the Tathāgata Ratnaketu-vajra, entered the samādhi called 'Diamond which is the Lamp of Knowledge' and pronounced this mantra which impassions:

*Oṃ sarvatathāgatānurāgaṇavajrasvabhāvātmako 'ham/*

"Oṃ. I am the self-existence of the anurāgaṇavajra of all the Tathāgatas."

Then the Lord, the Tathāgata Amoghasiddhi-vajra,

entered the samādhi called 'Unwasted Diamond' and pronounced this mantra of worship:

*Oṃ sarvatathāgatapūjāvajrasvabhāvātmako 'ham!*

"Oṃ. I am the self-existence of the pūjāvajra of all the Tathāgatas."

(2) One should continually and methodically worship the Buddhas with the five strands of desire (= sense objects). By the five kinds of worship he would speedily achieve Buddhahood.

So spoke the Lord Vajradhara, master of the Body, Speech, and Mind diamonds of all the Tathāgatas.

Then the Lord Vajradhara, master of the Body, Speech, and Mind diamonds of all the Tathāgatas, pronounced this secret mantra of all the Tathāgatas:

*Oṃ sarvatathāgatakāyavākcittavajrasvabhāvātmako 'ham!*

"Oṃ. I am the self-existence of the Body, Speech, and Mind diamonds of all the Tathāgatas."

(3) The one who has body as the mantra visualized should accomplish, exhorted by speech in the mind, the 'surpassing one', 'successful one', 'one satisfying the mind,' 'beloved one'.

(4) He should accomplish the selflessness of citta being visualized, (then) the contemplation of speech (*vācā*) and body, (then) the triple conjunction, (finally) the abode equal to space.

(5) The self-existence of body-, speech-, and mind-visualization is not reached by the praxis of mantra-body, nor is revelation in the absence of contemplation.

(6) Having pondered in brief this characteristic of body, speech, and mind, he should contemplate the samādhi 'Conjunction to revelation' as constructed by mantra.

(7) Then the glorious Vajradhara, accompanied by all the Tathāgatas, and most omniscient one among all the Buddhas, proclaimed the supreme contemplation.

(8) One should imagine a moon disk in the midst of the sky. Having contemplated an image of the Buddha, he should begin the 'subtle yoga' (*sūkṣma-yoga*).

(9) One should imagine a (minute) mustard seed at the tip of the nose and the moving and non-moving (worlds) in the mustard seed. He should contemplate the joyful realm of

knowledge as the (highest) secret that is imagined by knowledge.

(10) He should contemplate a solar disk in the midst of the sky, and having contemplated an image of the Buddha, superimpose it on that abode.

*Hūṃ!*

(11) One should contemplate a bright disk in the middle of the sky. (Then,) he should contemplate a lotus and a diamond in contact in the manner of an eye.

(12) He should contemplate a ratna disk in the middle of the sky and should perseveringly contemplate upon it the 'original yoga' (the syllables Oṃ, Āḥ, Hūṃ).

(13) [—omitted in Tibetan translation of the *mūlatantra* and in the explanatory tantra *Sandhivyākaraṇa*—]

(14) He should contemplate a light disk in the middle of the sky. He should project (thereon) a Buddha mark which is mild and in differentiation the retinue.

(15) He should imagine with perseverance at the tip of his nose a five-pronged (thunderbolt) appearing like a blue lotus petal and in the advanced degree the size of a tiny barley grain.

(16) With enlightenment his sole aim, he should contemplate vividly at the tip of his nose an eight petalled lotus with filaments and the size of a chick-pea.

(17) In the extraordinary case, he would construct therein (i.e. in the 'chick-pea') the contemplation of wheel and so on. (Then,) he would accomplish the ecstatic basis of enlightenment—the store of all (mundane) *siddhis* and the (eight supramundane) *guṇas*.

(18) He would project there in condensed manner what has been placed in the Buddha's enlightenment. He would draw forth the Dharma Word marked with body, speech, and mind.

(19) Then the glorious Vajradhara, the revealer of all the meaning of reality, expressed the sublime secret that issues from all the best praxis (*caryā*).

(20) The wise man, provided with forms, sounds, and tastes, should contemplate for six months; and should also contemplate by offering the great offering to the secret reality.

(21) The one desiring *siddhis* as fruit should perform by using excrement and urine as (imaginary) food. He would

accomplish the supreme reality and immaculate mind of enlightenment.

(22) He should imagine the great flesh as flesh for food. He would accomplish the mysterious body, speech, and mind that are in all *siddhis*.

(23) He should eat as food, the sublime flesh of elephant, horse, and dog, and not partake of other food.

(24) The wise Bodhisattva becomes dear to the Buddhas. Indeed, by this praxis one would quickly attain Buddhahood.

(25) He would become in the world Lord of the Realm of Desire (*kāma-dhātu*), the doer of deeds of the rank; the radiant, powerful leader, his handsome features gratifying the sight.

(26) He would assent to the world on sight, without being exhorted. This is what for all the Buddhas is the secret, the supreme enlightenment. This secret mantra is the reality transcending (the ordinary) body, speech, and mind.

Ended is chapter six, entitled 'Empowerment of Body, Speech, and Mind' in the Mahāguhyatantra 'Guhyasamāja' of the secret and the greater secret belonging to the Body, Speech, and Mind of the Tathāgatas.

## CHAPTER TWELVE

Then the teacher Vajradhara, who has accomplished the supreme Jñāna, proclaimed the diamond of speech which is the reality of the three diamond pledges.

(1) One should imagine this dance (*nāṭaka*) among the natures pure by intrinsic nature, which are equal to the sky and have the intrinsic nature devoid of discursive thought.

(2) One may accomplish the sum of all *siddhis* both in a spot of a great forest and in a secluded mountain adorned with flowers and fruits.

*Māṃ*

(3) The contemplation of the mañjuvajra in the diamonds of (one's own) body, speech, and mind, is comparable to the mañjuvajra which radiates in the body, speech, and mind (of the three realms).

(4) The pure self, adorned with all adornments, shines with a light of blazing diamond for a spread of a hundred yojanas.

(5) The gods Brahmā, Rudra, and so on, never see it. (Thus) the samādhi called 'Causing the disappearance of the highest samaya of the mañjuvajra.'

(6) Having caused what proceeds from the triple hook (i.e. the three lights) by means of the five *samayas* of excrement (=sense object) and urine (=sense organ) which arise from the inseparable triple vajra (i.e. the mind), he should contemplate it as cast into his mouth (=the Clear Light).

(7) He should contemplate therein the *citta* as inseparable from all the Buddhas. It would have from that moment a light like that of the mañjuvajra.

(8-9) Having contemplated by way of one's own mantra (Oṃ), and having imagined the wheel with the light of a firebrand as the abode of all the Buddhas, one would be like a Buddha. As many as be the atoms of the 36 Sumerus corresponding to that (wheel), they are all like Vajradhara. (Thus) the samādhi called 'Pledge of the Wheel'.

(10-11) Having contemplated by way of one's own mantra (Hūṃ), and (having contemplated) the Mahāvajra in the middle of the maṇḍala as the abode of all the vajras, one would be equal to the Cittavajra. As many as be the atoms of the 36 Sumerus, that many will be the ladies (*yoṣit*) who are its abode of merits (*guṇa*). Having made the obeisance of Rudra, he would be the Mahāvajra of the three realms. (Thus) the samādhi called 'Diamond equality'.

(12-13) Having contemplated by way of one's own mantra (Āḥ) the great eight-petalled lotus, one would be the store of all dharmas equal to Vajradharma. As many as be the atoms of the 36 Sumerus, the pure self causes them to take shape in the supreme maṇḍala of Buddha offerings. (Thus) the samādhi called 'Lotus equality'.

(14-17) He stays serving the triple-aeon pledge of the five knowledge-bearers. He meditatively worships the three secrets of all the Buddhas of the ten directions. He should contemplate his own mantra (Hā) as the sword with a light equal to the five rays. Holding it in his hand, wide-eyed, he would be a vidyādhara of the triple vajra. Worshipping with the great (mystic powers) of the three realms, having bowed to Brahmā, Indra and the Daityas, he, the solitary hero in the chiliocosm, would be the highest Guhyadhara. What one wishes with his mind of the vajrins of Body, Speech, and Mind—it confers such a *siddhi* created from the cittavajra. (Thus) the samādhi called 'Best of all swords'.

(18-19) Having meditated on the pellet of Oṃ, the size of a pea kernel, one should contemplate in its center the image of one's deity, imagining it in the 'mouth' (the brahmarandhra). Immediately he would have the same light as the bodhisattva, the same light as the Jambu river, appearing like the risen sun.

(20-21) Having meditated on the pellet of Āḥ, the size of a pea kernel, one should contemplate in its center the image of one's deity, imagining it in the 'mouth'. Immediately he would have the same light as the revelation-knowledge, the same light as the Jambu river, appearing like the risen sun.

(22-23) Having meditated on the pellet of Hūṃ, the size of a pea kernel, one should contemplate in its center the image of one's deity, imagining it in the 'mouth'. Immediately he would have the same light as the diamond body, the same light as the Jambu river, appearing like the risen sun.

(24-25) One should contemplate Vairocana stationed in the center of a clear sky. Having imagined a wheel in his hand, one would be a cakra-Vidyādhara. Having imagined the 'Great Wheel' family as the best praxis of Buddha body, one would enact with the knowledge diamond the best evocation (*sādhana*) of knowledge.

(26-27) One should contemplate a knowledge Akṣobhya stationed in the center of a diamond in the sky. Having imagined a thunderbolt in his hand, one would be a vajra-Vidyādhara. Having imagined the 'Great Diamond' family as the best praxis of Diamond body, one would enact with the knowledge diamond the best evocation of diamond.

(28-29) One should contemplate a Ratnavajra stationed in the center of a jewel in the sky expanse. Having imagined a ratna in his hand, one would be a ratna-Vidyādhara. Having imagined the 'Great Jewel' family as the best praxis of Jewel body, one would enact with the knowledge diamond the best evocation of jewel.

(30-31) One should contemplate an Amitābha stationed in the center of the dharma in the sky. Having imagined a lotus in his hand, one would be a padma-Vidyādhara. Having imagined the 'Great Lotus' family as the best praxis of Dharmakāya, one would enact with the knowledge diamond the best evocation of lotus.

(32-33) One should contemplate an Amoghāgra stationed in the center of the samaya in the sky. Having imagined a sword in his hand, one would be a khaḍga-Vidyādhara. Having imagined the 'Great Samaya' family as the best praxis of kāyasamaya, one would enact with the knowledge diamond the best evocation of samaya.

(34) The trident ( of Mahābala ), the knowledge-hook (of Ṭakkirāja), and the other (symbols of the Krodha-rāja-s), to be evoked by diversification of the vajra, are evoked with meditation of that (Akṣobhya) by means of the evocations of body, speech, and mind.

Thus spoke the Lord who is the vajra of siddhi-(revelation) belonging to the Great Pledge (mahāsamaya = the Diamond Vehicle).

(35) As a special (or distinguished) case, the performer should continually evoke the diamond attraction (of four lineages of goddesses) at a crossroads, a solitary tree, an ekaliṅga, or in a calm place.

(36-37) Having contemplated the 'incantation person' of triple yoga ( = born from the 3 syllables, Oṃ, Āḥ, Hūṃ) as the vajrin of triple yoga ( = having the stack of three sattvas), the hook for the (ordinary) body, speech, and mind, on the part of the 'Buddhas' (the jewel-like persons) who have jñānabuddhis (i.e. seek the non-dual knowledge); and having attracted, with the vajra arisen from the symbols ( = goddesses) of the ten directions, the supreme Buddha attraction that abides in the best windy maṇḍala, he would partake of that. (Thus) the attraction by the diamond of 'symbols in the sky' (khadhātusamaya = the goddesses).

(38) Having meditated on Vairocana, the 'Great Wheel' with the hook 'store of Buddhas', he should engage in the supreme attraction of the 'pledges' (samaya = the goddesses) by means of the thunderbolt (*vajra*), lotus (*padma*), and so on. (Thus) the attraction of the samaya (the yakṣiṇīs, etc.) of the three realms ('below the earth', 'upon the earth', 'above the earth').

(*39) He should contemplate a Buddha image endowed with the best of all aspects. And he should contemplate in its hand the hook and so on (the differentiation of the hook) of body, speech, and mind. Indeed, with this yoga he would be a performer of the rites of the 'place' (the rank of Vajrasattva).

(*40) He should contemplate the 'diamond of body' (one's own transfigured body) as endowed with the best of all aspects. Having meditated with the praxis (recitation of mantras) of diamond tongue, he would be equal to the Vāgvajra (i.e. Amitābha). When he offers the offering (i.e. one's own body) which is the best offering of the 'pledge' of the three secrets, he would be consummated.

(*41) This is the quintessence, the sum of secrets of all the Buddhas. Thus spoke the Lord, the great secret pledge.

(42) He should perfect the supreme triple vajra by the best pledge of 'great flesh' (the human corpse). He would become the Vidyādhara Lord by the best pledge of excrement and urine.

(43-44) He would obtain the five supernormal powers by the pledge-flesh of elephant. He would become the master of disappearance by the pledge-flesh of horse; the achiever of all *siddhis* by the pledge-flesh of dog, the supreme attraction of vajra by the best pledge of cow flesh.

(45) When he is unable to obtain any (such) (dead) flesh, having meditated upon any one (of them), he should mentally construct (the flesh). By this diamond praxis he would become empowered by all the Buddhas.

(46-47) He should contemplate the Vajrin of Body, Speech, and Mind (=the samayasattva) endowed with the best of all aspects; then in its heart (on a moon-disk) the Jñāna pledge (=the jñānasattva); and on (the latter's) crown, the holder of the best vajra (=the samādhisattva). This gratification of all the Buddhas is the supreme method of pledge. Enacting it by the best pledge (yields) the finest creation of every *siddhi*. (Thus) the samādhi called 'Partaking of all the vajras of samaya and jñāna'.

(48-49) Having meditated on the Vajrin (i.e. Akṣobhya) of Hūṃ when there is the best pledge-diamond of the tongue, and having enjoyed by the praxis of the five ambrosias, one may obtain the triple vajra. This (same) pledge of Āḥ (for Amitābha) and Oṃ (for Vairocana) is the supreme diamond method. Indeed, by this praxis one would become equal to Vajrasattva. (Thus) the samādhi called 'Ambrosia-garland of Vajrasamaya.'

(50) When he has the superior siddhi whose symbol (*samaya*) is the triple vajra (of Body, Speech, and Mind-the three lights), he would become the vajrin (possessor of the vajra) of three bodies (the Dharmakāya, Saṃbhogakāya, and Nirmāṇakāya). He would become the sea of wish-granting jewels belonging to all the Buddhas of the ten directions.

(51) The Diamond-soul shines on the worldly realm on all levels. When there is the superior *siddhi* of cakrasamaya (associated with Vairocana), it (the Diamond soul) becomes equal to the body of a Buddha.

(52) He would sport successful on all levels, numbering the Ganges sands. When there are all the superior samayas (ḍākinīs and ḍākas), he would become the Vidyādhara Lord.

(53) He shines alone in the chiliocosm during all disappearances (of speech activity and bodily members), he steals (the mystic powers) from all the Buddhas, enjoys the daughters of the best gods (such as Indra)—when he has the superior siddhi of all the samayas by reason of the potency of the kāya-vajra (= the Mahāmudrā).

(54) He sees with the diamond eye (the pure, refined divine eye), like a single myrobalan fruit in his hand, the Buddhas in the number of the Ganges sands, who are stationed in the triple vajra abode.

(55) He hears through the influence of supernormal faculty as though all around gathered to his ear as many sounds as are revealed in fields numbering the Ganges sands.

(56) He knows, in the form of a drama, the thought-announced character (the 160 prakṛtis) of body, speech, and mind of all the sentient beings in fields numbering the Ganges sands.

(57) He remembers, as though of three-days duration, the incidents of former lives occurring as he dwelt in saṃsāra through aeons numbering the Ganges sands.

(58) He emanates through the vajrin of magical power (*ṛddhi*) with bodies numbering the Ganges sands and adorned with clouds of Buddhas, for aeons numbering the Ganges sands. Thus spoke the Lord who has the supernormal faculty of

samaya, namely: the diamond eye, the diamond hearing, the diamond consciousness, the diamond abode, and the diamond magical power.

(59) When one has the success of goal that is the Buddha's supernormal faculty, then he becomes equal to the Buddha's body. He, the diamond of body and speech (and mind), would roam the worldly realm on all levels, surrounded by retinues as numerous as the Ganges sands.

(60-61A) There are four (steps): 1. occupation with the pledge of service, 2. arising of near-evocation, 3. evocation goal and the symbol, and 4. great evocation. Having understood them as a division of vajra, then one should accomplish the rites.

(61B-62-63) 1. He should contemplate the samādhi-praxis of service as the supreme revelation. 2. The deliberation on the bases of the vajras when there is foremost success is the near-evocation. 3. The contemplation of the lords of the mantras is said to be the exhortation when there is evocation. 4. At the time of great evocation, when he imagines the form of his own mantra-vajrin as the lord on the crown of his head, he is successful because of the jñāna-vajrin.

(64) One should create, everywhere and always, just with the knowledge nectar of service. For this brings to success the aim of mantra and of tattva, of all mantras.

(65) Success is always attained in spots of a great forest, places entirely clear of (other) persons, and abodes of mountain caves.

Thus spoke the Lord with the diamond of Mahāsādhana.

(66) Thus, the one of firm devotions (*vrata*) should perform the service by means of four vajras (the four in Chap. XVIII beginning with the 'revelation of voidness'). Contemplating through equality (of oneself) with the three vajra bodies (of Vajradhara), he reaches success.

(67) The wise man, having contemplated with the knowledge diamond of reciting Oṃ, that is, by union with the four temporal junctures (= the four goddesses) in five places (= the distinguished kind of the five sense objects), engages in the vow (= bliss).

(68) The siddhi is easily attained when one relies on the vajrasamaya (the Clear Light in sense objects) for seven days

(by one of superior organs), half a month (medium organ), a month or a half more (inferior organ).

(69) I have explained extensively by stressing the difference of days (for accomplishing siddhi in the Stage of Generation); (now) the siddhi that takes a half-month (the Mahāmudrā) is stated by sources (the Tathāgatas) of the high secret (the Clear Light).

Herein is the domain of the Upasādhana-vow :

(70-71) May the glorious holder of Buddha Body contemplated as the inseparable triple vajra, create for me today the place of blessing by way of the Diamond-holder of Body (Vairocana). May the Buddhas of the ten directions contemplated as the inseparable three vajras, create for me today the place of blessing characterized as body.

Herein is the domain of the Sādhana-vow :

(72-73) May the glorious speech-path of true-nature, contemplated as the inseparable triple vajra, create for me today the place of blessing by way of the Diamond-holder of Speech (Amitābha). May the Buddhas of the ten directions, contemplated as the inseparable three vajras, create for me today the place of blessing arising from the path of speech.

Herein is the domain of the Mahāsādhana-vow :

(74-75) May the glorious holder of the Cittavajra, contemplated as the inseparable triple vajra, create for me today the place of blessing by way of the Diamond-holder of Mind (Akṣobhya). May the Buddhas of the ten directions contemplated as the inseparable three vajras, create for me today the place of blessing, arising from mind.

(76) There is no doubt that if there is a Buddha (=yogin of Vairocana), a Vajradharma (=yogin of Amitābha), or a Vajrasattva (=yogin of Akṣobhya), then if the deluded self (*mohātman*) would go beyond, it would become rent asunder.

Ended is chapter twelve, entitled 'Instruction on the best evocation of the pledge' in the Mahāguhya-tantra 'Guhyasamāja' of the secret and the greater secret belonging to the Body, Speech, and Mind of all the Tathāgatas.

### III. Edited Pradīpoddyotana commentary on Chapter XII, 60-64, and English translation.

This portion of Candrakīrti's commentary is devoted to defining the four steps of *sādhana* constituting the 'Stage of

Generation' and then to explaining in detail the six members of yoga (*ṣaḍaṅga-yoga*) constituting the 'Stage' of Completion'. The part of the commentary on the six members of yoga is almost the same as is found in a work attributed to Nāgārjuna, the *ṣaḍaṅgayoga-nāma* (PTT, Vol. 85). Therefore, this comment by Candrakīrti may well have been a traditional commentary on the six members. At the end of the work ascribed to Nāgārjuna (meaning of course the tantric author), there is presented the lineage of the *ṣaḍaṅgayoga* of the *Guhyasamāja*: "Buddha Vajradhara; Ārya-Nāgārjuna; Nāgabodhi; Candrakīrti; Āryadeva; Śākyarakṣita; Ratnamitra; Dharmabhadra; Guṇamati; Mañjuśrījñāna; Amoghaśrī; Vīramati; Vijayakīrti; Varaprajñādharmabhadra; Śrībhadra; Dharmapāla; Śākyadhvaja; Vagīśvarakīrti; Ratnakīrti; Mahāsthavara; Śrīvanaratna; those are the chief ones. Also, from Śrīvanaratna to (the Tibetan) Gnam-gaṅ-rin-po-che; the chief one is Dharmabuddhi." However, the *Karmāntavibhāga* cited within the comment is by Kluḥi blo (*Nāgabuddhi) who might be the same person as the Nāgabodhi in the above lineage list.

Here I omit the verse numbers assigned in Bagchi's edition to the block of verses which Candrakīrti cites from the *Guhyasamāja*, Chap. XVIII. Candrakīrti does not include the verse line (Bagchi, XVIII, 144A) : *guhyatantreṣu sarveṣu vividhāḥ parikīrtitāḥ*; and the verse grouping thereafter diverges from the edited Sanskrit text. Otherwise, Candrakīrti's citation of the verses agrees for the most part with the edited text. But his line *guhyatrayaṃ vitarkaś ca vicāras tatprabhogataḥ* appears to be an improvement over the line *guhyaṃ tarkodayaṃ tarkaṃ vicāraṃ tat prayogataḥ* (Bagchi, XVIII, 144B). Nāropā's *Sekoddeśaṭika* (p. 30), when quoting the block of verses from Chap. XVIII, gives the line *guhyatrayodayas tarko vicāras tatprayogatā*, which at least verifies the reading *guhyatraya*.

The translation is somewhat expanded by extracts within parentheses of *Mcḥan ḥgrel* comments by Tsoṅ-kha-pa, PTT, Vol. 158, pp. 87-5 to 92-1.

*Edited Commentary on Chapter XII*, 60-64.

Idānīm utpattikramasādhanāṅgaṃ punaḥ spaṣṭayann āha/ sevetyādi/sevyate ālambyata iti sevā/tathatām eva samayaḥ/

tataḥ bhūbhāgādīnāṃ saṃyojanaṃ niṣpādanaḥ / sevāsamayasaṃyogaṃ / prathamam aṅgaṃ / śūnyatālambanaṃ sūryādyālambanam upasādhanaṃ / tad eva mantravinyāsaparyantaṃ sambhavatīty upasādhanasambhavo dvitīyaṁ / sādhanārthaṃ ca samayam iti/sādhanopasthāpanāyās taḥ adhyeṣaṇāṃ sādhanārthaḥ samaye sameti gacchatīti samayaḥ samādhi-sattvaḥ jñānasattvaś ca sādhanārthaś ca samayaś ca tṛtīyaṃ / avaśiṣṭasya maṇḍalarājāgrī karmarājāgrī paryantasya mahataḥ parārthasya sādhanaṃ mahāsādhanaṃ tac caturthakaṃ /

evam aṅgacatuṣṭayaṃ vijñāya vajrabhedena kulabhedena tatas tadantaraṃ karmāṇi vakṣyamāṇāni pūrvāṇyeva/sādhayed ity uddeśaḥ/sevāsamādhītyādinā uddiṣṭāny aṅgāni nirdiśate/ bodhicittālaṃbanaṃ/sevā saiva samādhīyate cetasi sthāpyata iti samādhiḥ / saṃyojanaṃ saṃyogaḥ / kiṃ tat bhūbhāgādiṃ maṇḍalacakraṃ paryantaṃ yādhimuktyā niṣpādayaḥ / sevāsamādhiś ca saṃyogaś ca sevāsamādhisaṃyogaṃ / tat kṛtvā oṃ śūnyateti mantrārthapravicāraṇ [otpāditāṃ] sambodhiṃ tathatālakṣaṇāṃ bhāvayed iti/

sūryacandrapadmādikrameṇaiva paryuparivyavasthāpya tadupari tryakṣaraṃ vinyasya sarvopagrahaṇena śaśāṅkamaṇḍalaṃ tadupari punas tryakṣaraṃ tadparāvṛttyā cihnaṃ cihnaparāvṛttyā mahāmudrārūpaniṣpādam upasādhanaṃ ya samīpe sādhya niṣpādya ta ity uktvā / siddhir mahāmudrāsiddhiḥ / tasyā agrātmādibhūtāḥ praṇavādayo mantrāḥ/ yasmin tad upasādhanam ity agraṃ / vinyastasamantamantrā [kṣaraṃ] mahāmudrārūpas tasmin vajraṃ / vairocanādisumbhaparyantāḥ teṣām āyatanāni rūpaskandhādayaḥ /

teṣāṃ tṛtīyavyavasthātikrameṇa nirnīya kāryakāraṇaparijñānaṃ vicāraṇī-sādhya tenādhiṣṭhānāyārādhyate yena tat sādhane codanaṃ proktam itiparyāyakathanaṃ kiṃ tu buddhakāyadhara ityādi/gāthādvayaḥ / mantrādhipativibhāvanam iti mantrā oṃkārādayaḥ / samādhisattvāḥ adhipatayaḥ jñānasattvāḥ mantrādhipatīnāṃ kulabhedena yathāsambhavaṃ dhyānaṃ mantrādhipativibhāvanam iti/

mahāsādhanetyādi yad uddiṣṭaṃ mahāsādhanaṃ tat saṃpādanakāleṣu jñānavajriṇaḥ / svādhidaivatayogavān mantrī vajrapadmasaṃskārapūrvikāṃ / samāpattiṃ kṛtvā svamantravajradṛgādayaḥ / tatsaṃbhūtā vajriṇas teṣāṃ viśvaṃ mahāmudrārūpaṃ dhyātvā mukuṭe 'dhipatiṃ dhyātveti/pañcatathāgatānām mahāmudrārūpasya jaṭimukuṭe mahāvajradharam adhipatiṃ pariśiṣṭe tatkulīnānāṃ mukuṭe vairocanādiḥ / dhyātvā siddhyate siddhim āpnoti/yathārutaṃ //

evaṃ caturyogakrameṇa vajrasattvasamārādhanaṃ pratipādyedānīṃ ṣaḍaṅgakrameṇa mahāvajradharaniṣpattim āha/ *Samājottare* :

*sāmānyottamabhedena sevā tu dvividhā bhavet/*
*vajracatuṣkeṇa sāmānyam uttamaṃ ṣaḍbhir aṅgataḥ//*

sevā jñānāmṛtenaiva kartavyetyādi sevyate mumukṣubhir abhyasyata iti sevā kim tat / pariviśuddhadevatāmūrtiḥ/ sā jñānāmṛtenaiva ṣaḍaṅgayogenaiva kartavyā niṣpādyā sarvataḥ/ sarvātmanā / sadā sarvakālaṃ / sarveryāpatheṣu evakāro 'vadhāraṇe eṣo hi jñānāmṛtākhyaḥ / ṣaḍaṅgayogaḥ / sarvamantrāṇāṃ sarvatathāgatānāṃ / mantrāḥ / sarpādayaḥ tattvaṃ devatātattvaṃ [*teṣām arthaḥ phalaṃ] tatsādhanān mantraṃ tattvārthasādhakaḥ/hi yasmād arthe yasmād evaṃ ṣaḍaṅgayogaḥ / tasmāt tenaiva sevā kāryeti/tāni pratyāhārādīni ṣaḍaṅgāni nirdiṣṭāni *Samājottare* :

*sevāṃ ṣaḍaṅgayogena kṛtvā sādhanam uttamam/*
*sādhayed anyathā naiva jāyate siddhir uttamā/*
*pratyāhāras tathā dhyānaṃ prāṇāyāmaś ca dhāraṇā/*
*anusmṛtiyoga(ḥ) samādhiś ca ṣaḍaṅga ucyate*

ity uddeśapadānāṃ nirdeśam āha /

*daśānām indriyāṇāṃ tu svavṛttisthaṃ tu sarvataḥ/*
*pratyāhāra iti proktaḥ kāmāhāraṃ prati prati/*
*pañcakāmās samāsena pañcabuddhaprayogataḥ/*
*kalpanaṃ dhyānam ucyeta tad dhyānaṃ pañcadhā bhavet/*
*vitarkaś ca vicāraś ca prītiś caiva sukhaṃ tathā/*
*cittasyaikāgratā caiva pañcaite dhyānasaṃgrahāḥ/*
*guhyatrayaṃ vitarkaś ca vicāras tatprabhogataḥ /*
*tṛtīyaṁ prītisaṅkāśaṃ caturthaṃ sukhasaṃgraham /*
*svacittaṃ pañcamaṃ jñeyaṃ jñānajñeyodayakṣayam /*
*sarvabuddhamayaṃ śāntaṃ sarvakāmapratiṣṭhitam /*
*pañcajñānamayaṃ śvāsaṃ pañcabhūtasvabhāvakam /*
*niścārya pdmanāsāgre piṇḍarūpeṇa kalpayet /*
*pañcavarṇaṃ mahāratnaṃ prāṇāyāmam iti smṛtam /*
*svamantraṃ hṛdaye dhyātvā prāṇam bindugataṃ nyaset/*
*niruddhe svendriye ratne dhārayed dhāraṇaṃ smṛtam /*
*nirodhavajragate citte nimittodgraha(ḥ) jāyate /*
*pañcadhā taṃ nimittaṃ tu bodhivajreṇa bhāṣitam /*

*prathamaṃ marīcikākāraṃ dhūmrākāraṃ dvitīyakam /*
*tṛtīyaṃ khadyotakākāraṃ caturthaṃ dīpavajjvalam /*
*pañcamaṃ tu sadālokaṃ nirabhragaganopamam /*
*sthiraṃ vai vajramārgeṇa sphārayet taṃ khadhātuṣu /*
*vibhāvya yad anusmṛtyā tadākāraṃ tu saṃsphare t /*
*anusmṛtir iti jñeyaṃ pratibhāsas tatra jāyate /*
*prajñopāyasamāpattyā sarvabhāvān samāsataḥ /*
*saṃhṛtya piṇḍayogena bimbaṃ madhye vibhāvayet /*
*ṛtiti jñānaniṣpattiḥ samādhir iti saṃjñitam /*

iti pratinirdesam āha / daśānām ityādi / indriyāṇi indriyārthāś ca indriyāni teṣāṃ daśānām indriyāṇāṃ viṣayaviṣayiṇāṃ svavṛttiḥ / yathā svagrāhyagrāhakasvarūpeṇa pravṛttiḥ / svavrttis tatra sthitaṃ svavṛttisthaṃ / sarvataḥ hīnamadhyottamabhedena kāmāhāraṃ prati pratīti / kāmyante abhilaṣyanta iti kāmā rūpādayas teṣām indriyair yadāharaṇaṃ grahaṇaṃ prati prati punaḥ punaḥ tadgrahyāhāra ityādyaṅgasya pratinirdeśam /

pratyāhāraviśodhanāya dvitīyam aṅgam āha / pañcetyādi/ pañca kāmā rūpādayaḥ / indriyāṇi viṣayabhūtāḥ samāsena / indriyair ekībhāvena pañcabuddhāḥ cakṣurādayaḥ taṃ teṣāṃ saṃyojanaṃ yojanaṃ / pañcabuddhaprayogataḥ / tasmād rūpādayaḥ ye pañcabuddhā(ḥ) ityevaṃvidhaṃ yat pariśuddhakalpanaṃ tad dhyānaṃ/tad vitarketyādibhedena pañcavidhaṃ bhavati vitarketyādi tadbhedakathanam / guhyatrayetyādi / indriyaviṣayendriyajñānāni guhyatrayaṃ / pañcendriyāṇi / indriyajñānāni / tadviśayāś ca pañcatathāgatātmaketi yat parikalpanaṃ sa vitarkaḥ / tasminn eva vicāraṇaṃ sthitivicāraḥ / evaṃ vicārayat sa tattvapraveśābhimukhyena yat saumanasyalakṣaṇaṃ tat prītīti saṃkāśaṃ tattve 'bhiniveśena kāyapraśrabdhyādilakṣaṇaṃ / yat prāptaṃ sukhaṃ tat sukhasaṃgrahaṃ / evam abhyasyataḥ prakarṣaparyantagamanāt/ jñānasya cakṣurādi/ṣaṭpravṛttir vijñānasya jñeye rūpādidharmadhātuparyante/udayo jñānajñeyodayaḥ / tasya kṣayaḥ/ cittasyagrāhyagrāhakaśūnyatvaparijñānalakṣaṇā cittaikāgratā svacittam ityuktaḥ tadevaṃvidhaṃ svacittaṃ yogena sarvabuddhamayaṃ śāntam iti grāhyādivikalpaśamanāt/śāntam/ bhāsamātraṃ tat sarvaśūnyataikaniṣṭhaṃ jāyate/pañcaprabhedaṃ dvitīyam aṅgaṃ /

pañcetyādi / ādarśādipañcajñānasvabhāvam adhaḥśvāsaṃ/ tam eva pṛthivyādyātmakaṃ svavajravivarān niścārya padma-nāsāgre piṇḍarūpeṇa bodhicittabindurūpeṇa dhyāyāt / tam evordhvapravṛttaśvāsaṃ pañcavarṇaṃ pañcatathāgatātmakaṃ tam eva mahāratnaṃ prāṇojjīvitaṃ āyāmeti dīrgha(ṃ) vistāryate yeneti sa prāṇāyāma iti smṛtaḥ jñāta(vya)ḥ/tam eva praveśādisvabhāvenāharniśaṃ jāpamānatvāt/svamantraṃ hṛdaye svahṛtpuṇḍarīke dhyātvā prāṇaṃ bindugataṃ samāhitam akṣataṃ nyaset iti tṛtīyam aṅgaṃ /

niruddhetyādi svarūpādaya indriye cakṣurādayaḥ asmin dvendriye nirodhe vilīne tato viṣayendriyādhārabhūte ratne cittaratne ca prāṇāyāmena saha nirodhe 'staṃgate yad dhārayet tad dhāraṇaṃ/kiṃ tat/bhūtakoṭiḥ/nirodhavajragate citte nimittodgraha(ḥ) jāyata iti/nirodhavajraṃ prabhāsvaraṃ tadbhūte tajjāte citte nimittānāṃ udgraho/nimittapratibhāsaḥ jāyate utpadyate / pañcadhātunimittaṃ tu bodhivajreṇa bhāṣitam iti pṛthivyā 'mbhasi layanān marīcikākāraṃ pratibhāsate/prathamaṃ nimittaṃ / evam ambhasas tejasi layanād dhūmrākāraṃ dvitīyaṃ / tejase vāyau layanāt khadyotakākāraṃ tṛtīyaṃ/sūkṣmadhātor ābhāsatrayagamanād dīpavadālokapuñjasvabhāva(ṃ) caturthaṃ / prakṛtyābhāsalayanān nirabhragaganavat satatālokaprabhāsavaramātraṃ bhavati pañcamaṃ / etāni pañcanimittāni nirvāṇa(ṃ) prāpayanti/, yathoktaṃ *Karmāntavibhāge*:

*prāṅ mahī salilaṃ gacchej jalaṃ gacchati pāvakam /*
*pāvako vāyum anveti vāyur vijñānam āviśet /*
*vijñānaṃ dhāraṇānvitvaṃ prabhāsvaram apy āviśed/iti/*

sthiram ityādinā / vajramārgeṇa 'laṅghanīyaṃ pañcanimittānupūrveṇa prabhāsvarapravesena khadhātuṣu lokadhātuṣu sphārayed vyāpayed dharmakāyarūpeṇa/etad dhāraṇāṅgam iti caturtham /

evam ātmānaṃ prabhāsvaragataṃ vibhāvya sākṣātkṛtvā yat pūrvaṃ anusmṛtyā marīcikādyākāreṇa bhūtakoṭiṃ prāpitam / tadākāreṇa tenaiva krameṇa saṃsphāret/utpādayet/etad anantaroktaṃ anusmṛtir iti jñeyaṃ jñātavyam / pratibhāsa saṃvit tatra pañcamam aṅgam anusmṛtir jāyate [*nānyatra]/

sarvabhāvāḥ prajñopāyasamāpattyā saṃvṛtiparamārthasatyayogena sthāvarajaṅgamaṃ sthitipiṇḍarūpeṇa mahāmudrārūpeṇa ekīkṛtya tasya sthāvarajaṅgamasya madhye yuganaddhātmakamahāvajradharabimbaṃ vibhāvayet/jānīyāt/ anena krameṇa ṛṭiti kṣaṇena jñānaniṣpattiḥ / jñānadehaniṣpattiḥ / samādhir iti ṣaṣṭham aṅgaṃ kathyate /

*Śrī-Māyājāle*' pīmam eva devatānispattibhedam udddyotayann āha

*yogas tu trividho jñeyo 'dhiṣṭhānaḥ parikalpaś ca/*
*niṣpannair cittabimbasya yogo buddhais tu varṇitaḥ/*
*adhiṣṭhānamātr [ā] haṃkāro yogo 'dhiṣṭhāna ucyate/*
*bodhicittaviśuddhis tu mantrabījodayo mahān/*
*kramān niṣpannabimbas tu mudrāganeṣu kalpitaḥ/*
*tatkalpiteti kathitayogaḥ kalpita ucyate/*
*sarvākāravaropetaḥ spʰaret saṃhārakārakaḥ/*
*ṛṭiti jñānaniṣpanno yogo niṣpanna ucyata iti/*

*Vairocanābhisaṃbodhitantre* 'pi/dvividhadevatāyogaṃ nirdiśate/ devatārūpam api guhyakādhipate dvividhaṃ pariśuddham aśuddhaṃ ca iti / **tatpariśuddham adhigatarūpaṃ** sarvanimittāpagatam apari[śuddha]ṃ sarvanimittaṃ rūpavarṇasaṃsthānaś ca/tatra dvividhena devatārūpeṇa dvividhakāryaniṣpattir bhavati/sanimittena sanimittā siddhir upajāyate/animittenānimittā siddhir iṣṭā jinavaraiḥ sadā animitte sthitvā vai sanimittaṃ prasādhyate/tasmāt sarvaprakāreṇa vinimittāni sevyata iti/saṃdhyā bhāṣā//

*Translation*

*The Stage of Generation*:

Now (*idānīm*) so as to clarify the (four) evocation member(s) of the Stage of Generation, he says 'Service' and so on. Because one serves and envisages, it is service (*sevā*), namely, just toward reality, as the 'pledge' (*samaya*). Pursuant to that, the undertaking and generation of the (diamond) spot of earth, etc. (generation of the palace from BHRUṂ, up to the Clear Light of conviction) is the 'occupation with the pledge of service' (*sevāsamayasaṃyoga*), the first member.

Having (in that way) voidness as meditative object, the meditative object of sun, and so on, is Near Evocation (*upasādhana*). Precisely the bringing to conclusion the depositing (in the body) of mantras (Oṃ, etc.) is the arising of Near Evocation (*upasādhana-saṃbhava*), the second (member).

Concerning 'the aim of the sādhana, and the symbol' (*sādhanārthaṃ ca samayam*), the aim of the *sādhana* means to solicit for establishing the evocation (of one's own three doors as the Buddha's Body, Speech, and Mind). 'Symbol' (*samaya*) means 'to get together', i.e. the symbol (one's own Symbolic Being), along with the Samādhisattva and the Jñānasattva, to wit, both the aim of the *sādhana* and the symbol are the third (member).

The accomplishment of the great aim of others, (accomplishment) which is the 'best victorious maṇḍala' and the 'best victorious rite' belonging to the remaining conclusion, is the Great Evocation (*mahāsādhana*). That is the fourth (member).

Having thus understood the four members as a division of *vajra*, i.e. as a division of 'family' (*kula*) (the five families), then, i.e. next, one should accomplish the rites to be stated subsequently precisely as the first.

(The first member :) Starting with the lines 'Sevāsamādhi ..., he expands upon the (four) members which were touched upon. The *bodhicitta* (in the void) as meditative object is service (*sevā*). Precisely that concentrates, i.e. halts in the mind, hence '*samādhi*'. Praxis (*saṃyoga*) means right application. That (imaginative) generation, by means of conviction (*adhimukti*), from the (diamond) spot of earth, etc. up to the *maṇḍala-circle*, which is both the service-*samādhi* and the praxis, is the *sevāsamādhisaṃyoga*. Having done that (much), he should contemplate the supreme revelation, possessing the character of thusness, which has arisen from pondering the meaning of the mantra, 'Oṃśūnyatā...'

(The second member:) (Then,) in the sequence of sun, moon, lotus, etc., one stacks successively higher, places the three syllables (ā, o, ha) upon that; then consolidates all that, and again imagines the moon-disk, and upon that the three syllables (Oṃ, Āḥ, Hūṃ). Then from the transformation of that, there arise the hand symbol(s) (of the six families). From the transformation of the hand symbol(s), there are completed the form(s) of Mahāmudrā (of the six families). What accomplishes and completes nearby, that is said to be (definition of) Near Evocation (*upasādhana*). The *siddhi* is the *siddhi* of *mahāmudrā* (body from the five *abhisaṃbodhis*). Its 'foremost' is the initial ones, the mantras Oṃ, etc. When that is present, the Near Evocation is foremost. Having placed all the mantra-syllables, there are the form(s) of the Mahāmudrā. Therein is the *vajra*, to wit, the (32) deities from Vairocana down to Sumbha(rāja). Their bases (*āyatana*) are the skandhas of form, etc.

(The third member :) Of those (members), one becomes certain by the stage of the third series (the Atiyoga) and accomplishes through pondering with thorough knowledge of cause (the placement of deities in the body) and fruit (of contemplating after that placement). Whereby (by inviting the deity host of the triple vajra and drawing them into oneself) one has pleased (the deities) for the sake of blessing (one's own three doors), thereby that 'is said to be the exhortation when there is evocation.' That is related by way of synonym (of evocation and exhortation). But why (the exhortation)? The two verses (Nos. 70-71) beginning '*buddhakāyadhara*'. The 'contemplation of the lords of the mantras' refers to the syllables Oṃ, etc. (i.e. when Vajradhara and Akṣobhya are the *maṇḍala*-rulers, Hūm; and the remaining four *samādhi-sattvas* by Oṃ, Svā, Āḥ, Hā). The Samādhisattvas are the lords; the Jñānasattvas belong to the lords of the mantras. The meditation on the various families according to their arising is the 'contemplation of the lords of the mantras.'

(The fourth member :) Regarding 'the great evocation (Mahāsādhana)..', what is pointed out as the great evocation belongs to the jñānavajrin-s at the time of generating it. The mantrins possessing the yoga of presiding deity, having aroused *samāpatti* preceded by instigation of the *vajra* and *padma* (of their own family), are their own mantras Vajradṛg, etc. (32 in no.), i.e. the vajrin-s arisen therefrom (i.e. as in a womb from the syllables Oṃ, etc.). To have imagined their totality as the form of Mahāmudrā (of the Victorious Maṇḍala), is stated as 'having imagined the lord on the crown of his head', that is, having imagined the lord Mahāvajradhara on the crown and twisted hair of the Mahāmudrā form of the five Tathāgatas, and (having imagined) Vairocana and the other Buddhas on the remaining crowns of their family deities (Locanā, etc.), one is successful, i.e. attains *siddhi*.

*yathārutam* /

*The Stage of Completion* :

Having thus explained the delighting of Vajrasattva (for the purpose of mundane siddhis) by the stages of four yogas (but with no treatment of 'Victory of the Rite, which belongs to Mahāsādhana), now (*idānīm*) he alludes to the completion of Mahāvajradhara by the stages of six members in the *Uttara-tantra* (Chap. XVIII) of the *Guhyasamāja* :

> By the distinction of 'shared' and 'superior',
> one posits two kinds of service: the 'shared'
> one by the four *vajras*, the 'superior' one by
> members six in number.

(Cf. XII, 64 :

> One should create, everywhere and always, just with the knowledge nectar of service. For this brings to success the aim of mantra and of tattva, of all mantras. )

As to the words, 'One should create just with the knowledge nectar of service', and so on, "One serves, having been studying with desire for liberation (the highest *siddhi*)", is (the definition of) 'service' (*sevā*). And why (the desired liberation)? The (yuganaddha) body of deity completely pure (of the two obscurations). That is to be created, i.e. completed, just with the knowledge nectar of service, i.e. just with the six-membered yoga. 'Everywhere' means in the nature of all. 'Always' means (those six) at all times and in all good postures. The expression 'just' (*eva*) is in the sense of restriction (to the particular instance). 'For this' (*eṣo hi*) refers to the knowledge nectar, i.e. the six-membered yoga. 'Of all mantras' means 'of all Tathāgatas'. 'Mantras' are SARPA ('serpent') and so on (diamond muttering of both *neyārtha* and *nītārtha* mantras). 'Reality' (*tattva*) means the god reality (of ultimate yuganaddha). Their aim (*artha*) is the fruit (*phala*). By accomplishing that (fruit, by means of the six members) one accomplishes the reality aim for the mantra. 'For', means wherefore in the sense of aim. For the reason the six-membered yoga is that way, for that reason the service is to create just with that (yoga).

Those six members, pratyāhāra, etc. are set forth in the *Uttara-tantra* of the *Guhyasamāja*:

> When one does the service with the six-membered yoga, he wins the supreme success. In no other way does the supreme *siddhi* arise.
>
> Pratyāhāra, dhyāna, prāṇāyāma, dhāraṇā, anusmṛti, and samādhi, are the six members.
>
> He expands upon those brief indications as follows (Chap.

XVIII, verses 141, ff. in Bagchi's numbering):

The dwelling upon interiorization of the ten sense bases on all levels severally directed toward the taking of desires, is called Withdrawal (pratyāhāra). The five desires are in condensation through the application to the five Buddhas. Meditation (dhyāna) is said to be imagination. And that Meditation is fivefold: Primary Conception (vitarka) is the secret triad, from the enjoyment of which comes Secondary Conception (vicāra). The vicinity of joy is the third, and the sum of pleasure is the fourth. One's own consciousness with removal of the upsurge of knowledge and knowables, is known as the fifth, with a peace composed of all Buddhas and abiding in all desires. Drawing forth the breath made of five knowledges and which is the self-existence of the five elements, one should imagine it in the form of a tiny ball on the tip of the lotus nose.

The great jewel of five colors is said to be prāṇāyāma. Having meditated on one's own mantra in the heart, one should place the prāna in its bindu form.

When one's sense organ and the jewel have ceased (to operate) one should retain. (That is) called Retention (*dhāraṇā*). When consciousness goes toward the diamond of cessation, the apprehension of signs arises.

Those signs have been explained by the diamond of enlightenment as fivefold. The first has the aspect of a mirage, the second the aspect of smoke. The third has the aspect of fire-flies, the fourth shines like a lamp, and the fifth is a steady light like a cloudless sky.

One should radiate that firm thing by the vajra path into the regions of the sky. Contemplating which, by Recollection (*anusmrti*) one should radiate those aspects. One should know about Recollection that there is the shining appearance, and that it (Recollection) is engendered therein.

Having drawn together by the equipoise of insight and means all states in condensation by the yoga of the small ball, one should contemplate the image in their middle. Instantly there is the consummation of knowledge called 'Samādhi'.

Explaining in detail, he states the verse 'of the ten' and so on. 'Sense bases' are the (personal) sense bases (of eye, etc.) and the objects (forms, etc.) of the sense bases. The 'interiorization' (*svavṛtti*) is of those ten sense bases which are the sense objects and the senses grasping them, to wit : according to the engagement with the intrinsic feature of the individual apprehended object and apprehending organ, there is interiorization. The abiding in that, is the dwelling upon interiorization. 'On all levels' means according to the distinctions of inferior, middling, and best (for each sense object), that is, 'severally directed toward the taking of desires'. 'Desires' according to the passage, "They desire and are attached to", are form, and so on (the five sense objects). 'Severally directed', i.e. again and again, toward that taking, i.e. apperception, of those (sense objects) by the sense organs, their apperception is the 'taking'. That is the detailed explanation of the initial member (which is the arcane body of purification 'afterwards obtained').

With the aim of purifying the Withdrawal, he states the second member with the verse 'the five' and so on. 'The five desires' are the sense bases of form, etc., i.e. the (five) sense objects. 'In condensation' means by unification (of the sense objects) with the sense organs. The 'five Buddhas' are the eye and other sense organs. The right conjunction of them (to their respective Buddha, Akṣobhya, etc.) is the conjunction 'through the application to the five Buddhas'. As a result, form and so on, are (also) those five Buddhas. In that fashion (of conjunction), whatever is the imagination purified (of ordinary appearance) is the 'Meditation'. That becomes fivefold by the division into 'Primary Conception' and so on. The verse 'Primary Conception' and so on, has the setting forth of its division. As to the verse 'the secret triad' and so on, the sense organ, the sense object, and the knowledge based on the sense, are the secret triad. The (rough) imagination that the five sense organs, the (five) knowledges based on the senses, and their sense objects have the nature of the five Tathāgatas, is Primary Conception. The deliberating (in detail) just on that, is Secondary Conception in location (those two are also arcane body of purification 'afterwards obtained'). When one is so deliberating (with those two), what has the characteristic of contentment through facing the entrance into reality, is the vicinity called Joy (*prīti*). What has attained the pleasure possessing the characteristic of body-cathartic and so on (the mind-cathartic), through adherence to reality, that is the sum of pleasure (*sukha-saṃgraha*). The one who thus has applied himself repeatedly so as to go to the pinnacle of excellence, has the removal of upsurge of knowledge and knowables, where the upsurge of knowledge is the six evolvements as eye, and so on, of perception (*vijñāna*), and where the upsurge in the knowables is in (the six) from form up to the *dharmadhātu* (which is the object of the sixth 'sense'); and where its removal is called 'one's own consciousness' (*svacitta*) as the voidness in consciousness of both apperceived and apperception,and as the one-pointedness of mind with the characteristic of complete knowledge.' One's own consciousness' of such fashion by reason of yoga is 'with a peace composed of all Buddhas'. The 'Peace' is through pacifying the discursive thought of the apperceived and so on. It is engendered (by successive dissolution of the three voids) as light-only and the ultimate that is one with universal void (the fourth void, the Symbolic Clear Light). That is the fivefold division of the second member.

Regarding the verse 'five' and so on, the downward breath has the intrinsic nature of the five knowledges, beginning with mirror-like, and is the individualizing factor of earth (and the other elements). Drawing it forth from the nostril of one's *vajra*, one should imagine it in the form of a tiny ball, i.e. in the form of the *bodhicitta-bindu*, on the tip of the lotus-nose (of the sacral place). Precisely that is the breath proceeding upward with five colors, the nature of the five Tathāgatas. Precisely that is the 'great jewel' (the 'drop of light' at the nose of the face, and which is recited). 'Prāṇa' is what envigorates; 'āyāma' is that by which it is spread far;—thus the explanation of prāṇāyāma to be known, because one should recite during day and night by way of the own-nature of making that (prāṇāyāma) enter and so on. 'Having meditated on one's own mantra (drop) in the heart', i.e. at (the nose of) the lotus (8-petalled) of one's heart, 'one should place' (*nyaset*) 'the *Prāṇa* in its *bindu* form' (the letter A, etc.) deposited, inviolable (*akṣata*). That is the third member.

Concerning the verse 'has ceased' and so on, the sense

bases are one's form, and so on (the five sense objects), as well as the eye, and so on (the five sense organs). When the pairs of sense bases have ceased, i.e. are not in evidence (as in death's sequence), then when the jewel which is the basis of sense objects and sense organs, and the jewel of consciousness (the *manovijñāna*, the sixth sense) have ceased along with *prāṇāyāma*, i.e. have set (*astaṃgata*), what one would retain, that is Retention. Why that? The True Limit (the gnosis of the Clear Light). (The verse states) "When consciousness goes toward the diamond of cessation, the apprehension of signs arises." The 'diamond of cessation' is the Clear Light (*prabhāsvara*). When consciousness has gone to it, it is born in it. The apprehension of signs i.e. the manifestation of signs arises, i.e. occurs (as prior signs). Regarding the passage, the signs of the five realms have been explained by the diamond of enlightenment (the details are as follows) : Through dissolution into water by earth (in the performer's body), the aspect of a mirage manifests—the first sign. Through the dissolution into fire on the part of water, the aspect of smoke—the second. Through the dissolution into wind of fire, the aspect of fire-flies—the third. Through the going into the three lights on the part of the subtle element (i.e. wind), the self-existence of the set of lights like a lamp—the fourth. Through the (sequential) dissolution of the (three) *prakṛti*-light(s), there is only the Clear Light, a lasting light like a cloudless sky—the fifth. Those five signs bring (consciousness) to Nirvāṇa, as is said in the *Karmāntavibhāga* : "First, earth goes into water. Water goes into fire. Fire passes into wind. Wind enters perception (*vijñāna*). Perception accompanied by Retention in turn enters the Clear Light". Then the verse 'that firm thing' (purified in the Clear Light) and so on (is as follows) : 'By the vajra path', (expansion of *buddhi* to the whole sentient world) i.e. by entering the Clear Light preceded by the indispensable ('non-evadible', *alaṅghanīya*) five signs, one should radiate, i.e. pervade with the form of the Dharmakāya, in the regions of the sky, i.e. the worldly realms. That, explaining Retention, is the fourth member.

'Contemplating', i.e. realizing in immediacy, that oneself has in that way gone into the Clear Light, 'by Recollection' that previously one has reached the True Limit by means of the aspects of mirage and so on, one should radiate, i.e. engender, in a sequence which is precisely by those aspects (in reverse order). Immediately after that was told, one should know, i.e. it should be known, about 'Recollection' that there is the shining appearance (*pratibhāsa*), which is right understanding (the gnosis of the Clear Light) and that therein is engendered the fifth member, Recollection, not anywhere else.

Having unified 'by the equipoise of insight and means', i.e. by the union of absolute and conventional truths, all states (*bhāva*), whether stationary (the receptacle worlds, *bhājana-loka*) or moving (the sentient life, *sattvaloka*), in the form of a tiny ball in location, i.e. in the form of Mahāmudrā (the divine body), (then) one should contemplate, i.e. should know, the image of Mahāvajradhara with the nature of yuganaddha in the middle of that, the stationary and the moving. In this sequence, instantly, i.e. in a moment, there is the consummation of knowledge, i.e. the consummation of the knowledge-body (the yuganaddha body), called 'Samādhi', i.e. explained to be the sixth member.

Besides, in the *Śrī-Māyājāla*, he clearly states the varieties in the generation of deity :

> Yoga should be known as of three kinds: with blessing and with imagination (on the Stage of Generation), and the yoga (on the Stage of Completion) of the *citta* image which is extolled by the perfected Buddhas.
>
> The ego of Blessing-only is said to be the yoga with blessing. When there is the pure *bodhicitta*, and the great source of mantra-seeds; and in sequence the perfected image, imagined in the set of mudrās—and when that (image) is imagined with the thought, "That is imagined", it is called the yoga with imagination.
>
> Endowed with the best of all aspects, and having consolidated (the deities) one should radiate (them). Instantly, there is the consummation of knowledge, called the completed yoga.

Also, in the *Vairocanābhisaṃbodhi* he sets forth the devatā-yoga as of two kinds:

> O master of the secret folk, there are two kinds of divine form—pure and impure. The pure kind is understood form, free from all signs. The impure kind has all signs,

with color-and-shape forms. Now, two purposes go with those two kinds of divine form. The kind with signs generates siddhi with signs; the kind without signs, the siddhi without signs. Besides, the holy Jinas have maintained that when one is always stationed in the signless kind, he can also bring to success (the siddhi) with signs. Therefore, by all means one should take recourse to the non-signed.

Saṃdhyā bhāṣā/.

PART TWO

# INTRODUCTIONS

## I INTRODUCTION TO BUDDHIST TANTRISM

### A. *Tantra* (*generalities*)

WHAT IS AN introduction to the ideas and practices of the Buddhist Tantras? Let me allude to the leading literature on the subject. It is well known that S. B. Dasgupta wrote a book entitled *An Introduction to Tantric Buddhism* (University of Calcutta, 1950). This has certainly been a helpful book for persons interested in the Buddhist Tantras. The Japanese scholars appreciated it especially since the kinds of Tantras which had been continued in Japan were of a quite different character from the works consulted by S. B. Dasgupta, and those scholars were also interested in the philosophical tenets which Dasgupta found in the tantric manuscripts which he consulted. It must also be admitted that Dasgupta was himself attracted to certain features of the manuscripts which he consulted, such as verses about the *cakras* (mystic centers) in the body, and the special way in which the male and female are regarded, suggestive of being compared with the Śākta movements that have been strong in Bengal. All the material which he brought forward is indeed authoritative data from those texts. Naturally he did not thoroughly represent the works he consulted; and besides they are replete with ritual details that are often tedious. Benoytosh Bhattacharyya made giant strides in opening up this subject by his various text editions; and of course he was well prepared to explain elements of the system, which he did in various publications with sympathy. I have frequently recommended to my students to consult G. Tucci's *Tibetan Painted Scrolls* for its Vajrayāna chapter; but this is an expensive work of restricted distribution. Then the late Professor F. D. Lessing of Berkeley and myself collaborated in the translation from Tibetan of the work now published (1968) as *Mkhas grub rje's Fundamentals of the Buddhist Tantras.* In conversations I have freely admitted that this is not an introduction for Westerners as it was for Tibetans, even though it presents the fundamentals of the four Tantra literature divisions with a considerable and convenient fund of information not hitherto available in any Western language. To answer the question posed above, an introduction should show what the Tantra is all about, the underlying suppositions, the leading instructions, to the extent of recreating the Tantra as a viable entity to be liked or disliked. The trouble with so much of the present writing on the Tantra is that the reader is, or should be, left with a feeling of distancy or bewilderment; he is neither genuinely for or against it, because he does not understand it. It is on this point that one can praise S. B. Dasgupta's work: he was not simply reproducing citations from texts; he tried to explain as he went along. But he could only explain when his own background allowed him, namely when these Buddhist Tantras overlapped the Hinduism with which he had a natural knowledge through his birthright and training.

Now, what is the relation of the Buddhist Tantra to Hinduism? This is hardly a one-directional influence. In fact, the Buddhist Tantra goes back in many of its leading ideas to the Brahmanism of the older Upaniṣads, and some of its ritual (e.g. the *homa*, or burnt offering) can be traced to old Vedic rites. In short, the Buddhist Tantra incorporated a large amount of the mystical ideas and practices that have been current in India from most ancient times, and preserved them just as did the Hindu Tantra in its own way, while both systems had mutual influence and their own deviations. The Buddhist Tantra is deeply indebted to certain later Upaniṣads such as the Yoga Upaniṣads, which were probably composed in the main form about 1st century B. C. to the beginning of the Gupta period, and which are a primitive kind of Hinduism. But these mystical practices were so thoroughly integrated with Buddhist dogma, that it is a most difficult matter to separate out the various sources of the Buddhist Tantra.

Then, with regard to the chronology, it is not my original idea to put the revealed Buddhist Tantras in the period of 4th and 5th centuries, A. D. (B. Bhattacharyya maintained such an early date for the *Guhyasamājatantra*). This certainly requires justification, and in the section 'Introduction to the Guhyasamājatantra' I shall present some arguments in its case. For the others I shall simply assert that there is no where else in Indian chronology to put the bulk of them: exactly in the same period which was the creative period of Hinduism and which cast the mold for the forms of Indian religion in the subsequent centuries. There are some notable exceptions just as there are for Hinduism; and in the case of the Buddhist Tantra certainly the expanded *Kālacakratantra* was composed much later. The Tantric revelations were kept in esoteric cults—for there must have been a tension between the orthodox Buddhist sects and these far-out tantric groups. This strict secrecy was continued up to around the 8th century when commentaries by named persons appear. Those commentaries continue through the 12th century, more and more coloring the public forms of Buddhism in its last Indian phase. However, we must look to other reasons for the disappearance of Buddhism; after all, the Hindus themselves are fond of Tantra and this has not caused Hinduism to disappear!

These tantric cults were introduced into China from India during the T'ang Dynasty but did not take root until the 8th century which saw the activity of the Indian masters Vajrabodhi and Amoghavajra (cf. Chou Yi-liang, *Tantrism in China*). The kind of Buddhist Tantras which prevailed in China gave rise to the two forms of Buddhist mysticism in Japan—the form handed down by the Tendai school (in which the Tantra is one of the topics of study) and that handed down by the Shingon School (in which the Tantra is the main thing). Buddhist Tantrism called the Diamond Vehicle, was brought to completion in Japan by Kôbô Daishi, founder of the Shingon. Japanese Tantrism is especially based on the works called the *Mahāvairocanasūtra*, also known as the *Vairocanābhisambodhi* (which yields the 'Garbha-maṇḍala') and the *Tattvasaṃgraha* (referred to in Japan as "Tip of the Thunderbolt" which yields the 'Vajramaṇḍala'). Forms of Tantra were also introduced and once apparently flourished in what is now called Java, where as Paul Mus has shown, the five levels of Borobudur symbolise the five Buddhas. But more than anywhere else the Buddhist Tantras came to flower in Tibet, starting with their implantation in the 8th century by the teachers Padmasambhava and Śāntarakṣita. After the cessation of composition in Sanskrit of the commentaries, they continued in the Tibetan language in an enormous literature.

There are serious problems in studying the Tantric literature. Because of the syncretic and deliberately mystifying nature of such texts as the *Guhyasamājatantra*, their sentences, although relatively simple in language complexity, continually need the guru's oral expansion and authoritative commentary. The problem is not with the individual words, which indeed mean what they ought; but rather in the fact that so many words, besides meaning what they ought, are employed in a range, of acceptable usages and then intend other senses in arbitrary analogical systems. Again, these texts are essentially practical, are concerned with doing things such as rites. And recipe books, even on the mundane level, are notorious for requiring a teacher to tell the missing steps. Then, in the case of the Tantras, the gurus have taken vows not to reveal the Tantras to the uninitiated ('immature') persons, and so the difficulty is compounded, even for those persons who are initiated. The style of writing is conducive to corruptions in the texts, certainly a fault in manuscripts of the *Guhyasamājatantra*.

It is understandable that the numerous difficulties of the literature might result in some unwarranted judgments. In fact, eminent authorities of the Tantras during their India period had disagreements with each other, and later investigators, such as the Tibetan gurus, decided that certain earlier authorities had misunderstood this or that important point. Therefore, it is right for us to be charitable in the event of seeming misinterpretations; but still they should be pointed out. In illustration, some questionable terms have been applied to the Buddhist Tantras. (1) There is no expression 'Dhyāni Buddhas' in the texts; one finds instead the words Tathāgata, Buddha or Jina, as in the compound pañcatathāgata ('five Tathāgatas'), (2) There is no terminology 'right and left hand paths' in the Buddhist Tantras, and no classification of the Tantras on that basis, insofar as classification by the tantrics themselves is concerned. The standard classification is into four classes, Kriyā-tantra, Caryā-tantra, Yoga-tantra, and Anuttarayoga-tantra. Of course, some Westerners may feel that certain Buddhist Tantras such as the *Guhyasamājatantra* teach practices which fit the category of 'left hand path' and there are statements in those Tantras which lend credence to such a theory. We should observe that the Hindu Tantras themselves use such terminology but in different ways, as shown in Chintaharan Chakravarti's work, *The Tantra: Studies on their Religion and Literature.* (3) The texts do not use the word śakti in the sense of the female consort power of a deity (of course, the word *śakti* can be and is used in the other meaning of a certain weapon). In the article, "Female Energy and Symbolism in the Buddhist Tantras" I gave the following list of generic words used for the goddesses or females in the class of Anuttarayogatantra *prajñā* ('insight'), *yoginī* ('female yogin'), *vidyā* ('occult science' or 'know how'), *devī* ('goddess' or 'queen'), *mātṛ* ('mother'), *mātṛkā* ('mother' or 'letters'), *ḍākinī* ('fairy'), *dūtī* ('female messenger'), *śūrī* ('heroine'), and *mudrā* ('seal' or 'gesture'). Of course, that use of the word śakti for the female consort of the Buddhist Tantras implies that this is what the tantrics mean by their consort. Later on, various scholars (S. B. Dasgupta especially) protested against the use of the word on the grounds that in these Buddhist Tantras, the '*prajñā*' (one of the most frequent of the words) is passive, not active like the Śaivitic śakti. That is one reason for my writing that article "Female Energy..", because when one goes into the texts he will find for the usage of the word *prajñā* that in the ordinary person who does not control his mind this is indeed a passive function, while the aim of the Buddhist praxis is to arouse the fiery potentiality of this function. How is it aroused? The *Mahāvairocanasūtra* has a celebrated verse about this matter, and which is correlated with mantra steps in the Shingon sect. Fortunately it is in Sanskrit, as cited in Kamalaśīla's (First) *Bhāvanākrama* (G. Tucci's *Minor Buddhist Texts*, Part II, p. 196 : vairocanābhisaṃbodhau coktam/tad etat sarvajñajñānaṃ karuṇāmūlaṃ bodhicittahetukam upāyaparyavasānam iti/ "And it is said in the *Vairocanābhisaṃbodhi* : '(Master of secret folk). The omniscient knowledge has Compassion for a root, has the Mind of Enlightenment for a motive, and has the Means for a finality'." In that passage 'omniscient knowledge' is equivalent to the Buddha's Perfection of Insight (*prajñāpāramitā*). Compassion provides this Insight with a root in the phenomenal world. The Mind of Enlightenment provides this Insight with a motive, the vow as cause. The Means provides this Insight with a finality, its fulfilment. At the first two levels, the Insight is still passive; it is with the Means that it appears in full flowering, its true active form.

When Insight (*prajñā*) is combined with the Means (*upāya*), it is no longer passive. Therefore, while it is not strictly correct to call Prajñā a śakti, the persons who applied this expression—and Benoytosh Bhattacharyya and Giuseppe Tucci had read widely in both Hindu and Buddhist Tantras—were closer to the truth than those who insist on the 'passive' interpretation.

This general problem of explaining the Tantras is so crucial that it is germane to dwell upon it some more. Fortunately, there is a master who expressed himself on this very point, the 8th century teacher Līlavajra, the teacher of Buddhaśrijñāna who heads one of the two lineages of Guhyasamāja interpretation. Līlavajra has written a commentary on the *Śrī-guhyagarbha-mahātantrarāja* (the *ṭikā-nāma*) (PTT, Vol. 82, pp. 248 and 249). He soon begins a section 'Method of Explaining the Tantra', which he says has three aims, in the sense of aims for the superior, intermediate, and inferior among candidates and sense organs. In the course of explaining for the aim of the superior candidate or sense organ, he includes that which is related to the form of meaning, which "has certainty about the reality of the *guhyagarbha*" (*gsaṅ baḥi sñiṅ po de kho na ñid ṅes paḥo*), regarding the chief words in the title of the Tantra on which he is commenting. Then he states that there are three kinds of *guhya* and three kinds of *garbha*. The three of *guhya* ('secret')) are (1) of the self existent (*raṅ bzhin=svabhāva*), (2) pregnant (*sbas pa=garbhin*), and (3) profound (*gab pa=gambhīra*). In explanation of the first kind, that of the self existent, he cites the text:

> Aho ! The *dharma* which is the utmost secret is the intrinsic secret (behind) diverse manifestation, highly secret through self existence; than which there is nothing more secret !

In summary of his commentary on this verse, it turns out that the utmost secret is the non-dual, self-originated Wisdom (*jñāna*), an effortless fount of good qualities while its own aspect is incognizable. It is an element located in the stream of consciousness (the *saṃtāna* or *saṃtati*), an incessant fountain of entities self appearing, but this element is obscured by discursive thought; it is both cause and effect as both consciousness and the imagined objective domain; there is nothing more central, and it appears through introspection (*svasaṃve-*

*dana*) but by reason of obscurations, men have sought it elsewhere. (This is certainly the 'embryo of the Tathāgata' theory from one stream of non-tantric Buddhism). The second kind of secret is the 'pregnant', so called because it is like the woman impregnated by another and with the embryo growing in privacy. This secret is deliberately given or withheld by the guru, and concerns the secret practice of the Tantra. Līlavajra says, "If one practices by praxis according to the word (of the Tantra) but lacks the *mantra*-precepts, this is a grievous fault" (sṅags kyi man ṅag med pa daṅ/sgra bzhin spyod pa rnams kyis spyad na/śin tu ñes pa che bas/ ). The third kind, the profound, is the perfect meaning of the Tantra (*rgyud kyi don phun sum tshogs pa*), and this is conferred by oneself through the two *pramāṇas*. He must mean Direct Perception (*pratyakṣa*) and Inference (*anumāna*). In summary of the three kinds of secret, the first of the self-existent is nature's secret, the second of 'pregnant' is conferred by another, the third of profound is conferred by oneself. When we think over Līlavajra's precepts, it strikes us that it is easy to be irrelevant about the Buddhist Tantra by treating as doctrine what in fact is a practice: as far as human secrecy is concerned, in Tantrism there is only 'pregnant' practice and profound doctrine. And that it is easy to go wrong by interpreting the literal words of the Tantra as the practice, while lacking the precepts of the guru which clarify what the practice should be. I have been told that this point is also stressed in the Shingon sect of Japan, and so this is a matter independent of whether the passage in question has 'sexual' symbolism. Lately some persons have found only a sexo-yogic topic to set forth as characteristic of the Anuttarayoga-tantra, but Līlavajra informs us that the most important issue and aim of the Tantras is that element hidden in the stream of consciousness, obscured by discursive thought (which plagues us all).

That man becomes interested in finding the element hidden in the stream of consciousness is probably the reason for the non-tantric teaching that Buddhahood is attainable only through a human body, which is a teaching continued in the Tantras (*Sṅags rim*, f. 460a-2):

> /dri med ḥod las/ skye ba ḥdi la saṅs rgyas ñid kyi ḥbras bu rab tu ster ba rgyud kyi rgyal poḥo/lha la sogs pa ḥgro ba lṅaḥi skye ba la ni ma yin no/zhes daṅ/It says

in the *Vimalaprabhā* : 'The phrase "grants the Buddhahood fruit in this life" means—the King of Tantras grants the Buddhahood fruit in this birth, which is a human birth; not in the birth which is one of the five (other) destinies (*gati*), god and the like.'

### B. *Definitions and varieties of Tantras*

The way of the Tantras is especially called the Vajrayāna ('Diamond Vehicle') or the Mantrayāna ('Mantra Vehicle'). Tsoṅ-kha-pa in his *Sṅags rim* cites the *Vimalaprabhā* : "The diamond (*vajra*) is the great 'insplittable' and 'unbreakable'; and the Great Vehicle (*mahāyāna*) which is precisely so, is the Vajrayāna : it combines the Mantra-way and the Prajñāpāramitā-way, which are (respectively) the 'effect' (or 'fruit') and the 'cause' " ( / rdo rje ni mi phyed pa daṅ mi cḥod pa chen po yin la de ñid theg pa chen po yin pa ni rdo rje theg pa ste/ sṅags kyi tshul daṅ pha rol tu phyin paḥi tshul ḥbras bu daṅ rgyuḥi bdag ñid gcig tu ḥdres par gyur paḥo). Hence in Tsoṅ-kha-pa's reform, non-tantric Buddhism (*pāramitāyāna*) must be mastered in preparation for the Tantras.

Concerning the expression 'Mantrayāna', the standard explanation is that in the *Guhyasamājatantra*, Chap. XVIII, p. 156 (two theoretical corrections with asterisks): The theoretical corrections were made by Professor Rasik Vihari Joshi and myself putting our heads together on this when he was teaching at Columbia University, Fall 1969. Compare S. Bagchi *Guhyasamājatantra*, XVIII, 70A, and Yukei Matsunaga, "The *Guhyasamājatantra*: A New Critical Edition," XVIII, 70B.

*pratītyotpadyate yad yad indriyair viṣayair manaḥ /*
*tanmano *man-itikhyātaṃ *trakāraṃ trāṇanārthataḥ //*
*lokācāravinirmuktaṃ yad uktaṃ samayasambaram /*
*pālanaṃ sarvavajrais tu mantracaryeti kathyate //*

Whatsoever mind arises in dependence on sense organs and sense objects, that mind is explained as the '*man*', the '*tra*' in the meaning of (its) salvation.

Whatever pledge and vow said to be free from worldly conduct has protection by all the *vajras*, that is explained as the *mantra* practice.

Nāgārjuna's *Aṣṭādaśa-paṭala-vistara-vyākhyā* (PTT, Vol. 60, p. 9-4, 5) explains the 'sense organs' and 'sense objects' as union of upāya and prajñā; and explains the words 'free from worldly conduct' as 'leaving off discursive thought about the ordinary body, and taking on the contemplation of the divine body' (tha mal paḥi lus rnam par rtog pa daṅ bral ba lhaḥi skur bsgom pa blaṅs nas). He does not comment on the words 'all the *vajras*'. In this literature, the multiplicity of vajras refers to the five Tathāgatas or Buddhas.

Besides, various Tantras may define the word 'Vajrayāna' in a way that characterizes the special subject matter of that Tantra. So we are led to understand *Guhyasamājatantra*, Chapter XVIII, p. 154:

> *moho dveṣas tathā rāgaḥ sadā vajre ratiḥ sthitā /*
> *upāyas tena buddhānāṃ vajrayānam iti smṛtam//*
>
> Delusion, hatred, and lust are always the repose lying in the *vajra*,
> Whereby the means of the Buddhas is called Vajrayāna ('Diamond Vehicle').

That verse presumably refers back to Chapter VIII, verse 2:

> *rāgadveṣamohavajra vajrayānapradeśaka/*
> *ākāśadhātukalpāgra ghoṣa pūjāṃ jinālaya//*
>
> May Thou, the diamond of lust, hatred, and delusion, who reveals the Vajrayāna;
> Thou, the best like the sky, the womb of the Tathāgatas—proclaim the worship (*pūjā*):

Candrakīrti's *Pradīpoddyotana*, and *Mchan ḥgrel* (PTT. Vol. 158, p. 62-1,2) first explain the passage according to the *neyārtha* comment with the usual meanings of the words (= the literal translation), and then go on to the *nītārtha* comment as follows: 'lust' is means (*upāya*), the 'spread of light' and its 40 prakṛtis; 'hatred' is insight (*prajñā*), the 'light' and its 33 prakṛtis; 'delusion' is nescience (*avidyā*), the 'culmination of light' and its 7 prakṛtis; 'worship' is the *yuganaddha* with non-dual knowledge. That terminology of the *nītārtha* comment will be explained in later sections.

As has been mentioned, the usual classification of the Buddhist tantra works is into four classes called Kriyā-tantra, Caryā-tantra, Yoga-tantra, and Anuttarayoga-tantra. This is the classification of the main corpus of Tantras translated into Tibetan and included in the collection called the Kanjur. The orthodox way of explaining this classification is either in terms of the candidates or in terms of the deities. *Mkhas grub rje's Fundamentals of the Buddhist Tantras* (p. 219) presents the candidate differentiation:

> Now, there are two methods laid down in the four Tantra divisions, namely, *outer action* (**bāhya-kriyā*), such as bathing, cleaning, etc.; and *inner yoga* (**adhyātma-yoga*). The Kriyā Tantra was expressed for subduing the candidates (*vineya*) who delight in *outer action*, while the Caryā Tantra was expressed for subduing the candidates who delight in practicing *outer action* and *inner yoga* in equal measure. The Yoga Tantra was expressed for subduing the candidates who delight in the *yoga of inner samādhi* with minimal outer ritual, while the Anuttara Yoga Tantra is the incomparable Tantra for subduing the candidates who delight in *inner-yoga*.

Mkhas grub rje alludes to the deity differentiation as the 'four Passion Families' (pp. 168-169), detailed in the notes thereto on the basis of the *Sṅags rim* :

> The mutual attraction of Insight (*prajñā*) and the Means (*upāya*) finds :
> some deities laughing — Kriyā Tantra;
> some deities gazing — Caryā Tantra;
> some deities embracing — Yoga Tantra;
> some deities in coition — Anuttara Tantra.

Tsoṅ-kha-pa emphasizes that this is not a description of the candidates of these Tantra divisions;...

Besides, it can be speculated that the fourfold grouping of Tantras (there were earlier groupings of six or more) is made with an eye to the four Siddhāntas. In later Indian Buddhism, it was standard to divide up Buddhist metaphysics into four viewpoints, called Siddhānta, that of the Vaibhāṣikas, Sautrāntikas, Yogācārins, and the Mādhyamikaṣ. That could be the implication of Paṇḍit Smṛti's commentary called *Vajravidāraṇā-nāma-dhāraṇī-vṛtti* (Tohoku no. 2684) to the effect that the four Tantras constitute four kinds of washing by four kinds of persons, namely, Śrāvakas, Pratyekabuddhas, Yogācārins, and Mādhyamikas, in the given order. In Mahāyāna terminology, the Śrāvakas and Pratyekabuddhas constitute the Hīnayāna saints, while Yogācārins and Mādhyamikas are followers of the two main philosophical Mahāyāna schools constituting the last two Siddhāntas. Also the first two Siddhāntas, those of the Vaibhāṣika and the Sautrāntika, are classified as Hīnayāna, with the Sautrāntika considered preparatory for the rise of Mahāyāna viewpoints. The relation set up by Paṇḍit Smṛti (also called Smṛtijñānakīrti) has an artificial tone, at best is an overgeneralization, and at the same time is suggestive.

In the Anuttarayoga-tantra, there is also a principal division into Father Tantras, such as the *Guhyasamājatantra* ; and Mother Tantras, such as the *Śrī-Cakrasaṃvara*, a division which Mkhas-grub-rje explains following Tsoṅ-kh-pa. In brief, a Father Tantra emphasizes the 'Means' side of the 'means-insight' union, and so deals especially with the topics so prominent in the present work of evoking the three lights followed by the Clear Light, and of introducing the Illusory Body into the Clear Light. A Mother Tantra puts emphasis on the 'Insight' side of the 'means-insight' union, and so treats the indissoluble bliss and void; in fact, insofar as material dealing with this topic is included in the present work, it was derived from the Mother Tantra literature. Besides, the *Guhyasamāja-tantra* is considered the chief Tantra of the Father class, as is the *Śrī-Cakrasaṃvara* of the Mother class, for the reason that the literature and cult for the two Tantras is the most extensive anddeveloped among the Tantras found in the Kanjur and Tanjur.

The *Guhyasamājatantra* (Chap. XVIII, 153, 6-7) also has its own definition and classification of tantra: "'Tantra' is explained as 'continuous series' (*prabandha*). That continuous series is threefold through the division—*ādhāra*, *prakṛti*, and *asaṃhārya*." The succeeding verse explains that *prakṛti* is the *hetu*, *asaṃhārya* is the *phala*, and *ādhāra* is the *upāya*. According to Mkhas-grub-rje, the Tantra of Cause (*hetu*) is the chief of candidates for the high goal of the Tantra. The Tantra of Means (*upāya*) is the Tantra of Path. The Tantra of Fruit (*phala*) is the rank of Vajradhara. Those explanations clarify the definition of 'Tantra' as 'continuous series'. Apparently what is meant is that the Tantra shows the continuous progress of a superior candidate (Tantra of Cause) along the Tantric Path (Tantra of Means) to the high goal of Vajradhara (Tantra of Fruit). Nāgārjuna's *Aṣṭādaśa-paṭala-vistarā-vyākhyā* (PTT, Vol. 60, p. 6-1) sets forth on the same basis three kinds of Vajradhara, causal Vajradhara, fruitional Vajradhara, and

Vajradhara of the means. The causal Vajradhara is Mahāvajradhara, the *ādinātha.* The fruitional Vajradhara is Akṣobhya and the other Tathāgatas. The Vajradhara of the means is of three kinds, guarding of the place, guarding of oneself, and guarding of yoga. Guarding of the place is the frightening away of the demons through emanation of the ten Krodha deities. Guarding of oneself is the contemplation of only Paramārtha-satya (supreme truth), by recollecting such mantras as "Oṃ śūnyatā.." Guarding of yoga is of two kinds; the collection of merit (arousing compassion and contemplating the four Brahmā-vihāra-s) and the collection of knowledge (contemplation of the four doors to liberation).

### C. *Some fundamentals of the Tantras*

Here we shall consider four fundamentals: analogical thinking, the subtle body, the three worlds, and initiation by the hierophant.

The first fundamental is analogical thinking : "As without, so within" (*yathā bāhyaṃ tathā 'dhyātmam iti*). The Sanskrit is from Abhayākaragupta's *Niṣpannayogāvalī* (ed. by B. Bhattacharyya, p. 4), where it applies to the *maṇḍala* of the 'Stage of Generation' (*utpatti-krama*). See *Mkhas grub rje's Fundamentals*.., Index under '*maṇḍala*' : the self existent *maṇḍala* is in the mind, and the reflected image *maṇḍala* is drawn outside in conformity. The outer rite must conform to the inner rite, and *vice versa.* One must clear defiled thoughts from a space within the mind and erect the meditative image in this space. In the external *maṇḍala*-rite, first one drives away the evil spirits from the selected area; in this consecrated space one will draw the *maṇḍala.* In Mkhas-grub-rje's work, probably the most intricate set of analogies is found in the chapter on the Yoga tantra. In the present work, the most remarkable analogies are those in the treatment of the 'hundred lineages' under the commentary of the 'Bhagavān Sarva' and 'Tathāgata' verses in Part Three. But the analogies are ubiquitous in the Tantras. The most important analogy of all is that of affiliation: the candidate should affiliate his body, speech, and mind with the Body, Speech, and Mind of the Buddha, called the three mysteries. According to Mkhas grub rje, it is this affiliation which establishes the superiority of the Diamond Vehicle (the Tantras) over non-tantric Buddhism. One affiliates his body by gesture (*mudrā*), his speech by incantation (*mantra*) and his mind by deep concentration (*samādhi*). *Mkhas grub rje's Fundamentals...* states, "In the Kriyā and Caryā (Tantras) one intensely contemplates the body as Great Seal (*mahāmudrā*), speech as Incantation (*mantra*), and mind as Reality (*tattva*)." This is the 'Quick Path' because all avenues of the being are operating for a common goal : the body, speech, and mind are not working at cross purposes.

In such a case, we might say of body, speech, and mind, what Ārya-Śūra wrote in his *Jātaka-mālā* in description of King Śibi (but in his case meaning the three types, *kāma*, *artha*, and *dharma*).

*tasmiṃs trivargānuguṇā guṇāughāḥ saṃharṣayogād iva saṃniviṣṭāḥ/*
*samastarūpā vibabhur na cāsu virodhasaṃkṣobhavipannaśobhāḥ//*

In him all forms having multitudes of virtues consistent with the three types appeared with common residence as though from merger of rivalries, and they had no loss of brilliance due to opposition and commotion.

In Hinduism it is believed that those three types when in harmony yield the fourth one, liberation (*mokṣa*).

To understand any system of Buddhist Tantra one must find out the basic correspondence system or systems and carry through accordingly. Fourfold correspondences are especially prevalent in the Yoga-tantra. Among Anuttarayoga-tantras, the *Guhyasamājatantra* regularly employs fivefold correspondences based on the five Buddhas, the five knowledges, the five personality aggregates, and so on. The *Kālacakra-tantra* uses sixfold correspondences, wherein the elements are increased to six by addition of 'knowledge element' to the five of earth, water, fire, wind, and space. Sevenfold correspondences can be noticed in commentaries of the *Śrī-Cakrasaṃvara-tantra*. An example especially pertinent to the present work is the Guhyasamāja set of four steps of *sādhanā* or spiritual culture. Once the praxis is established in four steps, then some other principal entities are put in correspondence; thus the four goddesses are identified with the four steps. This very principle is employed in the present work for grouping the forty verses which expand the *nidāna* of the *Guhyasamājatantra*.

Is there a particular philosophical position of Buddhism that fits this kind of analogical thinking? Mkhas-grub-rje reports the thesis of the school founded by his teacher Tsoṅ-kha-pa that the Prāsaṅgika Mādhyamika underlies all four classes of Tantra. This appears to stem from the acceptance of all four *pramāṇas* by the non-tantric Candrakīrti in his *Prasannapadā* commentary on the *Mūla-madhyamaka-kārikā*. There (in the commentary on the first chapter) Candrakīrti says, in agreement with the Hindu Naiyāyikas, that the four sources of knowledge (*pramāṇa*) provide a foundation for the knowledge of worldly objects. Therefore, this Buddhist school accepts *upamāna* (analogy) as an independent source of knowledge. However, the epistemology of this school may differ from that of the Naiyāyikas. Thus Candrakīrti (text, p. 75) goes on to modify his acceptance of the *pramāṇas* by insisting on their relativity, or mutual dependence: "There being the cognitions (*pramāṇa*), there are the cognizable objects (*prameyārtha*); and there being the cognizable objects, there are the cognitions. But, indeed, there is no intrinsic-nature kind of establishment for either the cognition or the cognizable object" (satsu pramāṇeṣu prameyārthāḥ/ satsu prameyeṣv artheṣu pramāṇāni/na tu khalu svābhāvikī pramāṇaprameyayoḥ siddhir iti..). In contrast, Asaṅga (as I pointed out in "The Rules of Debate According to Asaṅga") accepts only three *pramāṇas*, direct perception, inference, and testimony of authoritative persons. This appears to be consistent with Asaṅga's Yogācāra idealism, wherein the subjective consciousness has the upper hand over the objective domain. Because idealist philosophy does not admit an equal status of subject-object, it does not agree with the precept "As without, so within", and so does not admit analogy as an independent source of knowledge. The Buddhist logicians, as well known, accept only two *pramāṇas*, direct perception and inference.

A fundamental metaphysical postulate is that of the subtle body, which of course is a basic idea of the Hindu systems as well. Tsoṅ-kha-pa explains in his commentary on the *Pañcakrama* (PTT, Vol. 159, p. 41-5) that there are two kinds of 'mind-only bodies' (*sems tsam gyi lus*, *cittamātra-deha*), namely the body of 'states' (*gnas skabs*, *avasthā*) and the 'innate body' (*gñug ma paḥi lus*, *nija-deha*). The first of these is the 'body of maturation' (*vipākakāya*) formed during the ten states (*avasthā*), which are the lunar months of intrauterine life, and which is born, matures, and dies. The second of these is the body formed of winds and mind only, the 'mind only' including no five outer-sense based perception (*vijñāna*) and the 'winds' including only the basic five winds (*prāṇa*, etc.) and not the secondary five (*nāga*, etc.). According to *Mkhas grub rje's Fundamentals..*, the 'uncommon means body' (*asādhāraṇa-upāyadeha*), a kind of subtle body, is the basis for the tantric machinations; this body seems to be a development of the innate body (*nija-deha*). The Tantras believe that by praxis involving mystic winds and mental muttering, this innate body gradually becomes defined as separate though within the coarse body. A more advanced stage is when this body can appear separately as an illusory body and be made to enter an ultimate state called the Clear Light, thus returning to a condition from which it had fallen, and which is anterior to the male-female division. As this innate body is strengthened, first it brings out exceeding acuity of one or more senses. The supernormal sharpness of smell is a topic in the celebrated *Lotus Sūtra* (*Saddharma-Puṇḍarīka*) chapter XVIII on advantages of a religious preacher. Non-tantric Buddhism speaks of six supernormal faculties (*abhijñā*), while tantric Buddhism adds more, for example, the eight *siddhis*.

The remarkable occult physiology of the tantric books is really based on their theories of this subtle body. This body is said to have 72,000 'veins' (*nāḍī*), of which three are the chief ones located in the position of the backbone. These three, the chief conduits of the 'winds', are differently named in the Hindu and Buddhist Tantras:

| | *right* | *middle* | *left* |
|---|---|---|---|
| Hindu | Piṅgala | Suṣumnā | Iḍā |
| Buddhist | Rasanā | Avadhūtī | Lalanā |

Besides, the Buddhist Tantras superimpose on those three channels four *cakras* (suggesting how four-fold analogies may be superimposed on the three-fold ones). However, there are two systems, earlier and later. One primary group of four *cakras*, important for what is called the 'Stage of Completion' (*sampanna-krama*) and having affinities with Upaniṣadic teachings, corresponds to four of the Hindu system as follows:

| | *head* | *neck* | *heart* | *navel* |
|---|---|---|---|---|
| Hindu | Ājñā | Viśuddha | Anāhata | Maṇipūra |
| Buddhist | Mahāsukha | Saṃbhoga | Dharma | Nirmāṇa |

Here I may cite my article "Female Energy and Symbolism in the Buddhist Tantras" for observations stemming from Tsoṅ-kha-pa's commentary on the Guhyasamāja Explanatory Tantra *Caturdevīparipṛcchā* :

> The primacy in this system of four *cakras* for physiological manipulation in ascetic practices may well go back to the old Upaniṣadic theories of the four states of consciousness. The *Brahmopaniṣad*, one of the Saṃnyāsa Upaniṣads, later than the early Upaniṣads but preceding the Tantric literature as we now have it, teaches that the Puruṣa has those four states when dwelling in the four places, namely, waking state in the navel, sleep ( i.e. dream) in the neck, dreamless sleep in the heart, and the fourth, Turīya, in the head. In agreement, Tsoṅ-kha-pa writes : 'When one has gone to sleep, there is both dream and absence of dream. At the time of deep sleep without dream the white and red elements of the *bodhicitta*, which is the basis of mind, stay in the heart, so mind is held in the heart. At the time of dreaming, those two elements stay in the neck, so mind is held in the neck. At the time when one is not sleeping, they stay at the navel, so mind is held there. When the male and female unite, those two stay in the head.

The later system of four *cakras* is correlated with the theory of four elements deified as goddesses, and is important for the practice during the 'Stage of Generation' (*utpatti-krama*). Following the indications of the *Maṇimālā* commentary on Nāgārjuna's *Pañcakrama* (PTT, Vol. 62, p. 178-2) and the *Sarvarahasya-nāma-tantrarāja*, verses 37-39 (PTT, Vol. 5), the fire-disk at the throat (or neck) is shaped like a bow; the water-disk at the heart is circular in shape; the wind-disk at the navel is triangular; and the earth-disk in the sacral place is square. These are also the shapes of the four altars for rites of burnt offering (*homa*) aimed at certain mundane *siddhis* (see *nidāna* verse 15), and they are also the shapes of the four continents of Purāṇic mythology (compare the printed geometrical forms in the edition of the *Guhyasamāja*, Chap. XV). The elements supply the names for these *cakras* (frequently *māhendra* for earth, and *vāruṇa* for water). According to the *Sṅags rim* (Peking blockprint, 441a-5).

> */kha sbyor las/ /me ṅid gaṅ dan rluṅ daṅ ni/*
> */dbaṅ chen daṅ ni bzhin chu/ /ḥkhor lor sems*
> *kyi kun spyod pa/ /steṅ daṅ ṅos daṅ braṅ ḥog ḥgro/*
> *zhes gsuṅs pas me steṅ daṅ rluṅ bsegs daṅ sa thad kar*
> *daṅ chu ḥog tu ḥgroḥo /*
>
> It says in the *Sampuṭa* : 'Fire, wind, earth (*māhendra*), and water, are each the executors of consciousness in a (given) *cakra*, and move (respectively) upwards, at acute angles, forward, and downwards.' This means that the fire (vibration) moves upwards; the wind, at acute angles to the wave (*tiryak*); the earth, straight forward; and the water, downwards.

The earth disk is equivalent to the Hindu *Mūlādhāra-cakra*, said to lie below the root of the sex organs and above the anus. The series is increased in the Hindu Tantras with Sahasrāra at the crown of the head, where Buddhism places the Buddha's *uṣṇīṣa* (sometimes said to be outside the body); and with Svādhiṣṭhāna at the root of the penis, called in some Buddhist Tantras the 'tip of the gem' (**maṇy-agra*).

Then we must take for granted that there are three worlds full of gods and demons. In the *Guhyasamājatantra*, Chap. IV, p. 17, there is the line *atha vajradharaḥ śāstā trilokas tu tridhātukaḥ*, on which *Pradīpoddyotana* (*Mchan ḥgrel* edition, PTT., Vol. 158, p. 38.5) explains *triloka* as being *sa ḥog* (*pātāla*), *sa steṅ* (*bhūmi*), and *mtho ris* (*svarga*); and explains *tridhātuka* as being the 'realm of desire' (*kāmadhātu*), etc. The correspondences can be tabulated as follows:

| *Old Vedic words* | *Hindu period* | *Tibetan* | *Possibly the Buddhist three* |
|---|---|---|---|
| Dyaus | Svarga | sa bla = mtho ris ('superior world') | 'formless realm (arūpa dhātu) |
| Antarikṣa | Bhūmi | sa steṅ ('above the earth') | 'realm of form (rūpa dhātu) |
| Pṛthivī | Pātāla | sa ḥog ('earth and below') | 'realm of desire' (kāmadhātu) |

The Vedic *mantras* of the three worlds are also employed in the Buddhist Tantras, as in this passage of Tsoṅ-kha-pa's *Sṅagsrim* (f. 311b.4) :

> */bhūr ni rluṅ gi dkyil ḥkhor la sogs pa ḥkhor daṅ bcas paḥi sa ḥog go/bhuvaḥ ni sa steṅ gi hjig rten no/svaḥ zhes pa ni mtho ris te srid rtse mthar thug paḥo/.*
>
> *Bhūr* is the underworld accompanied by the circles of the wind disk (*vāyu-maṇḍala*) and so forth. *Bhuvaḥ* is the 'perishable receptacle' (*loka*) of 'above the earth'. *Svaḥ* is the ultimate pinnacle of existence, the superior world.

The females or goddesses in terms of the three worlds are especially treated in the *Śrī-Cakrasaṃvara-tantra* and its commentaries. How does one come in contact with any of those gods or goddesses? Mircea Eliade (*Yoga : Immortality and Freedom*, p. 208) cites the proverb 'a non-god does not honor a god' (*nādevo devam arcayet*). That means that one must awaken the senses of that particular realm and learn the rules. The child cannot make his way in the human world without human senses and without learning the human rules. Thus first one generates oneself into deity ('selfgeneration' in Mkhas-grub rje's work).

The last of these fundamentals is the topic of initiation (*abhiṣeka*) meant to confer power, explained as maturing the stream of consciousness. The power, including the permission to continue that tantric lineage, is conferred by the hierophant (*vajrācārya*). The *Pradīpoddyotana* on Chapter XVII (*Mchan ḥgrel*, p. 157-4) contains this passage :

> */ tathā cāha / mahāmahāyānaratnarājasūtre // bhagavān vajrapāṇiḥ / uḍḍiyānaparvate niṣaṇṇaḥ/sarvāṃś ca vajra-yānaśikṣitān āmantrayāmāsa// śṛṇuta nikhilavajrayāna-*

> *sikṣitāḥ tathāgataṃ parinirvṛtaṃ na paśyati/śāstāram api tu vajrācāryo vajraguruḥ / so'yaṃ śāstā bhavatīti/*
> And it is also said in the *Mahāmahāyānaratnarājasūtra*: The Lord Vajrapāṇi was seated on the mountain of Oḍḍiyāna, and addressed all the trainees of the Vajrayāna : "All you trainees in the Vajrayāna, listen! When one does not see the Teacher, the Tathāgata entered into Parinirvāṇa, then the hierophant, the diamond guru, will serve as his teacher."

Various passages stress that one should look upon the hierophant as upon the Buddha, to disregard his faults and notice only his virtues, in that way, he is able to play the role of master for the disciple.

Initiations are conferred in maṇḍalas and are accompanied by vows (*saṃvara*) and pledges (*samaya*). The 'Stage of Generation' has the five *vidyā* initiations as described in Mkhas-grub rje's work. They are called the '*vidyā*' because they are adversaries for the five forms of '*avidyā*' (nescience), also because they are in reality conferred by the goddess consorts of the five Buddhas. Mkhas grub rje points out that although the 'preceptor' and the 'hierophant' lift up the flask (all five rites are accompanied with 'sprinkling'), in fact the goddesses Locanā and so on hold the flask and conduct the initiation. In the transition to the Stage of Completion, there is the hierophant's initiation. Then there are three initiations proper to the Stage of Completion, the Secret Initiation, the Insight Knowledge Initiation, and the 'Fourth'. The initiating goddess is sometimes called the 'seal' (*mudrā*). The notes to Mkhas grub rje cite the verse: "The seal pledge is explained as solidifying the 'body made of mind' (*manomayakāya*); because it solidifies all the body, it is called a 'seal' (*mudrā*)." The fact that in each instance the goddess is imagined as the initiator, or is the female element behind the scenes, indicates the initiations as the step-wise progress in the solidification of the innate body of the tantras which non-tantric Buddhism calls the 'body made of mind', meaning the progress of that body to the pregenetic androgyne state and then to the Clear Light.

### D. *Winds and mantras*

A fundamental of the Buddhist Tantras that deserves

special treatment is the practice of mantras and machinations with winds. Such practices are very ancient in India, certainly of Vedic character. The doctrine of life winds is first worked out in the old Upaniṣads. The basic five winds are mentioned in *Chāndogya Up.*, III. 13 and V. 19, in the order *prāṇa*, *vyāna*, *apāna*, *samāna*, *udāna*. The winds are the 'breaths' resulting from 'water', as in the well-known 'Three-fold development' discussion of the *Chāndogya*; this is made clear in *Bṛhadāraṇyaka Up.*, 1.5.3. The functions ascribed to these winds continued to be speculated upon, and so came into the Buddhist Tantras in the theory of breath manipulation through *yoga* practice. Also a theory of five subsidiary winds developed, clarified later in *The Yoga Upaniṣads*; in the Buddhist Tantras these latter five are accorded the function of relating external sensory objects to the five sense organs, while the former five are attributed various internal functions. When ten breaths (*prāṇa*) are mentioned in *Bṛhadāraṇyaka Up.*, III. 9.4, Vedāntic commentarial tradition takes them to be the ten sensory and motor organs (*jñānakarmendriyāṇi*), thus explaining away the palpable reference to winds: but we can infer the real meaning to be that those winds vivify the sensory and motor organs. In the latter *Bṛhadāraṇyaka Up.* passage, modern translators have rendered the verb *rodayanti* with causative force ('make someone lament'), thus requiring an unexpressed object. A good Sanskrit grammar, such as the one by William Dwight Whitney, readily shows that the causative infix-*aya*-does not necessarily confer causative force upon a Sanskrit verb. So my translation of the Sanskrit passage:

> *katame rudrā iti. daśeme puruṣe prāṇāḥ ātmaikādaśaḥ; te yadāsmāt śarīrān martyād utkrāmanti, atha rodayanti, tad yad rodayanti, tasmād rudrā iti.*
>
> 'What are the Rudras ?' 'These ten breaths in the person with the *ātman* as the eleventh. When they depart from this mortal frame, they cry out ; and because they cry out, they are called Rudras.'

In the *Śatapathabrāhmaṇa's* celebrated account of the birth of Rudra (Eggeling's translation, SBE, Vol. XLI, pp. 157-161) we read : 'because he cried (*rud*) therefore he is Rudra.' The teaching that the winds make a sound as they depart is continued into the Buddhist Tantras, as in Tsoṅ-kha-pa's commentary *Bzhis zhus* on the *Guhyasamāja* Explanatory Tantra *Caturdevīpariprcchā* (Collected Works, Lhasa, Vol. Ca, 13b-5,6): "The reality of *mantra* tone which each wind has, is not revealed to the 'child' (*bāla*); its form, that is, its self-existence (*svabhāva*) or identity (*ātmaka*), is revealed to the *yogin*" (/rluṅ deḥi raṅ gdaṅs sṅags kyi de ñid du byis pa la mi gsal ba rnal ḥbyor pa la gsal baḥi gzugs te/raṅ bzhin nam bdag ñid can/).

In the *Guhyasamājatantra* tradition, the *Vajramālā* Explanatory Tantra, chapter 48 (PTT, Vol. 3, p. 221) holds that the phenomenal world is due to the two winds *prāṇa* and *apāna* identified with two mantra syllables A and HAM (*aham*, or egotism), which form the 'knot of the heart':

*/A nni srog gi rluṅ du bśad/*
*/de bzhin thur sel HAṂ du brjod/*
*/de gñis gcig gyur ḥkhor ba ste/*
A is explained as the *prāṇa* wind.
Likewise, *apāna* is said to be HAṂ
When those two unite, there is *saṃsāra* (the cycle of phenomenal existence).

In the full system of human life, there are, as was said, five principal and five subsidiary winds, generically '*vāyu*' or '*prāṇa*'. The five principal winds have the respective natures of the five Buddhas and are associated with the five *mantra*-syllables and body-*cakras* as follows:

| | | | |
|---|---|---|---|
| Oṃ | —Vairocana | —vyāna | —all over the body, or head |
| Āḥ | —Amitābha | —udāna | —throat |
| Hūṃ | —Akṣobhya | —prāṇa | —heart |
| Svā | —Ratnasaṃbhava | —apāna | —sacral region |
| Hā | —Amoghasiddhi | —samāna | —navel |

The four winds, leaving out *vyāna*, are held in basic time or ordinary life to breathe in and out cyclically through one or other nostril or both. Hence these four are *prāṇāyāma*. This word does not ordinarily signify in the Buddhist Tantra, 'restraint of breath' but rather *prāṇa*, in-breathing, and *āyāma*, out-breathing; or *prāṇa*, the passage of winds through the orifices, and *āyāma*, the out-going mental component that 'rides on the wind'. The *Pañcakrama*, in its first *krama*, called *Vajrajāpa*, cites the *Vajramālā* in regard to the ordinary outward passage of the winds:

19. *Dakṣiṇād vinirgato raśmir hutabhuṅmaṇḍalaṃ ca tat/*
*Raktavarṇam idaṃ vyaktaṃ padmanātho 'tra devatā//*
The ray leaving *via* the right nostril is the fire maṇḍala. This distinguished one of red color (i.e. the udāna wind) is the deity Padma-Lord (i.e. Amitābha).

20. *Vāmād vinirgato raśmir vāyumaṇḍalasaṃjñitaḥ/*
*Haritaśyāmasaṃkāśaḥ karmanātho 'tra devatā//*
The ray leaving *via* the left nostril is called 'wind maṇḍala'. With a yellowish-green appearance (i.e. samāna wind) it is the deity Karma-Lord (i.e. Amoghasiddhi).

21. *Dvābhyāṃ vinirgato raśmiḥ pītavarṇo mahādyutiḥ/*
*Mahendramaṇḍalaṃ caitad ratnanātho 'tra devatā//*
The ray leaving *via* both nostrils is the great radiance of yellow color—the earth maṇḍala (i.e. apāna wind) and this is the deity Ratna-Lord (i.e. Ratnasambhava).

22. *Adho mandapracāras tu sitakundendusaṃnibhaḥ/*
*Maṇḍalaṃ vāruṇaṃ caitad vajranātho 'tra devatā//*
Moving slowly downwards (but also leaving *via* both nostrils) is the water maṇḍala white like the Jasmine (i.e. the prāṇa wind), and this is the deity Vajra-Lord (i.e. Akṣobhya).

23. *Sarvadehānugo vāyuḥ sarvaceṣṭāpravartakaḥ/*
*Vairocanasvabhāvo 'sau mṛtakāyād viniścaret//*
The wind that proceeds throughout the body and evolves all activity (i.e. the vyāna wind) has the nature of Vairocana and departs (only) from the dead body (with blue color).

Recitation of the wind in the Stage of Generation (nidāna verse 12) means reciting according to the natural cycle of the winds. This recitation of winds is indicated, according to the *Pradīpoddyotana* commentary, as the meaning of the verses 9-14 (omitting 13) in Chapter Six ('Documents'). Verse 9 deals with meditation on the tip of the nose of the face; at this stage one must take the passage of the winds on faith. Then verse 10 mentions an image of the Buddha, which is Vairocana. But as the Vairocana wind, vyāna, does not enter into the inbreathing and outbreathing, the diamond recitation intended by the verse is in fact Amitābha's fiery udāna-wind. The text of Chapter Six interposes a 'Huṃ' before verse 11, hinting at the recitation of Akṣobhya's watery prāṇa-wind. Verse 12 mentions a ratna-disk which enables the knower of the system to assign here the recitation of Ratnasaṃbhava's earthy apāna-wind. Then verse 14 involves recitation of Amoghasiddhi's wind and black samāna-wind which is yellow green when passing out through the left nostril.

Then in Chapter Six, verses 15-18 state the advanced level of that recitation, as practiced in the Stage of Completion (nidāna verse 24). In the latter stage, the yogin moves those winds from their usual location in basic time to extraordinary combinations in fruitional time, as I summarized from Tsoṅ-kha-pa's *Rdor bzlas* in "Female Energy...", p. 88: Oṃ, the prāṇa wind of the heart cakra, the udāna wind of the neck cakra, and the *bindu* in the position of the *uṣṇīṣa*, is the thunderbolt of body at the Mahāsukha-cakra of the forehead. Āḥ, the initial prāṇa of the heart cakra, the apāna wind of the sacral center, along with the udāna of the neck center, is the thunderbolt of speech at the neck cakra. Hūṃ, the apāna wind of the sacral center, the udāna wind of the neck center, and the pervasive prāṇa (i.e. vyāna) normally in the forehead, is the thunderbolt of mind at the nave of the heart lotus. And the winds mixed that way dissolve the knots (*mdud*) of those centers. Accordingly, in fruitional time, the mantras have been reduced from five to three. This is meant to achieve three photism experiences called 'light', 'spread of light', and 'culmination of light'. The further reduction from three to one corresponds to the experience of the Clear Light which is free from the three.

Also, the Stage of Completion increases to three the noses meant by 'tip of nose', a teaching found in the *Vajramālā*, summarized in Tsoṅ-kha-pa, "Dkaḥ gnad", Lhasa collected works, Vol. Ca, 8a-2 :

> The three 'tips of nose' (*nāsāgra*) are 1. the 'tip of nose' of the sacral place; 2. 'tip of nose' of the face' ; 3. 'tip of nose' of the heart (sna rtse gsum ni/gsaṅ baḥi sna rtse, gdoṅ gi sna rtse, sñiṅ gi sna rtse). *Idem*: The three 'drops' (*bindu*) are 1. 'drop' of substance, 2. 'drop' of light, 3. 'drop' of mantra (thig le gsum ni/rdzas kyi thig le, ḥod kyi thig le, sṅags kyi thig le), *Ibid.*, f. 8a-6: The lustful person contemplates the 'substance drop' on the 'tip-of-

nose' at the sacral place; the hating person, the 'mantra drop' on the 'tip-of-nose' of the heart; the deluded person, the 'drop of light' on the 'tip of nose' of the face (*/ ḥdod chags can gyis gsaṅ baḥi sna rtser rdzas kyi thig le daṅ / / zhe sdaṅ can gyis sñiṅ gi sna rtser sṅags kyi thig le daṅ // gti mug can gyis gdoṅ gi sna rtser ḥod kyi thig le bsgom par bśad ciṅ /*)

See in this connection the explanation of *prāṇāyāma* among the six members of yoga in the *Pradīpoddyotana* commentary ('Documents'), where the contemplation of the three 'noses' seems not to go with three different persons but with the successive contemplation of a single person.

The relation between *prāṇa* and *mantra* is brought out in the discussion about the 'reality' (*tattva*) of the *mantra*. Thus *Pañcakrama*, 1st krama, verse 66; Śrī Lakṣmī, Vol . 63, p. 21-5 and 22-1 :

*mantratattvam idam vyaktam vāgvajrasya prasādhanam/*
*jñānatrayaprabhedena cittamātre niyojayet //*

This clear reality of *mantra* as the accomplishment of the speech diamond, is applied to 'Mind Only' by the variety of three gnoses.

Śrī Lakṣmī explains that *mantra* has two aspects, by distinction of cause and effect. "The cause is *prāṇa*, the effect is *mantra*; and their reality is the 'reality of *mantra*' " (/de la rgyu ni srog rluṅ daṅ / ḥbras bu ni sṅags ste/de dag gi de ñid ni sṅags kyi de ñid de/). The 'three gnoses' mean the three lights.

But then, do mantras have meaning ? See the discussion in *The Calcutta Review*, 137-1 (Oct. 1955), a portion of the serial translation by J. V. Bhattacharyya of the *Nyāyamañjarī*, here (pp. 7-13) discussing the validity of mantras. The opponents hold that the mantras do not convey meaning (p. 8) : "A mantra renders its assistance to a Vedic rite only by its recitation." Among their illustrations is the *mantra*, "Hear, oh slabs of stone !" (*śṛṇota grāvāṇaḥ*). They say (pp. 8-9): "This meaning is absurd since unconscious slabs of stone are never employed to listen to something." The author of the *Nyāyamañjarī*, when replying to their arguments, says of this particular example (p. 12) : "Śṛṇota grāvāṇaḥ is...a miraculous act by the influence of which slabs of stone can even hear." His chief answer is that the opponents have not taken ...pains to find out the meaning. In conclusion he states (p. 13): "Mantras, revealing their senses, render assistance to a sacrificial rite. But they do not help a rite by their mere recitation like the muttering of a mantra...." The viewpoint of the *Nyāyamañjarī* is quite consistent with that of the Buddhist Tantras, where the mantras do indeed have meaning. For example, one need only consult the Tanjur commentaries on the *Vajra-vidāraṇa-nāma-dhāraṇī*, to learn that each one of the mantra expressions is given its explanation in terms of functions of the various deities involved. The Buddhist Tantra also insists that mere muttering of the mantra is useless, since one must simultaneously make a *mudrā* and concentrate the mind accordingly. And it also agrees when the Buddhist Tantra speaks of success in the incantation as the state when the mantra seems to pronounce itself, thus assuming the role of a deity's body (*mantra-mūrti*). An interesting example of this is in the last chapter of the *Śrī Paramādya tantra* (PTT, Vol. 5, p. 171-5), understood with the help of Ānandagarbha's commentary (PTT, Vol. 73, p. 127-5). The Tantra states: "How is the Bhagavat the master of the deeds of 'diamond pride'? Because the best *mudrā* belongs to the great lord (*maheśvara*) who has the best of great *siddhis* and (she) greatly praises the diamond lord, the one who says 'I am the master of diamond pride' is the Bhagavat, the supreme primordial person." (/ de la rdo rje bsñems byaḥi bdag po bcom ldan ḥdas ci ltar yin zhe na // kun mchog dṅos grub chen po yi // dbaṅ phyug chen po phyag rgyaḥi mchog // rdo rje dbaṅ phyug cher bstod pas // rdo rje bsñems paḥi bdag po bdag ces bya ba ni bcom ldan ḥdas mchog daṅ poḥi skyes buḥo /). The idea here, as gleaned from Ānandagarbha's comments, is that 'diamond pride' is the name of a goddess and she is the best *mudrā*. Since she praises the Bhagavat, he is her master (*pati*). This alludes to the state when the *mudrā* coalesces with the *mantra* to reveal its sense (as the *Nyāyamañjarī* would say); and since its sense is 'diamond pride' (*vajragarva*) the mind united with that *mudrā* can be proud. She praises without any prompting: the incantation sounds by itself. She has her own deeds or functions.

However, some Western scholars have quite missed the point of how mantras acquire meaning. Take the celebrated mantra of the Buddhist Bodhisattva Lord Avalokiteśvara, *Oṃ maṇi padme hūṃ*. Scholars have ascribed this and that meaning to it; for example, "Oṃ, the jewel in the lotus, hūṃ." The implication of such an explanation is that the mantra has a meaning independent of the recitation, which is denied both by the Hindu *Nyāyamañjarī* and the Buddhist Tantras. When one goes into this cult of Avalokiteśvara, he finds out readily that this is called the six-syllabled formula. The six syllables are recited in the six times of day and night, along with fasting and correlated with gestures (*mudrā*), and the imagined six destinies of gods, men, etc. as associated with six colors. The meaning is the six Buddhas corresponding respectively to the syllables. By continual application to the cult with proper recitation of the six syllables in a correlation of body, speech, and mind, the yogin expects to identify himself with the Lord Avalokiteśvara who looks with compassion at the beings in the six destinies. Gradually the meaning is evoked by the recitation. While such a translation as "Oṃ, the jewel in the lotus, hūṃ" does not convey any intelligence of the cult; nevertheless, if one insists on a translation anyway in such form, it is proper to translate the 'maṇi padme' portion as "jewel in the lotus" because one would understand *maṇi* as the Middle Indic form equal to Sanskrit *maṇi* (*ḥ*), the nominative. In terms of mantra construction, because the initial and final syllables are Oṃ and Hūṃ, the middle portion 'maṇı padme' is equivalent to the syllable Āḥ, for these are the three heart syllables of the Buddhas corresponding to Body, Speech, and Mind, respectively Vairocana, Amitābha, and Akṣobhya. Accordingly, the middle portion stands for the Buddha Amitābha in the heaven Sukhāvatī.

The gods are literally *expressed* into manifestation; that is, they are called into phenomenal forms by mantra. In the Anuttarayoga-tantra cult, the syllables E-VA(M) serve for this expression. 'Evaṃ' (Thus) is the first word in the Buddhist scriptures, which normally begin "Thus by me it was heard" (*evaṃ mayā śrutam*). *Mchan ḥgrel*, PTT, Vol. 158, p. 13-3, states : "The syllable E is like a mother. Therefore, the 'insight' (*prajñā*) syllable (E) is symbolized as the sixteen vowels (*svara*). Va is like a father. The 'seminal drop' (*bindu*, *thig le*, *ṃ*) of Vaṃ makes manifest the vowels. Hence the 'means' (*upāya*) syllable (Vaṃ) is symbolized as the thirty-three consonants (*vyañjana*). Through their union arises, like sons, the host of words. Thus E is the womb (*ālaya*, *kun gzhi*) and Vaṃ the progenitor, of *pravacana* (the Buddhist scripture)." The *bindu* is also called in this literature the *bodhicitta* (mind of enlightenment).

## E. *The world of light*

In the article "Notes on the Sanskrit term Jñāna" I first tried to correlate the Guhyasamāja tradition of four lights (three light stages leading to or emerging from the Clear Light) with other systems of thought. Already it was apparent to me that the theory involved a reinterpretation of the old Buddhist formula of Dependent Origination (*pratītya-samutpāda*). With the researches of the present work behind me it is easier to detect the Upaniṣadic precursors of this theory (it would be hazardous to try to trace it back to the *Ṛg-veda*).

Perhaps the most discussed Upaniṣadic passage is the *Chāndogya Upaniṣad* from VI.2 to VI.6. This teaches a development order of 1. heat, becoming speech; 2. water, becoming breath; 3. food, becoming mind. By their respective colors of red, white, and black, they were later (Hindu period) identified with the three *guṇas* (employed extensively in the Buddhist Tantras), to wit: *rajas* (activity, passion), *sattva* (buoyancy, clarity), *tamas* (immobility, darkness), although the guṇa applicability to the Chāndogya text has been questioned. The *Bṛhadāraṇyaka Upaniṣad* I.5 portrays Prajāpati's production of the world as food for himself; and this suggestion of 'food' as the first produced is consistent with 1.5.3: "Mind, speech, breath, these he made for himself" (*mano vācaṃ prāṇam, tāny ātmane kuruta*), since we learn from the *Chāndogya* that 'food' becomes 'mind'. The *Bṛhadāraṇyaka* order is consistent with a tantric interpretation of Buddhist Dependent Origination, with my understanding of the *Varāhopaniṣad*, and with the Guhyasamāja-nidāna doctrine of three lights or three gnoses (*jñānatraya*). The *Varāhopaniṣad* is translated by T. R. Srinivasa Ayyangar and edited by G. Srinivasa Murti in *The Yoga Upaniṣads*. In the *Varāha* we read: "For says the Śruti, 'These are the five essential features, viz., Asti (there is), Bhāti (there shines forth), Preyas (whatever pleases), Rūpa (form) and Nāman (name). The first three are of the form of the Brahman. The two thereafter are the characteristics of the phenomenal world.'." If we rearrange the order of the *Chāndogya* terms and employ these other sources, a tabular comparison can be made as shown in Table I.

I. THE WORLD OF LIGHT : BRAHMANICAL & BUDDHIST

| Old terminology of *Chāndogya Up.* | Later terminology of *Varāha Up.* |
|---|---|
| **Brahmanism** | |
| 1. Black Food (kṛṣṇa-anna) | "It is" (asti) |
| 2. Red Heat (rohita-tejas) | "It shines forth" (bhāti) |
| 3. White Water (śukla-āpas) | Whatever pleases (preyas) |
| 4. Fire, Sun, Moon, Lightning | 4, 5. Name and Form |
| **Buddhism** | |
| Old terminology of Dependent Origination | Later tantric terminology |
| 1. Nescience (avidyā) | Culmination-of-Light (ālokopalabdhi) |
| 2. Motivations (saṃskāra) | Spread-of-light (ālokābhāsa) |
| 3. Perceptions (vijñāna) | Light (āloka) |
| 4. Name-and-Form (nāma-rūpa) | Phenomenal World |

Moreover, the relation of the tantric three lights to the first three members of Dependent Origination is plainly stated by *Mchan ḥgrel* on *Pradīpoddyotana* (Chapter III) in PTT, Vol. 158, p. 38-1. The *Pradīpoddyotana* quotes the *Saṃdhivyākaraṇa's* remark, 'said to be the doctrine of Dependent Origination' (*rten ciṅ ḥbrel ḥbyuṅ chos su grags*), to which *Mchan ḥgrel* adds, 'arising from the wind and mind only of the Clear Light' (*ḥod gsal gyi rluṅ sems tsam las skyes paḥi*).

Maryla Falk wrote a book entitled *Nāma Rūpa and Dharma-Rūpa*. It is undeniable that she hit upon the basic division by appreciating the significance of the research by the Geigers (p. 71, n.):

> One of the principal results of the long and detailed inquiry made by Mrs. M. Geiger and Prof. W. Geiger into the use of the term *dhamma* in the Pāli Canon (*Pāli Dhamma, vornehmlich in der kanonischen Literatur*, Abh. de Bayer. Ak. d. Wiss., Philos.-philol. u. hist. Kl., XXXI, 1. Munich 1921) is the conclusion that 'the concept *dhamma* takes in Buddhism the place of the *brahman* of older Vedānta' (p. 77). We have shown above that in Upanishadic thought, ever since its Vedic beginnings, the equivalence of both terms reflects the sameness of the entity they designate.

In short, the equivalence of Pāli *dhamma* and the old Indian term *brahman* leads to the equivalence Dharma-rūpa = Brahma-rūpa. This Dharma-rūpa is therefore the pre-genetic world, anterior to the phenomenal world denoted by Nāma-rūpa. The *Śatapatha-brāhmaṇa* (Eggeling's translation as quoted by Surendranath Dasgupta, *A History of Indian Philosophy*, I, p. 20) has the celebrated passage:

> Then the Brahman itself went up to the sphere beyond. Having gone up to the sphere beyond, it considered, 'How can I descend again into these worlds?' It then descended again by means of these two, Form and Name. Whatever has a name, that is name; and that again which has no name and which one knows by its form, 'this is (of a certain) form,' that is form: as far as there are Form and Name so far, indeed, extends this (universe). These indeed are the two great forces of Brahman; and, verily, he who knows these two great forces of Brahman becomes himself a great force.

The equivalent statement involving the equation Dharma = Brahman, and taking into account the *Pañcakrama* list of eighty *prakṛtis* in three sets (seven, forty, and thirty-three), each set constituting momentary dark spots obscuring three light realms, also called the triple vijñāna, can be expressed by Vijñāna (the (*Laṅkāvatāra's* 'body of the Tathāgata') descending into the womb by means of name-and-form, the fourth member of Dependent Origination. So also, when Gautama was meditating under the tree of Enlightenment, and according to the tradition found out the formula of Dependent Origination by working backwards from Old Age and Death, in each case thinking, 'What is the indispensable condition for this to arise?', he proceeded this way : That No. 11 'birth' is the indispensable condition for No. 12 'old age and death, and the whole mass of suffering'; and for No. 11 'birth'—No. 10 'gestation' (*bhava*); for the latter, No. 9 'indulgence' (*upādāna*); for the latter, No. 8 'craving' (*tṛṣṇā*); for the latter, No. 7 'feelings' (*vedanā*) (and 'ideas', *saṃjñā*); for the latter, No. 6, 'sensory contact' (*sparśa*); for the latter, No. 5 'six sense bases' (*ṣaḍāyatana*) ; for the latter, No. 4, 'name-and-form' (*nāma*-and-*rūpa*). And then, as we can see from the foregoing, in order for Gautama to answer the question 'What is the indispensable condition for name-and-form to arise?' he had to go to the sphere beyond, himself the Brahman, hence obtaining the Dharma-kāya. In this pre-genetic sphere, Gautama decided that 4. 'name-and-form' has 3. 'perception' (*vijñāna*) as its indispensable condition; the latter, No. 2 'motivations' (*saṃskāra*); and the latter, No. 1 'nescience' (*avidyā*). And—the *Guhyasamāja* tradition suggests—this is his way of stating in psychological terms, the 'white water', 'red heat', and 'black food' of the *Chāndogya Up.* vision, the atomic triad of the superior realm.

Since the correlation of the supramundane light stages of the *Guhyasamāja* commentarial tradition is associated with the first members of Dependent Origination, and with the developmental order of the *Bṛhadāraṇyaka Upaniṣad* (rather than with the *Chāndogya* order), it follows that if we are to acknowledge a feasibility that the formula of Dependent Origination is based on the Upanisads, we have to further admit that the *Bṛhadāraṇyaka Up.* is the one with which the Buddhist formula has the most affinity

Even if we accept that these three light stages may be traceable to such ancient sources as the old Upaniṣads, it must still be acknowledged that the theory of 80 prakṛtis superimposed on the three lights is a development after the rise of the Buddhist Tantras. The *Pañcakrama* commentary *Maṇimālā* cited under nidāna verse 6 explicitly mentions that the thirty-three female natures are generated by the wind in the left channel, the forty male natures by the wind in the right channel, and the seven neuter natures by the wind in the middle. This method of allotting mental states to three groups seems to be a development of the assignment of qualities to the three *guṇas* as we find in the *Bhagavadgītā*, Chapter 14, but of course in the present form a number of centuries after this Hindu classic. In contrast, as John Woodroffe, *Introduction to Tantra Shastra*, pp. 49, ff., points out, there are six *vṛtti* associated with the Svādhiṣṭhāna-cakra, ten *vṛtti* with the Maṇipūra, twelve *vṛtti* with the Anāhata, twelve *vṛtti* with the Viśuddha, sixteen *kalā* with the Sahasrāra, four *ānanda* with the Mūlādhāra; with no sets mentioned for the Ājñā-cakra. Thus, this kind of Hindu tantra assigns *vṛttis* to *cakras* rather than to the three *nāḍī*; and very few of the *vṛttis* can be identified with the *prakṛtis*.

As I perused the various commentaries on the *Pañcakrama* available in the Tibetan Tanjur, I tried to find some explanation for the numbers 'thirty-three' etc., and any suggestions of internal grouping within the three sets of natures, but to little avail. However, the *Pañcakrama* commentary called *Maṇimālā* attempts to rationalize the eighty *prakṛtis* in terms of the Buddhist Abhidharma set of fifty-one *caitasikadharmas* ('derivative mentals'), so in PTT, Vol. 62, pp. 186-187. I studied these pages with the help of the collaborated article by Dr. P. Cordier and L. de La Vallée Poussin, "Les soixante-quinze et les cent dharmas." For example, when this commentary analyses the set of thirty-three *prakṛtis* (see the list under nidāna verse 1) it includes nos. 1-3, three degrees of aversion, under *kaukṛtya* ('regret'); 4-5 (thinking) future and past, under *vitarka* and *vicāra* ('searching state of mind' and 'deciding state of mind')—*kaukṛtya*, *vitarka*, and *vicāra* being among the list of *aniyata-bhūmikas* ('indeterminate *caitasikas*'). It includes 11-13, three degrees of fear, under the three virtuous roots (*kuśalamūla*)—non-clinging (*alobha*), non-hating (*adveṣa*), and non-delusion (*amoha*), which are in the list of *kuśalamahābhūmikas* (mental elements present in every good conception); and so on. The attempt is obviously forced, but is significant for showing this author's belief that the *dharmas* are identical with the *prakṛtis*. This is a common theory that the conscious mind does not create a thought, but that the thought (here a *dharma* or a *prakṛti*) flows into the mind. Where does the thought come from? The Guhyasamāja system holds that the thought comes from one or other of three light realms. In terms of 'channels' (*nāḍī*), the archetypal world is called 'left', 'right', and 'middle'. A consistent theory was earlier stated in the *Bhagavadgītā* (Chap.

X, 4-5): "..the different states of being proceed from me alone."

Moreover, there is a curious resemblance between the thirty-three female *prakṛtis* and the five *sthāyi-bhāvas* as discussed by Edward C. Dimock, Jr., *The Place of the Hidden Moon*, and earlier in his article "Doctrine and Practice Among the Vaiṣṇavas of Bengal." There are informative annotations concerning them in Saraswati Goswāmi Thakur, *Shri Brahma-Saṃhitā*, pp. 10-3, 159-62, which represents the five as devotion of different individuals. The only source in the English language to my notice which presents these five in the form of stages of a single person to union with the Lord Kṛṣṇa, is Y. Jagannatham, *Divine Love and Amorous Sentiment*, a modern pamphlet picked up at Jayavelu's in Madras. When I studied these passages and added the advice of Mr. Kirpal Singh Narang about the five stages of the Sikhs (stated in his very words below) on the occasion of his Madison, Wisconsin visit on April 18, 1966, it occurred to me that the thirty-three *prakṛtis* of female consciousness to be presented under nidāna verse no.1 are roughly in five groups the fleeting moments of consciousness in the five stages of the devotee's 'female' soul becoming a Gopī (cow-girl) in union with the Lord. I give here in outline my merely tentative solution, observing that should it prove applicable, this would indeed provide a most important link between the *Pañcakrama* tradition and the early Vaiṣṇava Sahajiyā cult.

| *Sthāyi-bhāva* (*or Rasa*) | *Sikh Stages* | *Female Prakṛtis* |
|---|---|---|
| 1. Śānta, pacification of longing for the external world | Vairāgya ('aversion') | 1-3. degrees of aversion |
| 2. Dāsya, service to the Lord | Doing what is pleasing to the Lord | 4-9. thinking of future and past, sorrow and calmness |
| 3. Sakhya, being a friend to the Lord | Fear and Love | 10-22. *vikalpa*, fear, down to feelings |
| 4. Vātsalya, the Lord as a child | Knowing the Lord's Will | 23-30, intuition, down to affection |
| 5. Mādhurya or śṛṅgāra, the Lord Kṛṣṇa as a lover | Union | 31-33. worry, collecting, and jealousy |

In a comparable way, I noticed that the forty *prakṛtis* listed under nidāna verse no. 2 seem to be the very characteristics attributed to the Lord Kṛṣṇa in his various exploits, ranging from the Child Kṛṣṇa to the Divine Lover, and that the list seems easily to fall into five groups. Perhaps the forty *prakṛtis* of maleconsciousness derive from a Vaiṣṇava prototype.

The only way that occurs to me to reconcile the division of the eighty *prakṛtis* into three groups, with what seems to me to be an obvious division of the male and female ones into five groups, is to associate them with the right and left in five cakras starting with no. 1 at the base of the spine, no. 2 at the navel, and moving upward to union in the *ājñā-cakra* or *mahāsukha-cakra*. Admittedly, I have found no textual passage to support this theory.

## II. INTRODUCTION TO THE GUHYASAMĀJATANTRA

### A. *Texts, commentators, and history*

The Guhyasamāja literature falls into two distinct groups—the revealed texts in the Tibetan Kanjur and the exegetical literature in the Tibetan Tanjur. In *A Complete Catalogue of the Tibetan Buddhist Canons* (Tohoku catalog), the Kanjur works have numbers 442-447 (and disputed works 448-453), the Tanjur works 1784-1917 (cf. Alex Wayman, "Analysis of the Tantric Section of the Kanjur Correlated to Tanjur Exegesis," p. 121).

The chief revealed works in the Tibetan language with catalog titles are :

No. 442. Guhyasamāja mūlatantra : *Sarvatathāgatakāyavākcittarahasya-guhyasamāja-nāma-mahākalparāja.* Chaps. 1-17 of the Sanskrit text.

No. 443. Guhyasamāja uttaratantra : Chap. 18 of the Sanskrit text.

No. 444. Guhyasamāja-vyākhyātantra : *Sandhivyākaraṇa-nāma-tantra.*

No. 445. Guhyasamāja-vyākhyātantra : *Śrīvajramālābhidhānamahāyogatantra-sarvatantrahṛdayarahasyavibhaṅga-nāma.*

No. 446. Guhyasamāja-vyākhyātantra : *Caturdevīparipṛcchā.*

No. 447. Guhyasamāja-vyākhyātantra : *Vajrajñānasamuccaya-nāma-tantra* (However, from the Tibetan translation one would expect **Jñānavajra-*).

Tsoṅ-kha-pa writes in his commentary on the *Pañcakrama* called *Gsal baḥi sgron me* (Vol. 158, p. 175-5) : "Five Explanatory Tantras (*vyākhyātantra*) have been specifically mentioned by the 'noble father and sons' (i.e. the tantric Nāgārjuna as 'father' and the tantrics Āryadeva and Candrakīrti as 'sons'), that is, *Caturdevīparipṛcchā*, *Sandhivyākaraṇa*, and *Vajramālā* are stated to be Explanatory Tantras in the *Pañcakrama*; *Vajrajñānasamuccaya* is also said to be an Explanatory Tantra in the *Caryāmelāpakapradīpa*; and while the first two syllables of the *nidāna* (i.e.

E-VAṂ) are being explained in the *Pradīpoddyotana*, the *Devendraparipṛcchā* is specifically mentioned as the source;.... the Explanatory Tantra *Devendraparipṛcchā* was not translated (into Tibetan)." That passage in Tibetan : / ḥdus paḥi bśad rgyud du ḥphags pa yab sras kyis dṅos su gsuṅs pa na lṅa ste / rim lṅa las lha mo bzhis zhus daṅ / dgoṅs pa luṅ ston pa daṅ / rdo rje ḥphreṅ ba bśad rgyud du gsuṅs la / spyod bsdus las ye śes rdo rje kun las btus kyaṅ bśad rgyud du gsuṅs śiṅ / sgron gsal las gleṅ gzhiḥi yi ge daṅ po gñis ḥchad pa na lhaḥi dbaṅ pos zhus paḥi khuṅs dṅos su smos śiṅ.../ lhaḥi dbaṅ pos zhus pa bśad rgyud du gsuṅs te ḥdi ma ḥgyur ro / . The reason the Tibetan tradition accepted the *Devendraparipṛcchā* as an Explanatory Tantra is that immediately after the quotation from that work by title (reproduced in the materials for nidāna verses Evaṃ mayā..), Candrakīrti continued with a verse citation (reproduced in section B, next) which he introduced by the remark (*Pradīpoddyotana* MS): / mayetyādi vajrapadānām apy artho vyākhyātantrād avatāryate / "One can understand from the Explanatory Tantra the meaning of the diamond words '*mayā*' etc." Tsoṅ-kha-pa in his *Mchan ḥgrel* (p. 14-1) on the *Pradīpoddyotana* mentions, "Skal-ldan-grags-pa examined the *Vajramālā* carefully and could not find this therein." The thrust of the decision lies in the fact that the *Vajramālā* presents the forty nidāna verses in its chapter 59. Its brief chapter 58 is devoted to a treatment of the two syllables E-vaṃ. It is precisely the *Vajramālā* which should have had, but lacked the cited verses. Candrakīrti preceded his citation of the forty verses by citation of verses about the nidāna sentence but used other sources, first the named *Devendraparipṛcchā*, and then an unnamed work he calls an 'Explanatory Tantra'. The Tibetans (Tsoṅ-kha-pa, in any case) decided that Candrakīrti had treated the *Devendraparipṛcchā* with the authority ordinarily accorded an Explanatory Tantra, and identified that work accordingly. But that Tantra had not itself been translated; the *Pradīpoddyotana* passage apparently is the full extant portion of Sanskrit of this work (the *Subhāṣita-saṃgraha*, Part II, pp. 32-3, quotes the *Devendraparipṛcchā-tantra* by lines contained within the *Pradīpoddyotana* citation).

The *Vajrajñāna* also has a difficulty of literary history. It is a curious feature of Candrakīrti's *Pradīpoddyotana* that his classifying terminology used throughout this commentary on the *Guhyasamājatantra*, namely the 'Seven Ornaments' (*saptālaṃkāra*), is ascribed several times near the outset of his work to an Explanatory Tantra which he does not name, but which is none other than the *Vajrajñānasamuccaya*; and so Tsoṅ-kha-pa in turn cannot specify the *Pradīpoddyotana* for containing the name of this Explanatory Tantra. This silence regarding the title of the work from which he drew the material he popularized may mean that Candrakīrti had a hand in composing the *Vajrajñānasamuccaya*, the latter portion of it, or the expanded version (Toh. 450), to justify his commentarial position, as has been suggested by Yūkei Matsunaga in his article, "A Doubt to Authority of the Guhyasamāja-Ākhyāna-tantras."

Another mystery of Explanatory Tantras occurs in Candrakīrti's *Pradīpoddyotana* at the very end of chapter Four:

> */ yathoktaṃ bhagavatā vyākhyātantre /*
> *sarvāṅgabhāvanātītaṃ kalpanākalpavarjitam /*
> *mātrābindusamātītam etan maṇḍalam uttamam //*

As was said by the Bhagavat in the Explanatory Tantra:

> Transcending the contemplation of all portions (i.e. color and shape), free from both imagination and lack of imagination, transcending the upper sign and its *bindu* ̇, that is the supreme maṇḍala.

Tsoṅ-kha-pa in his *Mchan ḥgrel* (p. 41) mentions that an almost identical verse is found in the *Candraguhyatilaka* (another quotation from this work in the *Pradīpoddyotana* is reproduced in the initiation remarks in the section 'The two stages, initiations, and the clear light'; and Āryadeva appeals to this Tantra for the expression '100 lineages'). The only difference is where in the verse the compound *mātrābindu* is translated in Candrakīrti's work as *gug skyed thig le*, the *Candraguhyatilaka* Tibetan version has the words *ḥdren daṅ tshig* ('guide and letter'). Since the expression *mātrābindu* is difficult to interpret, it is possible that it is the original for those Tibetan words, with *ḥdren* = *bindu*, and *tshig* = *mātrā*. Tsoṅ-kha-pa left the matter open; he appears not to accept the evidence of one similar verse as final proof that Candrakīrti had this Tantra in mind. However, it so happens that this same verse is cited by Indrabhūti in his *Jñānasiddhi* (GOS ed., p. 83), and attributed to a chapter thirteen. On the preceding page he has cited the *Advayasamatāvijaya*, and his immediately succeeding quotation from a chapter nine, as well as that citation of chapter thirteen are presumably from that Tantra.

According to George Roerich, *The Blue Annals*, Part Two, p. 417, Bu-ston considered the *Advayasamatāvijaya* to be an Explanatory Tantra of the *Guhyasamājatantra*; he translated a version of that work in 22 chapters that was incomplete in the middle. Possibly this is the reason that Tsoṅ-kha-pa apparently ignores this work. Several centuries after his time, the Chinese version of this Tantra was used to fill out the missing portion of Bu-ston's translation, accounting for the present version in the Tibetan Kanjur. But if Bu-ston was serious about this *Advaya-samatāvijaya* as an Explanatory Tantra, I can find no confirmation of this in his own *Pradīpoddyotana* commentary in Collected Works (Part 9), where he freely cites the *Sandhivyākaraṇa* (in an older translation preceding the one now officially in the Kanjur), the *Vajramālā*, the *Vajrahṛdayālaṃkāra*, Yoga-tantras (on which he was the great authority), Āryadeva's various works, and other works, but not, as far as I could notice, the *Advayasamatāvijaya*.

Again, in his *Pradīpoddyotana* on chapter XIV, Candrakīrti quotes from an unnamed Vyākhyā-tantra an interesting prose passage with Vajrapāṇi as interlocutor (included in this work under 'Vān'). Finally, having mystified sufficiently the 'Explanatory Tantras,' Candrakīrti in his commentary on Chapter XVII cites the 'Mūla-tantra', which Tsoṅ-kha-pa identifies as the Mūla-tantra of the Yoga-tantra, namely the *Tattvasaṃgraha* (cf. the passage in the treatment of initiation). According to *The Blue Annals*, Book VII ('The Preaching of the Tantras'), there was a distinction of 'Outer' Yoga-tantra and 'Inner' Yoga-tantra, with the 'inner' variety becoming separately called 'Anuttarayoga-tantra'. One can therefore understand Candrakīrti's citation as indicating his adherence to this terminology, since the *Tattvasaṃgraha* is the *mūla-tantra* of the 'outer' Yoga-tantra. Indeed, there is much in common between the Yoga-tantra (such works as the *Tattvasaṃgraha*, the *Māyājāla*, *Sarvarahasya-tantra*, and *Śrī Paramādya*) and the 'Father' class of Anuttarayoga-tantra. Both classes of Tantra use the terminology of 'three samādhis', clarified in our Introduction III. C., although there are differences in definitions.

Candrakīrti's citation of both the *Sandhivyākaraṇa* and the *Vajramālā* as 'Ārya-vyākhyāna' shows that he took for granted the knowledge in his readers of those two works. By implication, when he cites a verse from the *Sarvarahasya-tantra* without any indication of source, those same readers are expected to know the work. Then, when he cites by name some other Tantras, such as the *Māyājālatantra*, the *Vajroṣṇīṣatantra*, the *Vairocanābhisaṃbodhi*, and the *Vajrahṛdayālaṃkāra*, we may infer that he gives the names because he cannot expect the followers of the Guhyasamāja to know those other Tantras by heart. But if this is indeed the case, it would also have to apply to his quotations from the named works *Devendraparipṛcchā* and the *Candraguhyatilaka*. So there are certainly many difficulties about the literary history of these works. Tsoṅ-kha-pa (PTT, Vol. 158, p. 175-6) rejects the view advanced by some that the *Vajrahṛdayālaṃkāra* and the *Māyājāla* are Explanatory Tantras, since some consistency with the *Guhyasamāja* does not qualify those works as 'Explanatory'. However, Tsoṅ-kha-pa, as Bu-ston before him, often cites the *Vajrahṛdayālaṃkāra-tantra* in commentarial material on the *Guhyasamājatantra*. His justification is suggested in his *Pañcakrama* commentary, PTT Vol. 158, p. 186-5, where he refers to the *Vajrahṛdayālaṃkāra* as a 'consistent means (*upāya*) tantra' (*phyogs mthun gyi thabs gyī rgyud*), that is to say consistent with one side of Guhyasamāja teaching.

According to Tsoṅ-kha-pa (PTT, Vol. 158, p. 177-1), while the Explanatory Tantra *Vajramālā* discusses some other matters, it principally teaches the 'arcane body', 'arcane speech', and 'arcane mind', and the illusory body (*māyā-deha*). He further explains (*ibid.*, p. 177-1, 2)) that the *Caturdevīparipṛcchā* principally teaches extensively the essentials of *prāṇāyāma*; and that the *Sandhivyākaraṇa* is consistent with the sequence of chapters of the *mūla-tantra* and is an Explanatory Tantra for the first twelve chapters of the *Guhyasamāja* and not for the remaining ones. He also mentions (*ibid.*, p. 176-1) that a larger and a smaller version of the *Vajrajñānasamuccaya* are stated in the commentary on the *Vajramālā*; these are numbered respectively 450 and 447 in the Tohoku catalog based on the Derge edition of the Kanjur-Tanjur (but the Peking edition of the Kanjur omits the larger version).

The principle of the 'explanatory tantras' seems to be a

consistency of terminology. Such works should employ the same names of deities and treat some major subjects of the basic tantra of the *Guhyasamāja*. The one which most qualifies as such is of course the *Sandhivyākaraṇa* because it does expand on the *Guhyasamāja* chapter by chapter for the first twelve chapters, and then itself comes to an end. Of course, other Tantras of the Anuttarayoga-tantra class have much material in common, but their departure in terminology makes it difficult to equate their subject matter. Tsoṅ-kha-pa, who commented on the chief Father Tantra, the *Guhyasamāja*, and the chief Mother Tantra, the *Śrī-Cakrasaṃvara*, frequently has remarks which correlate these two extensive sets of tantric literature. I made a modest attempt at this too in my "Female Energy. . . ." article, showing the equivalence of the Father Tantra vocabulary 'Mother,' 'Sister,' 'Daughter' with the Mother Tantra vocabulary 'Together-born female,' 'field-born female,' and 'incantation-born female'.

As we pass from those revealed tantric works to the exegetical literature, we should note that the former are written in strict anonymity and attributed to divine authorship, while in the case of the latter, the writers are pleased to attach their names to commentarial literature and elaborate rituals which have taken centuries to develop. Before it is possible even tentatively to ascribe dates to the revealed literature, we must do the same for the commentarial works, and here we note that some scholarly confusion already has set in. It simply is not possible yet to pinpoint with accuracy the date of Nāgārjuna as 645 A.D., the date given by B. Bhattacharyya in the introduction (p. xxx) to his edition of the *Guhyasamāja*. A helpful attempt is Rāhula Sāṅkṛtyāyana's geneological tree of the eighty-four Siddhas and list of the Siddhas in *Journal Asiatique*, Oct. Dec., 1934, pp. 218-225. Professor Giuseppe Tucci has given his lists and tentative dates of Siddhas in *Tibetan Painted Scrolls*, I, pp. 227-232. The Japanese scholar Hakuyū Hadano, in *Tohoku Daigaku Bungaku-bu Kenkyū-nempo*, No. 9 (1958), pp. 58-18, thoroughly discusses the traditions of King Indrabhūti.

Although the attempt involves trepidation, some chronological layers can be worked out through textual analysis and other considerations.

1. First come the revealed texts *Guhyasamājatantra*, the

three Explanatory Tantras named in the *Pañcakrama*, and the (uncertain) *Vajrajñānasamuccaya.* In a negative way, no works are extant composed with their names by the first persons in the Guhyasamāja lineage list (Tibetan tradition), namely Indrabhūti the Great, Nāgayoginī, and King Viśukalpa (per Tsoṅ-kha-pa, Vol. 158, p. 178-1, 2): i-ndra-bhu-ti chen po daṅ kluḥi rnal ḥbyor ma daṅ sa bdag bi-su-ka-lpas gzhuṅ mdzad pa ni ḥdi na mi snaṅ la /). There is a legendary account in *The Blue Annals* (I, pp. 359-60) :

> The adepts of the (Guhya)samāja agree that the Guhyasamājatantra had been preached by the Munīndra himself, following a request of Indrabhūti, the great king of Oḍḍīyāna, at the time when the Buddha had manifested himself in Oḍḍīyāna and initiated (the king). Thereupon the king and his retinue practised the Tantra by means of the prapañca-caryā (spros spyod) and became initiates (Vidyādhara—one who has attained spiritual realization or siddhi, grub pa), and the country of Oḍḍīyāna became deserted. After that a yoginī, who had descended from the realm of the Nāgas, heard it (i.e. the Tantra) from (king) Indrabhūti and taught it to king Viśukalpa of the Southern country. The mahā-brāhmaṇa Saraha heard it from him and taught it to ācārya Nāgārjuna. The latter had many disciples, but the chief ones were the four: Śākyamitra, Āryadeva, Nāgabodhi, and Candrakīrti.

Tsoṅ-kha-pa (*op. cit.*, p. 178-2), right after the mention of those first persons whose Guhyasamāja works do not exist (at least under their names), goes on to mention, what in this context should be the first work by an historical personnage, the *Guhyasiddhi*, whose authorship he assigns to Śrī-Mahāsukhanātha (*dpal mgon po bde ba chen po*). This name is undoubtedly drawn from the verse cited from a manuscript of this work by S. B. Dasgupta, *An Introduction to Tantric Buddhism*, p. 156, note: śrī-mahāsukha-nāthasya pāda-padmopajivinā / racitaḥ padmavajreṇa sarvasattvānukampayā // . The author is well known by the name Padmavajra (who also has the name Devacandra, per Tucci, Vol. I, p. 232). He might be different from the disciple of Buddhaguhya (2nd half, eighth century) who commented on the Yoga-tantra. Tsoṅ-kha-pa states that the

*Guhyasiddhi* establishes the meaning of the Samāja. It principally establishes the nidāna of the Guhyasamāja; and it teaches about the stages of the path : first, the Stage of Generation of placing syllables; second, on the basis of 'Victory of the Rite', one's own intrinsic nature symbolizing reality; third, for the sake of relying on that, the contemplation with recourse to the Jñāna-mudrā; fourth, the contemplation of mahāmudrā and abhisaṃbodhi togetherwith the fourfold praxis. *The Blue Annals*, I, p. 363, mentions besides this *Guhyasiddhi*, the work by King Indrabhūti, the *Jñānasiddhi*, as also based on the Guhyasamāja. Hence this must be a different Indrabhūti from the one who has no works on the Guhyasamāja. Tsoṅ-kha-pa also mentions that there exist no works by Saraha on the *Guhyasamājatantra*. About his time begin two lineages of Guhyasamāja commentarial tradition—the Ārya school (*ḥphags lugs*) and the Jñānapāda school (*ye śes zhabs lugs*).

(a) The Ārya school is headed by the tantric Nāgārjuna, whose most important works in the tantric field are his own compositions, the *Piṇḍīkṛta-sādhana* (especially for the Stage of Generation) and the *Pañcakrama* (for the Stage of Completion), which became authoritative for the sequence of *yoga*. Besides, his commentary *Aṣṭādaśa-paṭala-vistara-vyākhyā* on the 18th chapter (the Uttara-tantra) remained the most important of any commentary on that chapter, probably because Candrakīrti's *Pradīpoddyotana* does not cover this part. His commentary *Tantraṭīkā* on the mūla *Guhyasamājatantra* was overshadowed by the *Pradīpoddyotana*. His *Piṇḍīkṛta-sādhana* and *Pañcakrama* were based on the *Guhyasamājatantra*, first 12 chapters, especially chapter Six and Twelve ('Documents') and the Explanatory Tantras *Sandhivyākaraṇa* and *Vajramālā* (although he also refers to the *Caturdevīparipṛcchā*). He stressed the three lights and the Clear Light, the theory of eighty *prakṛtis* or *vikalpas* going with three *vijñānas*, interpreted with Yogācāra-type vocabulary probably adopted from the *Laṅkāvatāra-sūtra*. Nāgārjuna's *Tantraṭīkā* is an attempt to explain the *Guhyasamājatantra* on the basis of the *utpatti-krama* and *saṃpanna-krama*, as well as his five stages, to which he refers repeatedly, the latter under the title *Prakaraṇa* (*rab tu byed pa*) rather than *Pañcakrama*. So in PTT, Vol. 59, he mentions all five *krama* by name at p. 200-5 and again all five beginning with 'from the *Prakaraṇa*' (*rab tu byed pa las kyaṅ*) at p. 239-4; and has numerous quotations from Prakaraṇa at pp. 214-4, 218-5, 226-5, 236-2, 243-5, 289-1, 300-3, etc. Also, Bhavyakīrti's '*Prakāśikā*' commentary on *Pradīpoddyotana*, PTT Vol. 60, quotes the *Pañcakrama* twice on p. 257-4, 5 as '*Prakaraṇa*', suggesting that he was consulting Nāgārjuna's *Tantraṭikā* while writing his commentary on Candrakīrti's work. But the commentators on the *Pañcakrama* itself do not call it '*Prakaraṇa*'. An extensive commentarial literature arose on the basis of the *Pañcakrama*. I have mainly employed Śrī Lakṣmī's commentary, because it adheres closely to the text commented upon without wild speculations, has a beautiful flow of language, and uses the nidāna verses which are the basis of the present work. Another commentary which has supplied some important passages is the *Maṇimālā* which the colophon and accordingly the catalogs ascribe to Nāgabodhi. But this is hardly possible, because Nāgabodhi is among the earliest in the lineage. The *Maṇimālā* is the most developed of the Indian commentaries I examined. It employs the 'six alternatives' (*ṣaṭkoṭi*) terminology, which was popularized by Candrakīrti. It is full of opinionated speculations, such as (PTT, Vol. 62, p. 160-2) equating Nāgārjuna's five stages, *vajrajāpa*, etc., with the five paths (*mārga*), prayoga, etc. of the Prajñāpāramitā exegesis. The fact that the respective descriptions in the two different literatures have virtually nothing in common does not bother the author of the *Maṇimālā*, who makes up five reasons which need not be cited. A clue of identification is a certain frankness of language which the author has in common with Bhavyakīrti, the author of the *Prakāśikā* commentary on Candrakīrti's *Pradīpoddyotana* (see below). Thus in the *Maṇimālā* (*op. cit.* p. 155-3, 4, 5 and next page) the author takes up the problem of what is meant by the 'woman', 'man', and 'androgyne' of this literature. He mentions and rejects various opinions before giving his own. His remark about the usual theory of the 'woman' is precisely the remark given by Bhavyakīrti in the *Prakāśikā* (PTT, Vol. 61, p. 3-2), with alternate translation into Tibetan, where he rejects the view that a 'woman' is described by breasts and hair :

> If the feminine gender (*strī-liṅga*) has breasts and hair, then *mālā* ('garlands') and **svapnāsanī* ('beds') would not have feminine gender, because they do not have

> breasts and hair. And even when the (female) zones that do have hair are shaved, they have feminine gender. And it reduces to the absurdity that an actor impersonating a woman by means of attached breasts and wig, would have feminine gender" (*| gal te nu ma| daṅ skra can mo rtags yin na | deḥi tshe phreṅ ba daṅ ñal khri la sogs pa dag mo rtags su mi ḥgyur te|de rnams nu ma daṅ skrar mi ldan paḥi phyir ro || ḥbreg paḥi skra daṅ ldan paḥi sa phyogs dag kyaṅ mo rtags su ḥgyur ro| sbyar baḥi nu ma daṅ skraḥi cha lugs ḥdzin paḥi gar mkhan skyes pa yaṅ mo rtags ñid du thal bar ḥgyur ro|*)

There are other commentators on the Guhyasamāja system who are equally scornful of the vulgar interpretation of tantric symbols, of which our own generation has no monopoly. But it would take the same person to make the identical remark, given above, in two books.

In the Ārya school, the tantric Candrakīrti wrote the most eminent commentary on the mūla *Guhyasamājatantra*, called the *Pradīpoddyotana*. Its main contribution is to classify commentarial statements on the *Guhyasamājatantra* by a rigorous application of subdivisions of 'Seven Ornaments', a terminology stemming from the *Vajrajñānasamuccaya*, but which is merely referred to by Candrakīrti as the 'Explanatory Tantra' (see the Section C, *infra*, for a summary exposition of the full twenty-eight subdivisions) and to avoid Yogācāra terminology. The first commentary on his work may have been the primitive one by Lakṣmīṅkarā, sister of Indrabhūti, called the '*Viṣamapada-pañjikā*'. The main commentary on the *Pradīpoddyotana*, the '*Prakāśikā*' of Bhavyakīrti (according to the Tohoku catalog; PTT catalog incorrectly gives author's name as Āryadeva), seems intent on rebuking Candrakīrti by restoring the Yogācāra vocabulary pursuant to the indications of Nāgārjuna's works.

In this tradition the greatest work on important phases of tantric praxis is Āryadeva's *Caryāmelāpaka-pradīpa*. Āryadeva is a tantric writer, no more to be identified with the celebrated Mādhyamika author of the same name than are the tantrics Nāgārjuna and Candrakīrti. This tantric author Āryadeva also wrote a number of brief summary works of which now the most well-known is the *Cittaviśuddhiprakaraṇa* by reason of Prabhubhai B. Patel's edition. Of all the later writers of this

'Ārya' tradition of the Guhyasamāja cycle, Āryadeva gives the greatest literary impression of having actually 'done it'.

(b) The Jñānapāda school is named after Buddhaśrījñāna, whose teacher Līlavajra composed (in the Guhyasamāja class) only the *Nidānagurūpadeśa* and does not appear to have made a distinction between the 'Stage of Generation' and the 'Stage of Completion' (PTT, Vol. 158, p. 178-3; slob dpon sgeg paḥi rdo rjes rgyud kyi gleṅ gzhiḥi bśad pa tsam mdzad kyaṅ/ rim gñis kyi lam gyi srol zur pa mi snaṅ ṅo / ). Buddhaśrījñāna (see his legend in Roerich, *The Blue Annals*, I, pp. 367, ff.) wrote works exemplifying both Stages: the Stage of Generation in the *Samantabhadra-nāma-sādhana* (Tohoku No. 1855) and the Stage of Completion in the revealed *Mukhāgama* (Toh. No. 1853) and *Muktitilaka* (Toh. No. 1859) based on that revelation (PTT, Vol. 158, p. 178-3). Buddhaśrījñāna studied the Prajñāpāramitā under the celebrated specialist Haribhadra, and this part of his training is quite evident in his tantric works. He adopted an interpretive position in which at each point the explanations of the Guhyasamāja are tied in with Mahāyāna Buddhism, particularly of the Prajñāpāramitā type. That kept obviously Brahmanical doctrines from flowing into the syncretic tantric literature of his school. Perhaps partly due to his Buddhist piety, Buddhaśrījñāna had great fortune of disciples. One of his direct disciples, Buddhaguhya, became a celebrated commentator on the Caryā-and Yoga-Tantra classes of tantric literature. Another one, Dīpaṅkarabhadra is credited with a work of highest importance on ritual in the Stage of Generation, the *Guhyasamājamaṇḍalavidhi* (Toh. 1865), often referred to as the "Four-hundred-and-fifty verses," which has a *ṭikā* on it by Ratnākaraśānti (Toh. No. 1871). This Dīpaṅkarabhadra as well as Rāhulabhadra and some other direct disciples are credited in legend with advanced success in the yoga of the Guhyasamāja, it being hinted that they did better than Buddhaśrījñāna himself, who tried without success to generate the 'diamond body' (*vajrakāya*). Another disciple, named Vitapāda, wrote lengthy commentaries on the main works of the master. This school, at least as far as its literary products are concerned, does not bother with the topics of three lights and the Clear Light so prevalent in the works of the 'Ārya' school. If the Jñānapāda school comes across a term in the *Guhyasamājatantra* like '*prakṛtiprabhāsvara*', it would be prone to explain it just as in non-tantric Buddhism, to wit 'intrinsically clear' (said of the pure consciousness); while a writer of the Ārya school would be likely to say it means (in what is called the 'pregnant sense') 'the Clear Light along with the (80) *prakṛtis* (of the three lights'). However, it may well be the case that the Jñānapāda school does not deny that 'pregnant sense' but reserves it for the oral tradition, rigorously kept apart from the written works. The emphasis on the guru's precepts is shown by the very title of that work of Buddhaśrijñāna's, the *Mukhāgama* 'the tradition from the mouth'. Vitapāda's commentary on the master's *Muktitilaka* carries on this same stress by a number of consistent remarks (PTT, Vol. 65, p. 134-5): "from the mouth of one's own guru" (raṅ gi bla maḥi kha nas....); *ibid*, p. 135-2; " 'arisen in the lineage chain' means recourse to the errorless path of the illustrious gurus" (brgyud rims las byuṅ zhes pa ni bla ma dam paḥi ma nor baḥi lam du brten paḥo). Various commentaries on the *mūla-tantra* belong to the Jñānapāda school; probably the freedom from Candrakīrti's classifying terms in the later commentaries is the best indication of inclusion in that school. The Jñānapāda school took greater care with literary polish than the Ārya school. It has been preeminent in works on the Guhyasamāja ritual, especially on the praxis of *prāṇāyāma*; and the writer Smṛtijñānakīrti of this school wrote a commentary on the *Caturdevīparipṛcchā*, which is mainly devoted to *prāṇāyāma*. The towering tantric commentator of the last period of Indian Buddhism, Abhayākaragupta, is said to have belonged to the Jñānapāda lineage.

The author Ratnākaraśānti freely used both lineages in his own works, and his attitude is about what is found in Tibetan tantrism, where the followers of the Guhyasamāja cycle were glad enough to understand the Tantra and practice it in proper fashion, no matter which of the two lineages would contribute the most. In fact, both schools have an extensive literature on this Tantra, as extant in Tibetan translation. In the present work, products of the 'Ārya' school are chiefly utilized for the simple reason that it is this school which is built around the position found in the forty nidāna verses that are the main instigation of the current research. On the other hand, some important passages have been selected from texts of the Jñānapāda school.

The above summary prepares us to make some chronological observations. Tucci (I, p. 232) argues that we should accept the Tibetan tradition which makes Padmasambhava (middle eighth century) the disciple of a King Indrabhūti who therefore would fall in the period end of seventh to first half of eighth century. But Hadano (*op. cit.*) places Indrabhūti in the ninth century and Buddhajñānapāda in the eighth century. Of course, to reconcile the positions we should posit two Indrabhūti's. The first Indrabhūti would be the one associated with Oḍḍiyāna, who has no works on the Guhyasamāja, but could well be the author of the great commentary on the *Saṃpuṭa-tilaka* in the Mother Tantra tradition, just as Saraha, his junior, wrote commentaries on other Tantras, such as the *Buddhakapāla-Tantra*, but no distinguishable work on the Guhyasamāja. Saraha is placed by Sāṅkṛtyāyana as a contemporary of King Dharmapāla (769-809). The lama Tāranātha, in his tales of the Siddhas, calls the second Indrabhūti 'Indrabhūti the junior'. He could be the Indrabhūti of Orissa (Odivisa) whom Sāṅkṛtyāyana considered to be the only Indrabhūti. His master is Anaṅgavajra, and the latter's teacher Padmavajra. This would be the Padmavajra who wrote the *Guhyasiddhi*. His spiritual grandson Indrabhūti would be the one who wrote the *Jñānasiddhi*. Padmavajra would fall in the second half of the eighth century, just as do both the tantric Nāgārjuna of the Ārya school and Buddhaśrījñāna of the Jñānapāda school. In the ninth century comes Candrakīrti, author of *Pradīpoddyotana*, as well as the second Indrabhūti who has a sister Lakṣmīṅkarā; and also, probably, Āryadeva. This is easily the first half of the ninth, as maintained by (Miss) Malati J. Shendge, ed. *Advayasiddhi* (Baroda, 1964), p. 11, in agreement with Snellgrove and Sāṅkṛtyāyana. The Kashmirian Śrī Lakṣmī is probably not the same person as Lakṣmīṅkarā. Tilopa belongs to the tenth century because he is the *guru* of Nāropā who died in 1027, and the latter is a contemporary of Ratnākaraśānti. Guhyasamāja commentaries continued to be written through the twelfth century, as is deducible from translations into Tibetan. Thus, the Tanjur Guhyasamāja cycle of commentarial literature is composed between the eighth and twelfth centuries.

Once we place the commentarial literature, the way is open to approach the more tenuous clues for solving the problem of the revealed Tantras of the Kanjur. The tradition reported from Tāranātha that the Tantras were transmitted in utmost secrecy for 300 years before being rendered somewhat more public by the Siddhas (cf. B. Bhattacharyya, Intro. xxxv), would lead us to a fifth century A.D. time which is not unreasonable, even though we should be unhappy to have so little data to go on. The early fifth century is the creative period of Asaṅga (circa 375-430 A.D.), but I have rejected the never-substantiated attribution of the *Guhyasamājatantra* to his authorship in my *Analysis of the Śrāvakabhūmi Manuscript*, p. 39, on the basis of my studies in his known works (which include the Sanskrit prose commentary on the *Sūtrālaṃkāra*, but not the basic verses) and repeat my rejection here as a consequence of the intervening investigation of the Guhyasamāja literature. Not for the reason that the *Guhyasamājatantra* is unworthy of Asaṅga, rather that it is impossible of Asaṅga, and further—to mention an extrinsic reason—tantric commentators do not quote from Asaṅga's or his brother Vasubandhu's works to justify basic tantric ideas! Rather they quote the *Laṅkāvatāra-sūtra* for their Yogācāra-type vocabulary, and this *sūtra* was first translated into Chinese in 443 A.D. and in the fifth century had become so popular among Indian Buddhists that it was the chief text of Bodhidharma when he came to China in either 520 A.D. or 527 A.D. (the alternate dates of the Sino-Japanese tradition).

We can strengthen this tentative attribution to the fifth century by considering some further materials of the *Vajramālā* which, besides being the source of our nidāna verses, contains many other passages of supreme importance for understanding the Guhyasamāja cult. In my "Studies in Yama and Māra," pp. 70-73, I show from a work of Tsoṅ-kha-pa that the *Vajramālā* converts the Viṣṇu Avatār doctrine, at least the first five Avatārs, into a kind of esoteric embryology, namely that in the first five lunar months of uterine existence, the body has successively the forms of fish, tortoise, boar, lion, and dwarf. Now this doctrine is set forth in *Vajramālā's* Chapter XXXII, which also contains Yogācāra vocabulary tied in with the terminology of the *Laṅkāvatāra-sūtra*. As an example of this terminology in the *Vajramālā*, I may cite PTT, Vol. 3, p. 214-5, line 6 : "the secret state of the eight-*vijñāna* set" (/ rnam śes brgyad kyi tshogs dben pa / ). In that article, p. 71, note, I mention, "Miss Kamala Ray, 'The Ten Incarnations of Viṣṇu in Bengal', IHQ, Vol. XV (1941), pp. 370-85, explains that while the Avatāra theory is very ancient, the standard list is more modern, and (p. 373) 'Epigraphic evidences testify to the existence of this theory from the 5th century A.D. onwards (in Bengal).'" This suggests that at the time the standard list of ten incarnations became publicized, an esoteric tradition was developing concerning these incarnations as represented, at least the first five, by intra-uterine states.

Furthermore, in the previous introductory section, 'The world of light', I put forward the striking hypothesis that both the set of thirty-three female *prakṛtis* and forty male *prakṛtis* listed under nidāna verses nos. 1 and 2 can be interpreted as breaking down into five groups in each set, the first set especially going with the five stages of the Vaiṣṇava path to union with the Lord Kṛṣṇa (presuming there was once a faith in such a 'path'). If the sets of *prakṛtis* have their origin in a syncretism with Vaiṣṇavism, then the fact that later on the commentators on the *Pañcakrama* (from which the lists of *prakṛtis* are drawn) have no inkling, as far as the texts are concerned, of how to subdivide the sets of *prakṛtis*, indicates that some time must have elapsed between the adoption of this vocabulary in an esoteric oral way and the more public commentarial tradition. We must grant that any conclusion about this matter must be of a highly speculative nature, since the early syncretisms of Buddhism and Vaiṣṇavism are obscure, and since the erotic type of Kṛṣṇa worship is usually placed at a considerably later date than what we are now considering (fifth century, A.D.).

What I do maintain is that the *Vajramālā* has the earmarks of having been composed centuries before the tantric Nāgārjuna quoted it in his *Pañcakrama*, and I tentatively place it in the fifth century. The *Sandhivyākaraṇa* should tentatively be placed at about the same time, since it shows the same definite style of authoritative revealed literature. The other explanatory tantras can be roughly placed there also, subject to later investigations.

The above considerations leave open a date for the *Guhyasamājatantra* itself. This problem cannot be separated from the dating of all the main revealed Buddhist Tantras preserved in Tibetan translation in the Kanjur, because there is certainly a great deal of common material to be found in all these Tantras; as well as from the dating of the Śaivitic and Vaiṣṇava *āgamas*. I see no reason for denying it a century's priority to the *Vajramālā*; and so, on a purely tentative basis, ascribe the *Guhyasamājatantra* to the fourth century, A.D. But a decision on this matter requires solution of other problems of Indian literary history.

I am well aware that the kind of reasoning employed above might be challenged by the scholars who insist on a later date for the *Guhyasamājatantra*, in fact placed just prior to the historical commentaries on it. Therefore, I take the liberty of quoting extensively from my article in the Golden Jubilee Volume of the Bhandarkar Oriental Research Institute, "Early Literary History of the Buddhist Tantras, especially the Guhyasamāja-tantra":

"What is significant about the two commentarial traditions is precisely that there are two, with many differences within each of these traditions. Just as the Sautrāntika and Vaibhāṣika of non-tantric Buddhism could not have arisen fully-grown, in the form in which we know them, in the century immediately following the passing of the Buddha, so also the 'Ārya School' and the 'Jñānapāda School' could not have arisen in the century immediately following the composition of the *Guhyasamāja*, let alone the very same century! Indeed, any one who even partially surveys the *Guhyasamāja* literature as extant in Tibetan and notes the remarkable variance in explanation of a given passage of the basic Tantra, would experience at least a mild shock at the flimsy reasons given for a late dating of the *Guhyasamāja*. One example will be given to show what is meant, and this case is particularly chosen for a context where one would expect minimal variation between the commentaries because the expression to be explained is merely the 'three kinds' of each sense object as mentioned without explanation in the basic tantra of *Guhyasamāja*, Chap. 7:

*Ārya school*:

Nāgārjuna's *Tantraṭīkā* on *Guhyasamāja* (Derge ed., Sa, f. 105b-7); (form, the object of sight) 'has the nature of outer, inner, and both' (*phyi daṅnaṅ daṅ gñi gaḥi raṅ bzhin*).

Candrakīrti's *Pradīpoddyotana* on *Guhyasamāja* (Derge ed., Ha, f. 49a-5): (form, the object of sight) 'should be perceived and comprehended as inferior, intermediate, and superior' (*dman pa daṅ bar ma daṅ mchog gsum du rnam par śes śiṅ rtogs pa*) ; in Tsoṅ-kha-pa's *Mchan-ḥgrel* on the *Pradīpoddyotana* (PTT, Vol. 158, p. 55-3), we learn that the superior kind is the Buddha going with that sense object, e.g. Vairocana as form; (p. 56-1, form is also of three kinds, pleasurable, repulsive or displeasing, and neutral).

*Jñānapāda School*:

Praśāntajñāna's *Upadeśā-niścaya* on *Guhyasamāja* (PTT, Vol. 63, p. 64-5); the three kinds are superior (lust), intermediate (delusion), and inferior (hatred).

Celu-pā's *Ratnavṛkṣa-nāma-rahasya-samāja-vṛtti* (PTT, Vol. 63, p. 183-5): inferior, intermediate, and superior.

Jinadatta's *Pañjikā-nāma* on *Guhyasamāja* (PTT, Vol.63, p. 259-1) : "Because one discerns it as having the nature of superior, and so on, there are three kinds ; having the nature of outer, inner, and both, means "non-apprehension" (*anupalabdhi*), so one should understand it by the nature of three gates to liberation, of voidness, etc.' (mchog la sogs paḥi raṅ bzhin du brtags paḥi phyir rnam gsum mo / phyi daṅ naṅ daṅ gñi gaḥi bdag ñid mi dmigs pa ste / stoṅ pa ñid la sogs paḥi rnam par thar paḥi sgo gsum gyi ṅo bos rtogs par byaḥo /).

Ratnākaraśānti's *Kusumāñjali-guhyasamāja-nibandha-nāma* (Vol. 64, p. 127-1): the three kinds mean the respective offerings by the three kinds of yogins, the one of lust, of delusion, and of hatred.

Smṛtijñānakīrti's *Śrīguhyasamāja-tantrarāja-vṛtti* (PTT, Vol. 66, p. 132-3): 'The "three kinds" means that one knows (the object) as the three gates to liberation, the signless, etc.'

Ānandagarbha's *Śrī-guhyasamāja-mahātantrarāja-ṭīkā* (PTT, Vol. 84, p. 127-4, 5): 'The three kinds are outer, inner, and secret. That was explained by Ārya-Jñānapāda to mean fifteen in an external set, fifteen in a personal set, and fifteen in a secret set. Having cited his words,

I should here explain clearly his meaning.' (rnam pa gsum ni phyi daṅ naṅ daṅ gsaṅ baḥo / / de ḥphags pa ye śes zhabs kyis phyiḥi bye brag bco lṅa daṅ / naṅ gi bye brag bco lṅa daṅ / gsaṅ baḥi bye brag bco lṅar bśad paḥi don ḥdir sgrar draṅs nas gsal bar bśad par bya ste /). He goes on to take the outer as three, which multiplied by the five sense objects yields the number fifteen, and does the same for the inner or personal, and for the secret which involves the *prajñā-upāya* union. In each case, the three are the Buddha, the Bodhisattva, and the Devī, associated with that object by the triad of perception, sense organ and sense object, i.e. for form, the three are the Buddha Vairocana, the Bodhisattva Kṣitigarbha, and the Devī Rūpavajrā.

"There are three main sources for the various comments cited above. One is the Explanatory Tantra *Saṃdhivyākaraṇa*, which is a verse paraphrase, with slight enlargement, of the first twelve chapters of the *Guhyasamājatantra*. In its treatment of Chap. 7, it states (PTT, Vol, 3, p. 240-3):

*/ naṅ daṅ de bzhin phyi rol daṅ / gñi ga rjes su mi dmigs pa/*
*/ gzugs la sogs gsum de yin te / lha rnams la ni dbul bar bya//*

The three kinds of form and other sense objects are the non-apprehension of inner, outer, and both; one should offer those to the gods.

"The next source is the Explanatory Tantra *Vajramālā*, which states in what I call the '*nidāna-kārikā*', no. 19 :

*sthātavyaṃ viṣayeṣv asmād yoginādvayadarśinā /*
*hīnamadhyapraṇīteṣu jñānatrayanidarśanāt //*

Afterwards the *yogin* who sees the non-duality should be dwelling upon sense objects 'inferior', 'intermediate', and 'superior' by seeing the triple gnosis.

"The third source is the *uttara-tantra* (18th chap. of the Sanskrit text, p. 158) :

*rūpaśabdādayaḥ kāmāḥ sukhaduḥkhobhayātmakāḥ /*
*janayanti hṛdaye nityaṃ rāgadveṣatamodayam //*

The 'desires' (i.e. the 5 strands of desire, *pañcakāmaguṇa*) 'form', 'sound', etc.—pleasurable, painful, and neutral—continually generate in the heart, (respectively), the source of 'lust', 'hatred', and 'delusion'.

"With all that information at hand, it is easy to see that

some commentators relied especially on the *Vajramālā*, some especially on the *Saṃdhivyākaraṇa*, some especially on the *uttara-tantra*; and then some commentators tried to harmonize two different terminologies of 'three kinds'' by taking it as 'three times three', i.e. three each of each three. The *Saṃdhivyākaraṇa* expression 'non-apprehension' suggested to some commentators the non-tantric doctrines of 'Perfection of Insight' (*prajñā-pāramitā*) with its stress on voidness (*śūnyatā*), so they saw an opportunity to make contact with non-tantric Buddhism by the well-known set of Buddhism, the three gates to liberation (*trīṇi vimokṣa-mukhāni*), that is, the voidness (*śūnyatā-*), the undirected (*apraṇihita-*), and the signless (*animitta-*) gates. When one takes into account that these commentaries vary much more in most other places, where the *Guhyasamāja* passages are not restricted by such concrete objects as the sense objects, it is difficult to avoid the conclusion that some centuries of oral tradition have intervened between the basic *Guhyasamājatantra* and the eighth century when the 'historical' writers began to appear on the scene. Of course, if the basic Tantra had been concocted by the first commentator, or had been composed just prior to his writing activity, there should not have been any question of what the 'three kinds' were. Instead the commentators might have differed only in their metaphorical interpretation of the standard 'three kinds'."

Another conclusion one may draw from the evidence of the above extract is that it is hazardous to try to understand the *Guhyasamājatantra* just from reading it. Who, reading the phrase 'three kinds of form', would know what the three kinds are, unless someone told him?

Now turning our consideration to the forty nidāna verses, since they are a part of the *Vajramālā*, and no evidence has turned up to suggest their later addition, we may, pursuant to the above reasoning, place these verses also in the fifth century, A.D. Alaṃkakalaśa's commentary on the *Vajramālā*, which is extant in the Tanjur, does not comment all the way up to the chapter which contains the forty verses. The verses are cited in the *Pradīpoddyotana* without further explanation except for the classifying term 'pregnant sense' (*garbhy-artha*). The only Indian commentary on the *Pradīpoddyotana* translated into Tibetan that generously treats these verses with comments is Bhavyakīrti's *Prakāśikā*. This is a highly opinionated commentary, but I found it worthwhile citing in several places.

Later, in Tibet, Candrakīrti's work was highly prized. A commentarial tradition arose which did not neglect the 40 verses. The Tibetan Bu-ston's commentary on the *Pradīpoddyotana* (Vol. Ta of his collected works, published by Lokesh Chandra in Part Nine) must have been eagerly greeted by Tibetan monks when it first appeared, probably as the first native commentary on that work by an eminent authority on the Tantras. He continues the Mādhyamika tone of commentary in the same manner as the *Pradīpoddyotana* itself, that is, in a negative way by avoidance of the typical Yogācāra vocabulary found in many other commentaries, especially in the *Pañcakrama* tradition. Bu-ston has various disagreements with Bhavyakīrti's commentaries (the main one and the smaller one) and with Kumāra's commentary on the *Pradīpoddyotana*, as also with unnamed teachers ("Some persons say..."). Bu-ston comments topically, not sentence by sentence in the order of occurrence in Candrakīrti's work. This mode of commentary is not original, for some of the Indian commentaries are of this type. In line with this sort of commentary, he does not comment on the 40 verses in their order, but topically. So after some remarks for the first four verses, going with E-vaṃ ma-yā, he begins to jump around, although in the end accounting for almost all the verses. The Tibetan commentary on the Guhyasamāja by Kun-dgaḥ-don-ḥgrub (the "Man ṅag rim gñis gter mdzod"), recently reprinted in India, contains the 40 verses almost at the beginning, and in section KA, f. 37a-b (pp. 73-74), also treats the 40 verses topically and with extreme brevity. These topical groupings are of no help to me in the present work, because I shall treat the verses in their order, to fully bring out the author's intentions as an individual composition. The commentarial tradition on Candrakīrti's work culminated in Tsoṅ-kha-pa's *Mchan ḥgrel* (annotation in smaller writing in between the words or phrases) in the early fifteenth century. The *Pradīpoddyotana* had been first translated by the Indian pandit Śraddhākaravarma and the great Tibetan translator Rin-chen-bsaṅ-po (958-1055); Tsoṅ-kha-pa used this translation as well as 'the two new translations' (*Mchan ḥgrel*, p. 91-4). Tsoṅ-kha-pa's annotation has evidence that he had read Bu-ston's work and continued many of his ideas, but Tsoṅ-kha-pa's treatment is far advanced. He knew that in order for a commentary to be useful, it had to follow the order of the original work. So does his annotation (*Mchan ḥgrel*) on the *Pradīpoddyotana*, and his *Mthaḥ gcod* on the individual chapters. His *Don gsal ba* on the *Guhyasamāja* follows the order of the three *maṇḍalas* ; and his *Dbaṅ gi don* follows the order of the *maṇḍala*-rite. Thereby his works were of great convenience for me to consult, and it must have been the same for the Tibetans. There can be little doubt that the *Guhyasamājatantra* reached an advanced and mature interpretation in Tibet at the hands of the great teachers Bu-ston, Tsoṅ-kha-pa, and others.*

*After the present work was completed, I became indebted to Serkong Rimpoche, Assistant Tutor to H. H. the Dalai Lama, for allowing me to secure a copy of a text just reprinted in North India for restricted circulation. This is by Śes-rab-seṅ-ge, a disciple of Tsoṅ-kha-pa—a commentary on Candrakīrti's *Pradīpoddyotana* in its Tibetan version. This native work is a remarkable piece of popularization of a Tantric topic, which I believe was composed after the death of Tsoṅ-kha-pa, his teacher. The author appears to have taken as basis Tsoṅ-kha-pa's *Mchan ḥgrel* annotation on the *Pradīpoddyotana*, incorporating the annotation into the text commented upon in a lucid paraphrase which, however, omits thorny points and then adds citations from other works, Tantric and non-Tantric. The author constantly rationalizes with remarks like "don ni" ("the meaning is as follows"). In illustration, in the course of Chap. One commentary, his explanation of the forty verses is approximately a paraphrase of Tsoṅ-kha-pa's *Mchan ḥgrel* on those verses, but omits mention of Tsoṅ-kha-pa's difficult comment on *Śru*. In Sec. Ka, f. 45b to 46a-6, he has various ways of grouping the verses (which Tsoṅ-kha-pa did not present in his commentary), but gives no solution for the order of the verses from 1 to 40. In Sec. Nga, f. 41a, he points out that *pratyāhāra* and *dhyāna* (the first two of the six-membered yoga) are included in "arcane body" (T. *lus dben*)—which is Tsoṅ-kha-pa's position. It is this position that is the chief clue for solving the order of the forty verses, that is,if one tries to accommodate this position within the forty verses, especially with the *Kā-Ya* (Body) verses. It is good that this fascinating work is receiving its due appreciation from the Gelugpa Lamas who specialize in Tantra. Besides, the Tibetans have recently reprinted works by Mkhas-grub-rje and by the First Panchen Lama on aspects of the *Guhyasamāja* cult. I have made an important observation about the latter two works in my Appendix 2. In any case, my policy of relying on the Master Tsoṅ-kha-pa, rather than on the derivative literature of his followers, should be appreciated by the present-day Gelugpa monks, who can scarcely deny that Tsoṅ-kha-pa was as much a Lama (guru) as any that can be met today.

B. *The title of the work and its opening sentence* (*nidāna*)

The full title as found at the ends of chapters in the edited text is: *Sarvatathāgatakāyavākcittarahasyātirahasyaguhyasamājamahāguhyatantrarāja.* The following translation of the title will be justified: Great-secret King of Tantras—the 'Secret Union' of the secret and the greater secret belonging to the Body, Speech and Mind of all the Tathāgatas.

Vitapāda's commentary *Mukhāgama-vṛtti* (PTT, Vol. 65, p. 66-4) explains some of the construction of the title: "'Tantra of *samāja* by all the Buddhas' means Vajradhara because it is the union (*samāja*) by all the Buddhas in the manner of *paramārtha* and *saṃvṛti.* To show that, there is 'Thus' (*evaṃ*). 'Great secret' (*mahāguhya*) means the illusory (*māyopama*). 'Secret' (*rahasya*) means the Stage of Generation. 'Greater secret' (*atirahasya*) means the thusness of all modes. The great *āgama* which incomparably shows those matters, is the *Samāja*" (/ saṅs rgyas kun gyis ḥdus paḥi rgyud ces pa ni / saṅs rgyas thams cad don dam pa daṅ kun rdzob kyi tshul du ḥdus paḥi phyir rdo rje ḥchaṅ baḥo / de ston par byed pa la yaṅ de skad ces byaḥo / gsaṅ chen źes pa ni sgyu ma lta buḥo / gsaṅ la źes pa bskyed paḥi rim paḥo / ches gsaṅ ba źes pa ni dṅos po thams cad kyi de bźin ñid do / de rnams ston par byed paḥi goṅ na med paḥi luṅ chen po ni ḥdus paḥo / ). This commentary makes it clear that the compound *rahasyātirahasya* is a *dvandva*, to be understood by such pairs as *saṃvṛti-satya* and *paramārtha-satya*; Stage of Generation and Stage of Completion. By bringing in the expression 'Thus' (*evaṃ*), Vitapāda also indicates the relation between the title and the first sentence of the Tantra which begins with *evaṃ.*

The most important part of the title is the expression *guhyasamāja*, because this is the standard abbreviated form of the title, which in turn is abbreviated to *samāja.* Some light is shed on the abbreviated title by its chapter one, verse 3:

> *Bhāṣasva bhagavan tattvaṃ vajrasārasamuccayam* /
> *sarvatathāgataṃ guhyaṃ samājaṃ guhyasambhavam* //
> Lord, pray explain the *samāja*, the reality, sum of diamond essences, the all-tathāgata secret, and what arises from the secret!

The *Pradīpoddyotana* comments with various of its classifying signals, 'invariant sense' (*akṣarārthaḥ*), and so on: / *bhāṣasva* samājam iti sambandhaḥ / samājam iti dvayor ekībhāvaḥ samājam / akṣarārthaḥ // vajrapadmasamāyogaṃ samājaṃ/ samastāṅgaṃ // prajñopāyasamāyogaṃ samājaṃ / garbhī // saṃvṛtiparamārthasatyayor mīlanaḥ samājaṃ / guhyasambhavam iti saiva viśeṣaṇaḥ / guhyaṃ prabhāsvaraṃ tasmāt / sambhūtam advayajñānātmakaṃ mahāvajradharam iti yāvad/ kolikaḥ // sarvatathāgataṃ guhyam iti sarvatathāgatānāṃ *pāraṃparyeṇa gopanīyaṃ guhyaṃ / vajrasārās tathāgatāḥ teṣām ekībhāvalakṣaṇaṃ samuccayaṃ/ tattvaṃ yathābhūtaṃ// Translation (Mchan ḥgrel, p. 24): 'Pray explain the *samāja*' is the application. Concerning '*samāja*', the unification of a pair is *samāja* with invariant sense. The union of diamond and lotus is *samāja* with shared sense. Insight, the means, and their union is *samāja* with pregnant sense. The merger of the two truths, conventional and absolute, is *samāja*; what arises from the secret is precisely that as the extraordinary case, to wit, the secret is the Clear Light, and what arises therefrom goes up to Mahāvajradhara who is the non-dual knowledge; (*samāja*) with ultimate sense. The all-tathāgata secret is the secret, to be preserved of all the tathāgatas, handed down in succession (of master and disciple). The diamond essences are the Tathāgatas; their sum has the characteristic of unification. The reality is as it really is.

The words 'Body, Speech, and Mind' run through a gamut of usages, of which the most comprehensive list is ten in number (see Ratnākaraśānti's exposition in C, below). The invariant sense is that the Diamond of Body is Vairocana, the Diamond of Speech is Amitābha, and the Diamond of Mind is Akṣobhya. To these three Tathāgata families are added Amoghasiddhi and Ratnasaṃbhava to make a total of five Tathāgatas, the usual meaning of 'all the Tathāgatas'.

In the second paragraph after verse 3 of chapter one, there occurs the expression *sarvatathāgatānāṃ kāyavākcittaguhyaṃ*, on which the *Pradīpoddyotana* comments (*Mchan ḥgrel*, p. 24):

> / sarvatathāgatānāṃ kāyavākcittaguhyaṃ samayasaṃvarādikulatrayapariṇāmaḥ / akṣarārthaḥ // sarvatathāgatānāṃ kāyavākcittaguhyaṃ vyañjana [trayam] / samastāṅgaḥ // sarvatathāgatānāṃ kāyavākcittaguhyaṃ jñānatrayaprakṛtyābhāsavāyuvāhanaṃ / garbhī // sarvatathāgatānāṃ kāyavākcittaguhyaṃ jñānamayadehaḥ/kolikaḥ//

'The secret of the body, speech and mind of all the Tathāgatas' means the extending to the three families of pledges, vows, and so on; invariant sense. 'The secret of the body...' means the three syllables (for generating the deities); shared sense. 'The secret of the body...', means the wind-vehicle for the appearance of the (eighty) *prakṛtis* upon the three lights; pregnant sense. 'The secret of the body...', means the body made of knowledge; ultimate sense.

The foregoing should demonstrate the multiple levels of interpretation that can be, and were extended to the words of the title.

The length of the opening sentence (*nidāna*) is established by theory that it demonstrates the 'five perfections', that is to say, of the teaching, the retinue, the time, the teacher, and the place. Naturally we give much weight to the tradition of the Explanatory Tantra *Vajramālā*, as found in Alaṃkakalaśa's *Śrī-vajramālā-mahāyogatantra-ṭīkā-gambhīrārthadīpikā* (PTT, Vol. 61, p. 164-1):

> / bsdus don źes bya ba ni phun sum tshogspa lṅa daṅ ldan pa ste / de la ḥdi skad ces bya ba la sogs pas bstan paḥi bya ba phun sum tshogs paḥo // bdag gi thos pa źes bya ba la sogs pas ni ḥkhor phun sum tshogs pa mdor bstan paḥo// dus gcig na źes bya ba la sogs pas ni dus phun sum tshogs paḥo // bcom ldan ḥdas źes bya ba la sogs pas ni ston pa po phun tshogs paḥo / / de bźin gśegs pa thams cad kyi sku daṅ gsuṅ daṅ thugs kyi sñiṅ po rdo rje btsun moḥi bha-ga rnams bźugs ste / źes bya ba la sogs pas ni gnas phun sum tshogs pa gsuṅs so /
>
> The 'concise meaning' is possession of five perfections. Among them, by way of *evaṃ*, there is the perfection of what is to be taught. By way of *mayā śrutam*, there is the perfection of the retinue, in brief. By way of *ekasmin samaye*, there is the perfection of time. By way of *bhagavān*, there is perfection of the teacher. By way of *sarvatathāgatakāyavākcittahṛdayavajrayoṣidbhageṣu vijahāra*, there is perfection of the place.

On the other hand both Vajrahāsa's *Tantrarāja-śrīguhyasamāja-ṭīkā* and Līlavajra's *Guhyasamājatantra-nidāna-gurūpadeśabhāṣya* (PTT, Vol. 66, p. 75-5 and p. 97-2) explain the application of five perfections (*phun sum tshogs*) in this manner : 1. the teacher (*ston pa*) indicated by *bhagavān*; 2. compiler (*sdud pa po*), by *evaṃ mayā śrutam ekasmin samaye*; 3. place (*gnas*), by *sarvatathāgata..vijahāra*; 4. retinue (*ḥkhor*) by *anabhilāpyānabhilāpyaiḥ* (text, chap. I, p. 1, line 3) down to *saṃdṛśyate sma* (text, p. 2, line 12); 5. *tantra*, i.e. the discourse (*rgyud*), by *evaṃ*. Therefore, the intention of these two authors (obviously closely affiliated) is to extend the *nidāna* down through the naming of all auditors to the discourse. The same allotment of the text to perfection of the retinue is apparently given by the writer Kumāra in his *Pradīpadīpa-ṭippaṇī-hṛdayādarśa* (PTT, Vol. 60, p. 220-1). However, as the *nidāna* verses are found in the *Vajramālā*, I accept Alaṃkakalaśa's explanation especially since the forty syllables going with the *kārikās* amount to the length as stated by Alaṃkakalaśa. The *nidāna* thus established is as follows :

> Evaṃ mayā śrutam ekasmin samaye bhagavān sarvatathāgata-kāyavākcittahṛdaya-vajrayoṣidbhageṣu vijahāra.
>
> Thus by me it was heard—on an occasion—the Bhagavat ('the Lord') was dwelling in the *bhagas* of the diamond ladies of the heart belonging to the Body, Speech, and Mind of all the Tathāgatas.

Smṛtijñānakīrti's *Śrī-guhyasamāja-tantrarāja-vṛtti* (PTT. Vol. 66, p. 125-5) makes a distinction of 'shared' and 'unshared' sense to apply to defining the *nidāna* itself. He says, "Among those words, *evaṃ* comprises all aspects of sound ; hence it is the form of the 'unshared' *nidāna*, which symbolizes the adamantine state of the 'mind of enlightenment' (*bodhicitta*)" ( / de la ḥdi skad ces pa ni sgraḥi rnam pa mthaḥ dag bsdus pa ste/ des thun moṅ ma yin paḥi gleṅ gźiḥi ṅo bo byaṅ chub kyi sems rdo rje ñid mtshon paḥo / ). Furthermore, "The words *mayā śrutam*, etc. express the form of the 'shared' *nidāna*" (/bdag gis thos pa źes pa la sogs pas ni thuṇ moṅ gi glen gźiḥi ṅo bo gsuṅs te /). His subsequent comments show that by 'shared *nidāna*' he means the part which succinctly expresses the five perfections. According to his commentary, 'by me' (*mayā*) is the perfection of the auditor (in other texts, the perfection of the retinue); 'was heard' (*śrutam*), the perfection of the teaching; 'on an occasion' (*ekasmin samaye*), the perfection of the time; 'the Bhagavat' (*bhagavān*), the perfection of the teacher ; and the remaining words down to 'was dwelling in the *bhagas*'

(...*bhageṣu vijahāra*), the perfection of the place. His explanation leaves the *nidāna* the same length as my acceptance. However, no other commentary that I examined mentions such a divison of the words as made by Paṇḍit Smṛti.

The meaning of the *nidāna* as a coherent sentence can be considered on several levels. There is the simple paraphrase, with a few words added, as in Tsoṅ-kha-pa's *Mchan ḥgrel* on the *Pradīpoddyotana* (bracketted expressions from *Mchan ḥgrel*, pp. 11 and 12):

> Thus by me it was heard (directly, not from an intermediary; but not yet comprehended)—on an occasion (not with another element of consciousness; not at another time; and in a single instant)—the Bhagavat (having the six allotments, lordliness, etc.) was dwelling (with the dress of a *cakravartin*) in the *bhagas* (destruction of defilement) of the diamond ladies (the *prajñā* view of voidness attended with great ecstasy, *mahāsukha*) of the heart (Mahāvajradhara) belonging to the Body, Speech, and Mind of all the Tathāgatas.

That paraphrase is consistent with Indrabhūti's explanation in his *Jñānasiddhi* (GOS, p. 81): / evaṃ mayā śrutam ekasmin samaye bhagavān sarvatathāgatakāyavākcittahṛdayavajrayoṣidbhageṣu vijahāra ekasminn eva kāle / bhagavān aiśvaryādiguṇayuktatvāt / hṛdayaṃ jñānaṃ tad eva vajrayoṣit abhedyaprajñāsvabhāvatvāt, tad eva bhagaṃ sarvakleśabhañjanāt, teṣu sarvatathāgatakāyavākcittahṛdayavajrayoṣidbhageṣu vijahāra / "Thus by me it was heard—upon an occasion—the Lord was dwelling in the *bhagas* of the diamond ladies of the heart belonging to the Body, Speech, and Mind of all the Tathāgatas" :—'on precisely that occasion, the Lord, because endowed with the (six) merits of lordliness and so on; was dwelling in those *bhagas* of the diamond ladies of the heart belonging to the Body, Speech, and Mind of all the Tathāgatas, where the diamond ladies are precisely the heart-knowledge, because of the self-existence of non-dual insight, and where the *bhaga* is precisely the same, because of destroying all defilement."

The Explanatory Tantra of the *Guhyasamāja* called *Saṃdhivyākaraṇa* re-tells the *nidāna* in this revealing manner (PTT, Vol. 3, p. 231-4), labelled '*kolika*' (ultimate sense) for the portion cited in *Pradīpoddyotana* (*Mchan ḥgrel*, p. 17-5 to p. 18-1):

/ punar aparam ārya-vyākhyānam āha /
evaṃ mayā śrutaṃ tattvam ekasmin samaye sphuṭe /
bhagavān guhyavajreśas trivajrasamayottama(ḥ) //
sarvatathāgate jñāne acintyaguṇasaṃpadi /
sadasadubhayātīte asthānasthitisaṃjñini //
ākāśaikasvabhāve'smin sarvajñajñānabhāvini /
jagaddhṛdi viśuddhākhye vijahāra mahāmuniḥ //
(end of quotation).

/ ma rig pa daṅ ḥdu byed daṅ /
/ rnam par śes daṅ miṅ daṅ gzugs /
/ skye mched drug daṅ reg pa daṅ /
/ tshor ba daṅ ni sred pa daṅ //
/ ñer len srid pa skye ba daṅ /
/ rga śi śes bya rig ma yin //
/ ṅa rgyal che baḥi ṅa rgyal daṅ /
/ ṅaḥo sñam ṅa rgyal mṅon ṅa rgyal /
/ gźan yaṅ ṅa rgyal las ṅa rgyal /
/ cuṅ zad ṅa rgyal log par bcas //

Furthermore, the 'Ārya-Vyākhyāna' states :

Thus, the Reality, was heard by me on a certain time extraordinary.

The Bhagavat, diamond lord of mysteries, with the supreme pledge of the triple *vajra*,

Was dwelling as the Mahāmuni in the pure heart of the world, in this unique self-existence of sky having the modes of omniscient knowledge, in the all-Tathāgata gnosis having the inconceivable perfection of merits; beyond existence, non-existence, and both, called 'place of no location'.

The wisdom (*vidyā*) (there) is the knowable of nescience (*avidyā*), motivations (*saṃskāra*), perceptions (*vijñāna*), name-and-form (*nāma-rūpa*), six sense bases (*ṣaḍāyatana*), contact (*sparśa*), feelings (*vedanā*), craving (*tṛṣṇā*), indulgence (*upādāna*), gestation (*bhava*), birth (*jāti*), old age and death (*jarā-maraṇa*); and (that 'place of no location') has pride (*māna*), haughty pride (*atimāna*), 'I am'-pride (*asmimāna*), assuming pride (*abhimāna*), pride over pride (*mānātimāna*), begrudging pride (*ūnamāna*), along with the perverse kind (*mithyāmāna*).

The *Saṃdhivyākaraṇa* represents the place where the Bhagavat was dwelling to be the 'Nirvāṇa without fixed abode' (*apratiṣṭhitanirvāṇa*); his consort, the *vidyā*, to be the instantaneous vision of all twelve members of Dependent Origination (*pratītya-samutpāda*) headed by nescience (*avidyā*); and his pride, the standard seven kinds mentioned by *Abhidharma-kośa* (V. 10). Apparently what is meant is that ordinary persons can have one pride or several in combination, but it is superhuman to have all seven. The pride thereby becomes the 'divine pride' (*devatā-garva*).

Another re-telling of the *nidāna* is quoted by Candrakīrti from an (unnamed) Explanatory Tantra (understood in Tibetan tradition to be the *Devendraparipṛcchā*)—it was immediately preceded by the *Devendraparipṛcchā* passage on E-vaṃ—and is here edited from the *Pradīpoddyotana* manuscript and translated with some *Mchan ḥgrel* (p. 14-1,2) expansion :

mayā śrutam iti proktaṃ cakravartisvarūpiṇā /
bījarūpeṇa yat sṛṣṭaṃ devatācakram uttamam //
paramānandakālo'sau ekaṃ samaya ucyate /
aṣṭaiśvaryeṇa bhagavān mahāsukhapade sthitaḥ //
sarvatathāgatāḥ proktāḥ pañcaskandhā jinair iha /
tadātmakāyavākcitto hṛdvajro'sau mahāsukhaḥ //
yoṣitsusaṃskṛtā mudrā bhagaṃ padmaṃ susaṃskṛtam /
vijahāra sthitas tatra bindurūpeṇa vajradhṛk //

The words 'by me was heard' are pronounced by the true form (the *bodhicitta* in father-mother union) of the Wheel-turner (cakravartin). What is emitted by that seed-form is the chief divinity-circle (=the Vijaya-maṇḍala generated in the mother-lotus).

That time of supreme bliss is said to be 'on an occasion'. The Lord abides in the place (the *bhaga*) of great ecstasy with the eightfold lordliness.

'All the Tathāgatas' are pronounced by the Conquerors to be the five personality aggregates in this world. That 'diamond of the heart' with great ecstasy has the 'body, speech, and mind' of the (practitioner's) self.

The 'lady' is the well-finished Mudrā (i.e. the *karma-* or *jñāna-mudrā* as a result of having been generated into a goddess and having had the gods placed in her). The *bhaga* is the well-finished lotus. The Vajra-holder 'was dwelling' therein (i.e. in the *bhaga*), abiding in the form of the *bindu*.

A pregnant implication of the 'winds' is brought in by the formulation in the *Śrī-Vajrahṛdayālaṃkāratantra* (PTT, Vol. 3, p. 255-5) : "Thus by me it was heard—on an occasion—the Bhagavat was dwelling in five-part manner within the circle of the ten ladies of the heart belonging to the Body, Speech, and Mind of all the Tathāgatas." (/ ḥdi skad bdag gis thos pa dus gcig na / bcom ldan ḥdas de bźin gśegs pa thams cad kyi sku daṅ gsuṅs daṅ thugs kyi sñiṅ po bud med bcuḥi dkyil na cha śas lṅa baḥi tshul du bśugs so / ). 'In five-part manner' presumably means as five Tathāgatas; and 'circle of ten ladies', the five principal and five ancillary winds. The pregnant sense of the *nidāna* in terms of 'winds' is further borne out by *Guhyasamājà*, Chap. I, p. 3: / atha khalu akṣobhyas tathāgataḥ sarvatathāgata-kāyavākcittahṛdaya-vajrayoṣidbhageṣu caturasraṃ virajaskaṃ mahāsamayamaṇḍalam adhiṣṭhāpayām āsa /

/ svacchaṃ ca tatsvabhāvaṃ ca nānārūpaṃ samantataḥ /
/ buddhameghasamākīrṇaṃ sphuliṅgagahanajvalam /
/ svacchādimaṇḍalair yuktaṃ sarvatathāgataṃ puram //

The translation is aided by *Mchan ḥgrel* (p. 20-4, 21-1, 2, and 81-4) :

> Then, you know, (the officiant = ) Akṣobhya Tathāgata ( = *vijñāna-skandha* and lord of the three lights or the three *jñānas*) blessed the four-cornered dustless *maṇḍala* of 'Great Pledge' in the *bhaga-s* ( = the Clear Light resorted to by illustrious persons) of the diamond ladies ( = the Clear Light) of the heart belonging to the Body, Speech, and Mind of all the Tathāgatas—'on all levels with diverse forms, both clear and the self-existence, of clarity, pervaded by a Buddha-cloud that thickly blazes with (five) tongues of flame ( = the five ancillary winds), (each) full of all the (five) Tathāgatas associated with the *maṇḍalas* of clarity ( = Light), etc. ( = Spread-of-Light and Culmination-of-Light).'

Here the rays of the five ancillary winds are each multiplied by five, to be compared with the twenty-five twisted threads called *jñāna-sūtra* in the *maṇḍala*-rite described in *Mkhas grub rje's Fundamentals of the Buddhist Tantras*. Each Buddha is associated with a certain color and symbolized by a thread of that color.

On the other hand, the literal form of the *nidāna* is doubtlessly challenging, since the word *bhaga* often has the meaning of 'female organ'. Therefore, the *Vajrajñānasamuccaya* (PTT, Vol. 3, p. 253-1) has this passage :

> The Bhagavat spoke: 'The Śrāvakas and so on, unliberated from the discursive impressions of practising the law free from passion (*virāgadharma*), became astonished to hear the diamond words (*vajrapāda*) of the Mahā-yoga-tantras—"was dwelling in the *bhaga*(s) of the ladies" —which exemplify the doctrine of lust (*rāgadharma*). The explanation which does not conflict with their aspirations is said to be the explanation as the shared sense.

The last sentence (smon par byed pa de rnams daṅ mi ḥgal baḥi sgo nas bśad pa de ni spyiḥi don du bśad pa gsuṅs paḥo) can be clarified with Candrakīrti's classifying terms, as set forth below. The Tantra is here alluding to the sense shared with non-tantric Buddhism. Assuming an explanation of the *nidāna* is forthcoming concordant with ordinary Buddhism, we assume such is the explanation in Tsoṅ-kha-pa's paraphrase presented above and Indrabhūti's brief expansion. The *Saṃdhivyākaraṇa's* re-telling seems also to represent the 'shared sense'. The explanations in terms of winds and in terms of the three lights and Clear Light should be considered as the unshared sense, especially unshared with non-tantric Buddhism.

### C. *The seven ornaments and subdivisions*

Also fundamental to this tantric system is that there are levels of interpretation of the basic Tantra, a difference of explanation in accordance with the listeners, and a determined categorization of the sentences of the Tantra. Herein lies the great contribution of Candrakīrti's *Pradīpoddyotana* employment of the classificatory twenty-eight subdivisions of the 'Seven Ornaments', a terminology stemming from the *Vajrajñānasamuccaya-tantra.* Some examples of this classification have already been presented in the foregoing sections, especially 'pregnant sense'. At the end of the *Pradīpoddyotana*, Candrakīrti suggests the reason for adopting this terminology by recalling the Buddha's dilemma immediately after his enlightenment, when he hesitated to teach his doctrine since it was too profound for people at large. Yet the Buddha did begin to teach on the basis that persons were like lotuses—some were still in the mud, others had a stem reaching up, and a few had blossoms on the surface which needed sun warmth. So also, in the case of the Tantra, one had to adapt the explanation to the particular stage of the candidate. Accordingly, the master had to know multiple explanations, so he could answer a disciple to his temporary satisfaction.

For presenting below the gist of the classification, I employ the *Pradīpoddyotana* manuscript which is somewhat chaotic at the beginning, Tsoṅ-kha-pa's *Mchan ḥgrel* on that work, and Śraddhākaravarman's **Vajrajñānasamuccaya-tantrodbhava-saptālaṃkāra-vimocana* (restored title) (PTT, Vol. 60, pp. 138-139). Yūkei Matsunaga has also studied this terminology in an article in Japanese, "On the Saptālaṃkāra" (March 1963).

The seven ornaments are : 1. Introduction (T. *gleṅ bslaṅ ba*), 2. Way (T. *tshul*), 3. Alternatives (T. *mthaḥ*), 4. Explanation (T. *bśad pa*), 5. Grouping (the auditors) (T. *bsdus pa*), 6. Persons (T. *gaṅ zag*), 7. Purpose (T. *dgos pa*).

The first ornament, of Introduction, has five sections : 1. name, i.e. Mahāyogatantra (the commentarial reference to the *Guhyasamājatantra*, which however lacks that appellation in its formal title); 2. for whom, i.e. for the ocean of candidates (*vineya*); 3. composer, i.e. Vajrasattva, the sixth Buddha; 4. extent, i.e. seventeen chapters and twenty rites (*cho ga ñi śu*), continuation tantra (*uttara-tantra*) in one chapter, and explanatory tantras of such-and-such extent; 5. requirement, i.e. the 'Stage of Generation' (*utpatti-krama*), the 'Stage of Completion' (*saṃpanna-krama*), the ordinary and the superior, etc.

The second ornament, of Way, constitutes two interpretations of four parts, 1. lineage (*saṃtāna*, *rgyud*), 2. underlying cause (*nidāna*, *gleṅ gźi*), 3. true word (*nirukti*, *ṅes paḥi tshig*), 4. impulse (*hetu*, *rgyu*). As to the two interpretations, the *Pradīpoddyotana* passage (*Mchan ḥgrel*, Vol. 158, p. 4) states that there are four parts to the Way of becoming a Buddha according to the doctrine free from lust (*virāgadharma*) and four parts according to the doctrine of lust (*rāgadharma*), as in the following tabulation:

| *four parts* | *as virāgadharma* | *as rāgadharma* |
|---|---|---|
| 1. lineage | birth of the man (in a fortunate place) | generating the Buddhas of the five families in the Stage of Generation |
| 2. underlying cause | rearing in the circle of women | unification of those families in the Stage of Completion |
| 3. true word | the teaching according to the Vinaya | *dhāraṇīs* such as (the incantation) '*vajra*' |
| 4. impulse | (zestful) practice of the Law with desire for the fruit (Enlightenment) | practices such as the 'erotic' (*śṛṅgāra*) |

The Virāgadharma is of course based on the biography of Gautama Buddha. In his case, the '*saṃtāna*' is the solar lineage (*sūryavaṃśa*) through his father King Śuddhodana and mother Queen Māyā. The '*nidāna*' is his early life in the palace, reared by the nurses and then surrounded by the harem women, toward whom he had '*virāga*' (aversion) and from whom he left for the religious life. The four parts seem to agree with the order of superintendence of the four goddesses who in chapter XVII implore the Lord to emerge from the Clear Light (see the section 'Diamond Ladies of the Heart'); that is, they implored in the order Mind, Body, Speech, Acts.

The third ornament, of Alternatives, amounts to six (*ṣaṭkoṭi*) in three pairs, which are : 'hinted meaning' (*neyārtha, draṅ baḥi don*) and 'evident meaning' (*nītārtha, ṅes paḥi don*); 'twilight language' (*samdhyā bhāsā*) and 'non-twilight language' (*no saṃdhyā bhāṣā*); 'standard terminology' (*yathāruta*), e.g. '*maṇḍala*', and coined terminology (*no yathāruta*), e.g. '*kotākhya*' (pseudonym for one of the ten winds). There has been much scholarly discussion in the past on the meaning of the term *saṃdhyā bhāṣā* (of which *saṃdhi-bhāṣā* is a form), and in the Renou memorial volume I defended my interpretation that it is 'twilight language'.

The fourth ornament, of Explanation of the sense of a given passage, is of four kinds (1) 'invariant sense' (*akṣarārtha, yig don*), (2) 'shared sense' (*samastāṅgārtha, spyi don*), (3) 'pregnant sense' (*garbhy-artha, sbas don*), (4) 'ultimate sense' (*kolikārtha, mthar thug don*), in further explanation and breakdown as follows :

1. 'invariant sense', i.e. literal meaning.
2. 'shared sense', of two sorts :
   (a) sense shared with non-tantric Buddhism,
   (b) sense shared with the three lower Tantras.
3. 'pregnant sense', of three sorts :
   (a) pregnant sense clarifying the doctrine of lust (rāgadharma-prakāśana-garbhin),
   (b) pregnant sense revealing 'conventional truth' (-Illusory Body) (saṃvṛti-satya-sambodhagarbhin),
   (c) pregnant sense considering the three gnoses (jñānatraya-vicintana-garbhin).

4. 'ultimate sense', of two sorts :
   (a) ultimate sense clarifying the Clear Light (prabhāsvara-prakāśa-kolika),
   (b) ultimate sense revealing the paired-union (yuganaddha-prabodhana-kolika).

The fifth ornament, of Grouping (the auditors), is of two kinds :—an assembly, to which 'invariant sense' and 'shared sense' among the four Explanations are taught; and disciples, to whom 'pregnant sense' and 'ultimate sense' among those four are taught.

The sixth ornament, of Persons, means the five kinds of persons who receive initiation (*abhiṣeka*) and adhere to pledges (*samaya*) and vows (*saṃvara*). They are called 'jewel-like person' (*ratna-pudgala*), the 'blue-lotus' (*utpala*), the 'white-lotus (*puṇḍarīka*), the 'red-lotus' (*padma*), and the 'sandalwood' (*candana*), each of which is defined in the *Pradīpoddyotana.* In the notes to *Mkhas grub rje's Fundamentals of the Buddhist Tantras*, pp. 218-9, Bhavyakīrti's commentary was cited : "The 'sandalwood-like' is in the family of fools; the 'blue-lotus-like' has inferior faculty (*indriya*); the 'white-lotus-like' has intermediate faculty; the 'red-lotus-like' has keen faculty ; the 'jewel-like' has the most excellent of faculties." The notes also cited the *Thob yig gsal baḥi me loṅ* (of Blo bzaṅ ḥphrin las) showing the difference of instruction in terms of the six alternatives: the evident meaning, standard terminology, and twilight language are expressed to the 'jewel-like person'. The other three alternatives are expressed to the other four types of persons. In Śraddhākaravarman's terminology of three kinds of Tantra, the five persons are called 'causal tantra' (*hetu-tantra*) because they are like seeds. Upon receiving initiation, they enter the 'tantra of means' (*upāya-tantra*). First they attentively listen to the Tantra with 'listening insight' (*śrutamayī prajñā*) then study to attach meanings to the words with 'thinking insight' (*cintāmayī prajñā*), whereupon with 'cultivation insight' (*bhāvanāmayī prajñā*) they conceptualize in the 'Stage of Generation' and then do the praxis in the 'Stage of Completion'. The discussion about these persons in Tsoṅ-kha-pa's *Mthaḥ gcod* (on Chapter One) (PTT, Vol. 156, p. 33-2, 3) makes it clear that it is precisely in terms of these three levels of 'insight' that the terminology of 'faculty' (inferior, etc.) is employed.

The seventh ornament, of purpose (*kārya*), is the third kind of Tantra, called 'fruitional tantra' (*phala-tantra*), and is of two kinds, ordinary and superior. The ordinary kind is the attainment by the four kinds of persons, exclusive of the 'jewel-like person', of the eight great *siddhis* at the limit of the Stage of Generation, whereupon they go no further. The superior kind is the attainment by the 'jewel-like person' of the rank of Vajradhara, because that person having arrived at the limit of the Stage of Generation, rejects the ordinary *siddhis*, and goes on to the Stage of Completion for the high goal.

Ratnākaraśānti illustrates the classificatory vocabulary of the *Pradīpoddyotana* in the *Piṇḍīkṛta-sādhanopāyikā-vṛtti-ratnāvalī*, PTT, Vol. 62, p. 69-3, 4 :

> */ sku rdo rje ni rnam par snaṅ mdzad do / / gsuṅ rdo rje ni ḥod dpag tu med paḥi / / thugs rdo rje ni mi bskyod pa ste / / yi geḥi don to / / sku rdo rje ni yi ge oṃ mo / / gsuṅ rdo rje ni yi ge āḥ ḥo / / thugs rdo rje ni yi ge hūṃ ste / / spyiḥi don to / / sku rdo rje ni rus sbal gyi rtsa daṅ / gsuṅ rdo rje ni zla baḥi rtsa daṅ / thugs rdo rjc ḥdod paḥi gdugs kyi rtsa ste / sbas paḥo / / sku rdo rje ni chags pa daṅ / gsuṅ rdo rje ni chags pa daṅ bral ba daṅ/ thugs rdo rje chags pa bar ma ste / mthar thugs paḥo / / sku rdo rje ni khrag daṅ / gsuṅ rdo rje ni śu-kra daṅ / thugs rdo rje ni dri chab ste / dgoṅs pas bśad paḥo / / sku rdo rje ni snaṅ baḥo/ / gsuṅ rdo rje ni snaṅ ba mched paḥo / / thugs rdo rje ni snaṅ ba ñe bar thob pa ste / dgoṅs pa ma yin paḥo / / sku rdo rje khru ñi śu paḥi dkyil ḥkhor daṅ / gsuṅ rdo rje ni khru bcu drug paḥi dkyil ḥkhor daṅ / thugs rdo rje ni khru bcu gñis paḥi dkyil ḥkhor te / sgra ji bźin paḥo / / sku rdo rje ni tshaṅs paḥo / / gsuṅ rdo rje ni dbaṅ phyug chen po daṅ / thugs rdo rje ni khyab ḥjug ste / sgra ji bźin ma yin paḥo / / sku rdo rje ni źi ba daṅ / gsuṅ rdo rje ni dbaṅ daṅ / thugs rdo rje ni mṅon spyod de / draṅ baḥi don to / / skuḥi rdo rje ni skuḥi dkyil ḥkhor daṅ / gsuṅs rdo rje ni gsuṅ gi dkyil ḥkhor / daṅ thugs rdo rje ni thugs kyi dkyil ḥkhor te / ṅes paḥi don to /*
>
> The Diamond of Body is Vairocana; the Diamond of Speech is Amitābha; the Diamond of Mind is Akṣobhya; *invariant sense.* The Diamond of Body is the syllable Oṃ; the Diamond of Speech is the syllable Āḥ; the Diamond of Mind is the syllable Hūṃ; *shared sense.* The Diamond of Body is the vein of the tortoise (*kūrmaka*) (the right *nāḍī*);

the Diamond of Speech is the vein of the moon (*śaśāṅka*) (the left *nāḍī*); the Diamond of Mind is the vein of love's umbrella (*madanātapatra*) (the middle *nāḍī*); *pregnant sense.* The Diamond of Body is desire; the Diamond of Speech is aversion; the Diamond of Mind is indifference; *ultimate sense.* The Diamond of Body is blood; the Diamond of Speech is semen; the Diamond of Mind is scented water; *twilight language.* The Diamond of Body is Light; the Diamond of Speech is Spread-of-Light; the Diamond of Mind is Culmination-of-Light; *non-twilight language.* The Diamond of Body is the *maṇḍala* of twenty-*hasta* size; the Diamond of Speech is the *maṇḍala* of sixteen-*hasta* size; the Diamond of Mind is the *maṇḍala* of twelve-*hasta* size; *standard terminology.* The Diamond of Body is Brahmā; the Diamond of Speech is Maheśvara; the Diamond of Mind is Viṣṇu; *coined terminology.* The Diamond of Body is an appeasing rite (*śāntika*); the Diamond of Speech is a controlling rite (*vaśikara*); the Diamond of Mind is a destroying rite (*ābhicārika*); *hinted meaning.* The Diamond of Body is the *maṇḍala* of Body; the Diamond of Speech is the maṇḍala of Speech; the Diamond of Mind is the *maṇḍala* of Mind; *evident meaning.*

### D. *Importance of the forty verses*

Perhaps no more eloquent testimony can be made on behalf of the verses than what is presented in the *Pradīpoddyotana* itself immediately after its citation of the forty verses from the *Vajramālā.* Insofar as I can make out the manuscript at this point (Plate 2A, fol. 1, line), it appears to read :

> / *vijahārapadaṃ so'rthaḥ śrīsamājaparisphuṭeḥ* /
> / *vyākhyātaḥ mañjughoṣeṇa vajramālām upārata iti* /
>
> There is a verse : "To the sentence *vijahāra*, this meaning resting on the *Vajramālā* has been explained by Mañjughoṣa so as to elucidate the Glorious *Samāja.*"

The *Prakāśikā-nāma-vyākhyā-ṭīkā* (PTT, Vol. 60, p. 296-1) comments : "explained the meaning to the sentence *vijahāra*, i.e. the meaning to the sentence of the *nidāna*" (bźugs paḥi tshig don ni gleṅ gźiḥi tshig don bśad pa yin źes pa ni). The verse represents the Bodhisattva Mañjughoṣa as the pronouncer of the forty kārikās in the *Vajramālā* to elucidate the *nidāna* and therefore the whole *Guhyasamājatantra*. Tsoṅ-kha-pa explains it this way in his commentary on the *Pañcakrama* called *Gsal baḥi sgron me* (PTT, Vol. 158, p. 176-5 to p. 177-1) : "(But) the main thing is that the *Pradīpoddyotana* has stated that all the meaning of the (*Guhyasamāja*) Tantra is comprised by the *nidāna* of forty syllables E-vaṃ ma-yā, etc., and that in this (*Vajramālā* Explanatory Tantra) the meaning of each syllable is explained respectively by forty verses starting with the verse ' "E" signifies the Noble Woman (*satī*) Prajñā'." ( / gtso bo ni E-vaṃ ma-yā la sogs paḥi yi ge bźi bcuḥi gleṅ gźis rgyud kyi don thams cad bsdus par sgron gsal las gsuṅs pa de rgyud ḥdir / E ni śes rab dam pa ste / / źes sogs tshigs bcad bźi bcuḥi tshigs bcad res yi ge reḥi don ḥchad pa ḥdi yin no / ).

While I am indeed far from having mastered the various Tanjur commentaries and sub-commentatries on the *Guhyasamājatantra*, on its *Pradīpoddyotana*, or on the *Pañcakrama*, I did scan a considerable number for the research embodied in the present work; and the only quotations of the forty verses I could find were in the beautiful Tanjur commentary on the *Pañcakrama* by Śrī Lakṣmī, called *Pañcakrama-ṭīkā-kramārtha-prakāśikā*. She quotes at least verses nos. 7, 12, 18, and 40—the nos. 7 and 18 as from the *Vajramālā*, the other two without name of source; and at other places uses language reminiscent of still other verses among the forty. The reason, the quotations are easy to recognize, is that the translator into Tibetan of her text, recorded as Mantrakalaśa, who is not the translator of the *Vajramālā* or of the *Pradīpoddyotana* wherein the translation of the forty verses into Tibetan differs triflingly and in only a few cases, has employed the identical translation of those four verses as among the forty verses cited in the *Pradīpoddyotana*. Presumably Mantrakalaśa (12th cent., A.D. ?) had memorized the whole group of verses, as Tibetan followers of the *Guhyasamājatantra* may still do today. And in consideration of the kind of passages Śrī Lakṣmī ordinarily quotes, namely famous, well stated, and appropriate lines, I draw the conclusion that when she quotes *nidāna* verses 12 and 40 without naming the original work, she expects the reader to know the forty verses by heart, as she herself obviously does. Candrakīrti also knows them well since he quotes the block of forty verses in Chapter One of his great work. This does not prove that all Indian followers of the *Guhyasamāja* memorized the forty verses and then received explanation of them from the *gurus*, but it does suggest this to be the case for followers of the *Guhyasamāja* in the light of the *Vajramālā*, and subsequently in the light of the *Pradīpoddyotana*, hence for followers of the '*Ārya*' school or tradition.

If this memorization of the forty verses for centuries took place as stated above, there must be a good reason to be ascertained from the content or implications of the verses themselves. The section 'Introduction to the Yoga of the *Guhyasamāja-tantra*' leads up to the solution that the *nidāna* verses can be grouped in conformity with the major steps of the Stage of Generation and the Stage of Completion. One must therefore admit that, given sufficient insight into each verse and into the groupings of the verses, it would be theoretically possible to arrange underneath these verses, or to present in introductions to groups of the verses, every important statement of *Guhyasamāja* 'pregnant' practice. And since the Tantras are a practice rather than a philosophy, the verses thereby elucidate the entire *Guhyasamājatantra*.

It might be objected, that if this is so, why are not these verses more widely quoted, and a number of independent commentaries written? The answer is that their very breadth of coverage renders these verses less practical for the candidates of the cult, who need specialized treatises or explanations for the particular phase of the cult in which they are engaged. A similar situation is found with the celebrated formula of Dependent Origination in non-tantric Buddhism. It is admitted that this formula sums up Buddhist doctrine, and theoretically everything of doctrinal importance can be arranged under one or other of the twelve members of the formula. But in practice the Buddhist monks wanted specialized treatises; and there are a number of important works of Buddhist doctrine that barely take account of Dependent Origination.

There is another reason. It turned out in the course of gathering materials for the present commentary on the verses that they touch upon a number of disputed points in terms of the steps of *yoga*. It may well be the case that in classical times the commentators did not wish to argue for their respective positions while writing such a commentary. Candrakīrti takes the lead in this silence about the verses, since he refrains from making any comments on them other than appending his signal 'pregnant sense' and adding the verse cited at the opening of the present section.

But since the present work is not meant to teach anyone how to proceed through the intricacies of the Guhyasamāja cult, but rather to show what the *Guhyasamājatantra* is all about, these forty verses with appropriate introductions serve admirably to advance this understanding.

It may well be the case during the time when this cult flourished in India, that the master would expect the disciples to understand these verses more and more as they progressed in the praxis (*caryā*), and that the *guru* would provide oral explanation coordinated with the disciple's level of attainment. As soon as the Guhyasamāja literature was rendered out of its original Indic language into Tibetan, the necessity to have 'bird's eye' views of the literature made the *nidāna* verses even more important, and led to Tsoṅ-kha-pa's invaluable annotation.

## E. *The maṇḍala of the Guhyasamāja*

The word *maṇḍala* is uniformly defined as an inner content (*maṇḍa*) bounded by an enclosing element (*-la*). For example, the extract from the *Saṃdhivyākaraṇa* in this sub-section illustrates the meaning of the word by the inner content as 'knowledge' with an enclosing element as the non-tantric statement of the path. There is also a ritual sequence of two kinds of *maṇḍala*, the *maṇḍala* of residence (*ādhāra-maṇḍala*) and the *maṇḍala* of the residents (*ādheya-maṇḍala*); the former is the palace and the seats for the gods; the latter is the group of gods who take their places in that palace. The palace is the inner sanctum of the maṇḍala. In the case of the Guhyasamāja-maṇḍala, the full complement of deities seated in the palace totals thirty-two. They are the cast of the Guhyasamāja drama.

The dramatis personae amount to the following characters; and any other deities mentioned in the Guhyasamāja cycle are held to be aspects or aliases of these thirty-two primary ones:

5 Buddhas : Akṣobhya, Vairocana, Amitābha, Ratnasambhava, Amoghasiddhi.

8 Bodhisattvas : Maitreya, Kṣitigarbha, Vajrapāṇi, Khagarbha, Lokeśvara, Sarvanivāraṇaviṣkambhin, Mañjuśrī (or Mañjughoṣa), Samantabhadra.

9 Yoṣits : Locanā, Māmakī, Pāṇḍarā, Tārā; and Rūpavajrā, Śabdavajrā, Gandhavajrā, Rasavajrā, Sparśavajrā.

10 Krodhas : Yamāntaka, Prajñāntaka, Padmāntaka, Vighnāntaka, Acala, Ṭakkirāja, Nīladaṇḍa, Mahābala, Uṣṇīṣacakravartin, Sumbharāja.

The following diagram of the Guhyasamāja maṇḍala deities with assigned numbers shows their places in the palace in the event of the Aksobhya-maṇḍala :

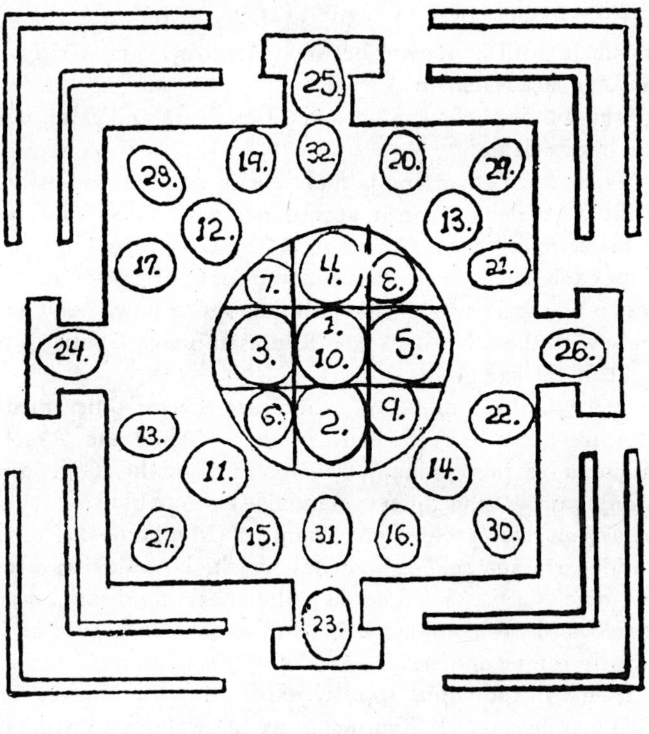


In the center : 1. Akṣobhya and 10. Sparśavajrā. In the inner circle : 2. Vairocana (E.), 3. Ratnasambhava (S.), 4. Amitābha (W.), 5. Amoghasiddhi (N.); 6. Locanā (S.E.) 7. Māmakī (S.W.), 8. Pāṇḍarā (N.W.), 9. Tārā (N.E.). In the second circle : 11. Rūpavajrā (S. E.), 12. Śabdavajrā (S.W.), 13: Gandhavajrā (N.W.), 14. Rasavajrā (N.E.).

In the third circle : 15-16. Maitreya and Kṣitigarbha, on the two sides of the East Gate on the Eastern (white) *paṭṭikā*; 17-18. Vajrapāṇi and Khagarbha, on the two sides of the South Gate on the Southern (yellow) *paṭṭikā* ; 19-20. Lokeśvara and Mañjughoṣa, on the two sides of the West Gate on the Western (red) *paṭṭikā*; 21-22. Sarvanivāraṇaviṣkambhin and Samantabhadra, on the two sides of the North Gate on the Northern (green) *paṭṭikā*.

In the four gates : 23. Yamāntaka (E.), 24. Prajñāntaka (S.), 25. Padmāntaka (W.), 26. Vighnāntaka (N.). In the intermediate directions : 27. Acala (S.E.), 28. Ṭakkirāja (S.W.), 29. Nīladaṇḍa (N.W.), 30. Mahābala (N. E.).

In the zenith : shown between Maitreya and Kṣitigarbha, 31. Uṣṇīṣacakravartin.

In the nadir : shown between Lokeśvara and Mañjughoṣa, 32. Sumbharāja.

When the Guhyasamāja-maṇḍala is painted and Akṣobhya is the chief deity; then in accordance with Tucci's indications in his article, "Some Glosses upon the Guhyasamāja," p. 343, Vairocana, being in the east and in front of the Akṣobhya image, has to be represented in the painting upside down; and accordingly with the other deities. Ratnasambhava (south) is to the right of the image.

In the Guhyasamāja cult, there are several different deities that are taken as the central deity. While the Akṣobhya-maṇḍala is predominant, there is also the Guhyasamāja Mañjuvajra (the first maṇḍala in Abhayākaragupta's *Niṣpannayogāvalī*), based on Mañjuśrī (Mañjughoṣa). Also the Buddhaśrījñāna school had rites in which Avalokiteśvara was the chief deity. Fortunately, the most important *maṇḍala*, the Akṣobhya-maṇḍala, exists in Sanskrit in a precise form, namely the second *maṇḍala* in the *Niṣpannayogāvalī*.

In his introduction (pp. xvii-xix) to the edition of the *Guhyasamājatantra*, B. Bhattacharyya has well stated with brevity from the first chapter the procedure by which the Lord (as Mahāvajradhara) first emanated the deities. In the terminology of the *Pradīpoddyotana*, this is a 'restricted circle of deities' (*pratibaddhadevatācakra*), because only the five Buddhas, four yoṣits, and four krodhas are specifically indicated in that emanation. According to Ratnākaraśānti's *Kusumāñjali-guhyasamāja-*

*nibandha-nāma* (PTT, Vol. 64, p. 96-1), this involves the three secrets of the Buddha, the secret of Body, of Speech, and of Mind. "In brief, the secret of body is the lord Vairocana, and so on; the secret of speech is Locanā, and so on; the secret of mind is Yamāntaka, and so on" ( /de la mdor bsdu na / skuḥi gsaṅ ba ni bcom ldan ḥdas rnam par snaṅ mdzad la sogs paḥo // gsuṅ gi gsaṅ ba ni / spyan la sogs paḥo / / thugs kyi gsaṅ ba ni gśin rje gśed la sogs pa ste / ). In that emanating role Mahāvajradhara is called 'Bodhicittavajra' (Diamond of the Enlightenment Mind') because all the deities emanate from *bodhicitta*. But, as was mentioned, in the present case, only thirteen of the deities are emanated. Also G. Tucci, *The Theory and Practice of the Maṇḍala*, has included his translation of chapter one from the beginning. Therefore, it is not necessary to repeat here the whole process; but the essential details should be mentioned.

The Lord first shifted from the role of Vairocana and adopted the role of Akṣobhya Tathāgata, in which form he blessed the four-cornered dustless maṇḍala of 'Great Pledge' in the *bhaga*-s of the diamond ladies, according to the passage translated with annotation in our preceding discussion of the *nidāna* sentence. Then the Lord Mahāvajradhara in the center of this maṇḍala began the emanation. The Lord's first *samādhi* involved a mystical generation called 'the body of the great incantation person' (*mahāvidyāpuruṣamūrti*) (the passage is translated with annotation under *nidāna* verses on 'Tathāgata'). When the Lord blessed this body, the Lord was seen by all the Tathāgatas to have three heads. This is the stage called Mahāsādhana, and according to Tsoṅ-kha-pa, the phase of it called 'Victorious maṇḍala' (*vijaya-maṇḍala*). The Lord thus appeared in the role of the hierophant to teach the procedure to the disciples (in this case, the Tathāgatas). Then, the Lord, in the appropriate *samādhi*, uttered the heart-mantra 'Vajradhṛk' of the Hatred Family and took on the black, red, and white (headed) appearance of Akṣobhya, thus situated in the center of the maṇḍala. In another *samādhi* the Lord, uttering the heart-mantra 'Jinajik' of the Delusion Family, transformed himself into Vairocana, also black, red, and white, seated in front (east). He continued with 'Ratnadhṛk' of the Cintāmaṇi Family and Ratnaketu (=Ratnasambhava), seated in the south; 'Ārolik' of the Vajrarāga Family and Amitābha, seated behind (west);

and 'Prajñādhṛk of the Samaya Family and Amoghavajra, (=Amoghasiddhi), seated in the north. The Lord, in another *samādhi*, emanated five goddesses as consorts of the five male deities. They are all called *rati* ('love') because they love their particular lord (whose family purifies the respective defilement of hatred, etc.). Thus he first transformed himself into the goddess Dveṣarati (=Māmakī) in the center with Akṣobhya; then Moharati (=Buddha-Locanā) in the east with Vairocana, Īrṣyārati (=Māmakī again) in the south with Ratnasambhava, Rāgarati (=Pāṇḍarā) in the west with Amitābha and finally, Vajrarati (=Samayatārā) in the north with Amoghasiddhi. Then the Lord, through a series of four *samādhis*, transformed himself successively into the Krodha deities, fierce directional guardians: by the mantra 'Yamāntakṛt', the fierce Yamāntaka at the east gate; 'Prajñāntakṛt', Prajñāntaka at the south gate; "Padmāntakṛt', Padmāntaka at the west gate; 'Vighnāntakṛt'. Vighnāntaka at the north gate. The basic maṇḍala was now complete: the Lord had finished his masterful show to the assembly.

While that projection or spill-out of the deities is the goal to be achieved (step four), the human performer has to start in a more humble manner. He is given a meditational sequence in which he first ascends to the plane of the void (step one). There he imagines germ syllables, which transform themselves into hand symbols (step two), and finally into the bodies of the deities (step three), thus the 'body maṇḍala'. He can then proceed with his own spill-out as a maṇḍala (the *utsarga-maṇḍala*, infra) (step four). For the human performer the full set of thirty-two deities is stipulated in the case of the Akṣobhya-maṇḍala, available in Sanskrit, as was mentioned, in the *Niṣpannayogāvalī*. This maṇḍala is based on Nāgārjuna's *Piṇḍīkrama* (or *Piṇḍīkṛtasādhana*). Following is my translation of Abhayākaragupta's text :

*The Akṣobhyamaṇḍala*

Concerning the *maṇḍala* stated in the *Piṇḍīkrama* it (involves procedures) like the foregoing (Mañjuvajra-maṇḍala) up to (creation of) the palace. Now we shall mention the particulars of the fierce deities. In the middle of the palace is a fierce black Akṣobhya ; his right and left face (resp.) white and red; holding in his right hands the *kula* (=Krodhavajra), wheel, and padma ; holding in his left hands the bell, the wishing-gem, and sword ; and embracing a Sparśavajrā like himself. In the directions east, etc., of him are Vairocana, etc., and in the intermediate directions south-east (*āgneya*), etc. are Locanā, etc.

Among them, Vairocana is white, mild; has white, black, and red faces ; holds the wheel, *vajra*, white lotus, bell, gem, and sword. The hand symbols (*cihna*) in four hands, as abovementioned (for Vairocana) and below stated for other Buddhas are in the respective order, in the upper, then the lower, right hands, and in the lower, then the upper left hands. The colors are assigned to the three faces by the order—basic, right, left faces.

Ratnasambhava is yellow ; his faces (in order), yellow, black, and white; holds the *gem*, the *vajra*, wheel, bell, yellow lotus, sword.

Amitābha is red; his faces red, black, and white ; with his left hand, holds at his heart a staff having a red lotus together with a bell here following Tibetan ; with his right hand holds a full-blown lotus; and with his other hands, a *vajra*, wheel, *ratna*, and sword.

Amoghasiddhi is green; has faces green, black, white; holds the sword, the *viśvavajra*, the wheel, the bell, green lotus, and gem.

Those five Tathāgatas and the other deities to be described below, down to Samantabhadra are adorned with *jaṭājūṭa* (twisted matted head hair), jewel diadem, and various jewels.

Locanā is like Vairocana, but has a white *utpala* in place of the white *padma*.

Māmakī is like Akṣobhya, but has a reddish-blue *utpala* in place of the *padma*.

Pāṇḍarā is like Amitābha.

Tārā is like Amoghasiddhi and holds the *viśvavajra*, wheel, yellowish-blue *utpala*, bell, (maṇi-)jewel, and sword.

In the second circle, in the S. E. corner is Rūpavajrā, like Locanā, but with her first two hands holding a red mirror. In the Southwest is Śabdavajrā, yellow, with faces yellow, black, white; her first two hands playing a blue *vīṇā*; her remaining hands holding the *vajra*, blue *utpala*, *ratna*, and sword. In the Northwest is Gandhavajrā, like Pāṇḍarā; her first two hands holding a yellow perfumed conch-shell. In the Northeast is

Rasavajrā dark blue, her faces dark blue, black, white; her two hands holding a red savory chest (*rasa-bhāṇḍa*); with the remaining hands, holding the *vajra*, wheel, *ratna*, sword.

In the third circle, on the Eastern *paṭṭikā* (strip) are (the Bodhisattvas) Maitreya and Kṣitigarbha. On the Southern *paṭṭikā* are Vajrapāṇi and Khagarbha. On the Western *paṭṭikā* are Lokeśvara and Mañjughoṣa. On the Northern *paṭṭikā* are Sarvanivāraṇaviṣkambhin and Samantabhadra. These eight are like the lords of their own families, but Maitreya's basic arm holds a Nāgakesara flower along with its branch marked with a wheel.

At the gates of East, etc., and in the intermediate directions of Southeast, etc., also in the zenith and in the nadir are the 10 krodhas in sequence. Among them, Yamāntaka is black his faces black, white, and red; holds a *vajra* club, the wheel, the *vajra*, at his heart a threatening gesture (*tarjanī*) along with a noose, the bell, and axe.

Prajñāntaka is white; faces white, black and red; holds a *vajra*, a white staff marked with a *vajra*, the sword, and at his breast the *tarjanī* along with noose, the bell and axe.

Padmāntaka is red; faces red, black, white; holds a red *padma*, a sword, club, bell, and axe.

Vighnāntaka is blue; faces blue, white, red; holds the *viśvavajra*, wheel, club, *tarjanī* along with noose, bell, and axe.

Acala is blue; faces blue, white, red; holds the sword, *vajra*, wheel, *tarjanī*, and axe.

Ṭakkirāja is blue; faces blue, white, red; with two hands he adopts the *vajra-hūṃkāra* (gesture); with the remaining hands he holds the *vajra*, the sword, the noose, and the hook.

Nīladaṇḍa is black; faces black, white, and red; holds a blue staff marked with a *vajra*, a sword, a wheel, against the chest a *tarjanī* along with noose, a *padma*, and an axe.

Mahābala is black; faces black, white, and red; holds a black staff marked with a *vajra*, a sword, and wheel, at the heart a *tarjanī* along with noose, the *padma* and axe.

Uṣṇīṣacakravartin is black; faces black, white, and red; with his two basic arms grasps the *uṣṇīṣa* on his head; with his remaining arms holds the *vajra*, the *padma*, the *tarjanī*, and the sword. His two hands execute the *uṣṇīṣa-mudrā* called by some Samantāvabhā, called by some otherwise, made as follows :

the palms stretched out together facing upwards; the two thumbs held on the nails of the two ring fingers; the small fingers to a point; likewise the nails of the two middle fingers together coming to a point; the two forefingers on the middle fingers, forming a cone.

Sumbharāja is black; his faces black, red, white; holds a *vajra*, a wheel, a *ratna*, at his breast a *tarjanī* along with a noose, a *padma*, and sword.

These (32) deities beginning with Akṣobhya are three-faced, six-armed, all upon a *viśvapadma*, and individually seated in their respective order, on a (1-5) (the five Buddhas, to wit:) five-pronged *vajra*; (goddesses, Locanā, etc.) (6) wheel, (7) nine-faced emerald, (8) red lotus, and (9) *viśvavajra*; (goddesses, Rūpavajrā, etc. down to Sparśavajrā:) (10) wheel, (11) *vajra*, (12) *padma* (13) *viśvavajra*, and (14) Nāgakesara flower; (eight Bodhisattvas, to wit :—) (15) wheel, (16) *vajra*, (17) *ratna*, (18) *padma*, (19) *vajra*, (20) *viśvavajra*, (21) *vajra*, and (22) staff; (the ten krodhas, to wit:—) (23) *vajra* , (24) red lotus, (25) *viśvavajra*, (26) staff with sword, (27) *vajra*, (28) blue staff marked with *vajra*, (29) black staff, (30) *vajra*, and (31-32) sun and moon each situated on a *vajra*.

Furthermore, they are composed of jewels coloured like their own deity (-progenitor). Among them, Vairocana, the goddesses, and the Bodhisattvas are located on a moon. The others are located on a sun. (Tathāgatas) such as Akṣobhya are in *vajraparyaṅka* (leg position). The Krodhas have their left leg extended, their right one retracted; on each face three eyes, each red and round; are howling and blazing; have especially frightening forms, and are called the fearful *rakṣācakra* ('protective circle').

Here only the maṇḍala lord is together with his *prajñā* (goddess consort). The other male deities, down to Sumbharāja, are without prajñā. Yamāntaka and the others in the *rakṣācakra* are together with a *prajñā* looking like themselves (or : 'their own light', *svābha*) in order:—(1) Vajravetālī, (2) Aparājitā, (3) Bhṛkuṭī, (4) Ekajaṭā, (5) Viśvavajrī, (6) Viśvaratnī, (7) Viśvapadmā, (8) Viśvakarmā, (9) Gaganavajriṇī, (10) Dharaṇīdharā.

In the heart of Akṣobhya is a 'Knowledge Being' (jñānasattva), two-armed, with a red *prajñā*. In its heart is a black

Hūṃ. Oṃ in that of Vairocana; Svā in that of Ratnasambhava; Āḥ in that of Amitābha; Hā in that of Amoghasiddhi : Lāṃ Māṃ Paṃ Tāṃ (respectively) in those of Locanā and the other goddesses. (The officiant utters : ) Jaḥ Hūṃ Vaṃ Hoḥ. Khaṃ in that of Sparśavajrā. Mai-thliṃ in those of the Bodhisattvas, Maitreya, etc. Oṃ Oṃ Oṃ Hūṃ Oṃ Saṃ Hūṃ in those of the ten Krodhas. The heart mantras of the deities are stated in the *Vajrāvalī* (another work by Abhayākaragupta).

The *kuleśa* (family master) is the previously-mentioned Vajrasattva of Akṣobhya and Samantabhadra, but holds a *vajra*, wheel, *padma*, bell, gem, sword, and embraces a Vajradhātvīśvarī looking like himself.

Akṣobhya belongs (as their essence) to the Tathāgatas, Māmakī, Vajrapāṇī, Mañjughoṣa, Uṣṇīṣa-, and Sumbharāja.

Vairocana belongs to Locanā, Rūpavajrā, Maitreya, Kṣitigarbha, Yamāntaka, Acala.

Ratneśa (=Ratnasambhava) belongs to Śabdavajrā, Khagarbha, Prajñāntaka, Ṭakkirāja.

Amitābha belongs to Pāṇḍarā, Gandhavajrā, Lokeśvara, Padmāntaka, Nīladaṇḍa.

Amoghasiddhi belongs to Tārā, Rasavajrā, Sparśavajrā, Viṣkambhin, Vighnāntaka, Mahābala.

So ends the Akṣobhya-maṇḍala stated in the *Piṇḍīkrama*.

* * *

The foregoing translation leaves some matters to be explained. The six hand symbols of Vajrasattva are set forth by Ratnākaraśānti in the *Piṇḍikṛta-sādhanopāyikā-vṛtti-ratnāvalī* (PTT. Vol. 62, p. 77-5) as the signs of the six families: The *vajra* is the emblem of Akṣobhya, being the intrinsic nature of the five knowledges. The wheel is the emblem of Vairocana, being the intrinsic nature of contemplating the 'wheel of the doctrine' (*dharmacakra*). The red lotus (*padma*) is the emblem of Amitābha, being the intrinsic nature of *prajñā* not adhered to by the mud of lust, etc. The bell (is the emblem of Vajrasattva), being the intrinsic nature of *prajñā* that is the purity of gestation (*bhava*). The 'wish-granting gem' (*cintāmaṇi*) is the emblem of Ratnasambhava, being the knowledge which fulfills all hopes. The sword is the emblem of Amoghasiddhi, being the *prajñā* (that severs) the corrupt practice. ( / de la rdo rje ni mi bskyod paḥi phyag mtshan te /

ye śes lṅaḥi raṅ bźin no / / ḥkhor lo rnam par snaṅ mdzad kyi phyag mtshan te / chos kyi ḥkhor lo bsgom paḥi raṅ bźin no // pa-dma ni ḥod dpag tu med paḥi phyag mtshan te / ḥdod chags la sogs paḥi ḥdam gyis mi gos paḥi śes rab kyi raṅ bźin no / / dril bu ni srid pa rnam par dag pa śes rab kyi ṅo bo ñid do / yid bźin nor bu rin chen ḥbyuṅ ldan gyi phyag mtshan te / bsam pa thams cad rdzogs par byed paḥi ye śes so // ral gri ni don yod par grub paḥi phyag mtshan te / ñon moṅs pa spyod paḥi śes rabbo/). That attribution of emblems to the individual Tathāgata families plus important elements from the translation of the Akṣobhya-maṇḍala can be clarified with correspondential significance in tabular form, as in Table II.

Concerning the remark 'Vajrasattva of Akṣobhya and Samantabhadra', Nāgārjuna's *Piṇḍīkṛta-sādhana*, 52 B-53, states: "Then he should enterprise the Atiyoga : Following upon Akṣobhya he should develop a Vajrasattva, three-faced, radiant with six hands, and shining with sapphire light" (....atha atiyogaṃ samārabhet / akṣobhyānupraveśena trimukhaṃ ṣaḍ bhujojjvalaṃ / indranīlaprabhaṃ dīptaṃ vajrasattvaṃ vibhāvayet / ). Nāgārjuna, in the subsequent verses, shows that this involves placing the Guhyasamāja deities in spots of the body maṇḍala. Ratnākaraśānti (*op. cit.*, p. 77-4, 5) comments : " 'three-faced' because the purity of the three liberations; and 'six-handed' because the purity of the six perfections" (rnam par thar pa gsum rnam par dag pas źal gsum pa / pha rol tu phyin pa drug rnam par dag pas phyag drug pa). (The three liberations are through voidness, wishlessness, and signlessness; the six perfections are giving, morality, forbearance, striving, meditation, and insight). It appears that Vajrasattva is the yogin possibility of a person, as the essence of the Tathāgatas, Akṣobhya, and as their enlightenment-pledge, Samantabhadra; who has advanced, equivalent to the non-tantric progression of the Bodhisattva during the first seven stages, to the last three Bodhisattva stages, as indicated by his embracing Vajradhātvīśvarī ('Queen of the Diamond Realm'), who is drawn from the yogin's own heart, according to the verse cited under nidāna verse 33.

## II. CORRESPONDENCES OF AKṢOBHYA-MAṆḌALA

| *Tathāgata Families (with colors)* | *Emblem* | *Prajñā (and seat)* | *Vajrā (sense object goddess)* | *Bodhisattvas* | *Krodhas* |
|---|---|---|---|---|---|
| Akṣobhya (black) | Thunderbolt (vajra) | Māmakī | Sparśavajrā | Vajrapāṇi and Mañjughoṣa | Uṣṇīṣacakravartin and Sumbharāja |
| Vairocana (white) | Wheel (cakra) | Locanā (on wheel) | Rūpavajrā holding mirror | Maitreya and Kṣitigarbha | Yamāntaka and Acala |
| Ratnasambhava (yellow) | Wish-granting gem (cintāmaṇi) | (Māmakī) (on nine-faced emerald) | Śabdavajrā, playing a vīṇā | Khagarbha | Prajñāntaka and Ṭakkirāja |
| Amitābha (red) | Red Lotus (padma) | Pāṇḍarā (on red lotus) | Gandhavajrā, holding a conchshell | Lokeśvara | Padmāntaka and Nīladaṇḍa |
| Amoghasiddhi (green) | Sword (khaḍga) | Tārā (on crossed thunderbolt, viśvavajra) | Rasavajrā, holding savory chest | Viṣkambhin | Vighnāntaka and Mahābala |
| Vajrasattva | Bell (ghaṇṭā) | Vajradhātvīśvarī | | Samantabhadra | |

The utterances 'Jaḥ, Hūṃ, Vaṃ, Hoḥ' also require explanation. They represent the four mantra stages of attracting toward the yogin, drawing in, and bringing about non-duality with the 'knowledge beings'. Cf. *Sādhana-mālā*, No. 110, pp. 230-231; Oṃ vajrāṅkuśī ākarṣaya Jaḥ, Oṃ vajrapāśī praveśaya Hūṃ, Oṃ vajrasphoṭa bandhaya Vaṃ, Oṃ vajrāveśe vaśīkuru Hoḥ. "Oṃ, May the diamond hook attract, Jaḥ !" "Oṃ, May the diamond noose drawn in, Hūṃ !" "Oṃ, May the diamond chain tie, Vaṃ !" "Oṃ, May the diamond bell subdue, Hoḥ !"

So far the data about the maṇḍala has involved the deities who are the residents of the palace. Now I shall turn to the theory of the Guhyasamāja maṇḍala as the residence. An interesting statement about the symbolism of the Guhyasamāja maṇḍala is presented in the *Saṃdhivyākaraṇa* on *Guhyasamāja*, Chapter IV, verses 9-18, of which verse 9 is as follows :

> *dvādaśahastaṃ prakurvīta cittamaṇḍalam uttamam /*
> *caturasraṃ caturdvāraṃ catuṣkonaṃ prakalpayet //*
>
> One should construct the supreme maṇḍala of consciousness, measuring twelve hastas. One should imagine it with four sides, four corners, and four gates.

On that verse of the basic *Guhyasamāja-tantra*, the *Pradīpoddyotana* cites this commentary as from the'*Ārya-vyākhyāna*', which in this case means the *Saṃdhivyākaraṇa* :

> *athātaḥ kathayiṣyāmi maṇḍalaṃ cittam uttamam /*
> *vajrajñānapratīkāśaṃ kāyavākcittamaṇḍalam //*
> *navātmakam idaṃ śreṣṭhaṃ suniyuktaṃ tathoditam /*
> *dvividhāgamam aṅkitaṃ supramāṇaṃ tad ucyate //*
> *saṃvṛti paramarthaṃ yad advayaṃ śobhanaṃ mataṃ /*
> *prajñā sūtram idaṃ tasyās tad upāyānuvarttitam //*
> *prajñopāyaikasūtreṇa dharmaṃ sambhogam uttamam /*
> *sūtritaṃ maṇḍalaṃ caitaṃ pratītya dvādaśaṅgatah //*
> */ satyāryaṃ caturasraṃ syād brahmavihārakoṇakaḥ /*
> */ dvārasaṃgrahavastvākhyaṃ pratyekaṃ turyasaṃjñakaḥ //*
> */ dharmatattvārthaṃ aṅkitaṃ cakrādyantaramaṇḍalam /*
> */ abhedyajñānacihnaṃ tad vajrendranīlamudrakam //*
> */ pañcakāraprabhedākhyaṃ śūlaṃ saṃsāranāśakam /*
> */ prāktād ādarśarūpaṃ tu cakraṃ jvālārcibhūṣitam //*
> */ samantasamatājñānaṃ ratnaṃ yāmyaikasaṃjñitam /*

*| pratyavekṣaṇapadmākhyaṃ padmarāgārciṃ paścimam ||*
*| uttarottaracittaṃ yaj jagadvikalpadālanam |*
*| kṛtyānuṣṭhānakhaḍgaṃ syād raśmijvālāsamaprabham ||*
*| āgneyyāṃ netraṃ maitrīṃ tu nīlameghasamaprabham |*
*| nairṛtyāṃ karuṇākhyā syān māmakīkulavajrakaḥ ||*
*| vāyavyāṃ padmasaṃjñā tu muditāsusthitānanā |*
*| aiśānyutpalam ābhāti sopekṣā nīlasannibhā ||*
*| dānapūrvaṃ tathā dvāre mudgaraṃ kāntisuprabham |*
*| tathaiva priyavādyākhyaṃ daṇḍaṃ vajrārcisuprabham ||*
*| arthacaryāṃ tu padmākhyaṃ paścime hayakanthare |*
*| vajraṃ samānacaryārthaṃ vajrakuṇḍalivajriṇaḥ ||*
*| tad itthaṃ kathitaṃ samyak mudrāvinyāsalakṣaṇaṃ |*
*| yathāsaṃsthānataḥ pūjā bhavet trividhabhāvanaiḥ |*
*| mahatvapūrvakaṃ tv etaṃ mudrā maṇḍalam ucyate ||*

Translation (*Mchan ḥgrel*, pp. 40-41):

Now I shall relate the supreme maṇḍala of consciousness, the maṇḍala of Body, Speech, and Mind, resembling the (non-dual) Knowledge of Diamond.

This best one, made of nine (five personality aggregates and four elements), thus expressed as well-constructed, is that one said to be of goodly authority marked by lineage of two kinds.

What as convention (saṃvṛti = illusory body) and supreme (paramārtha = Clear Light) is the non-dual loveliness, that is this thread (for the maṇḍala outline) as the insight of which it is applied by the means.

By the single thread of insight and means, there is the supreme Dharma (-body) (insight—Clear Light) and Sambhoga (-body) (means—illusory body), threaded as the maṇḍala of mind by twelve members (= 12-hastas measurement) in dependence.

The Noble Truths are the four sides; the Sublime Abodes (i.e. love, compassion, sympathetic joy, and impartiality), the corners; the articles of conversion (i.e. giving, pleasing words, acts in accordance, and exemplary conduct), the gates—in each case by fours.

The inner circle of wheel, and so on, symbolizes the meaning of dharma-reality. The symbol of the indivisible knowledge is the diamond-sapphire seal.

It has facets of five kinds ( = the five knowledges). The tip destroys (the habit-energy of) the phenomenal world. In the east is the form of mirror (-knowledge), its disk adorned with blazing light.

The sameness knowledge all around is the jewel whose one name is 'southern'. West is the lotus of discriminative (-knowledge) with the light of a ruby.

What is the best mind of the north destroys the discursive thought of living beings. The procedure-of-duty sword would have the same light as blazing rays.

In the south-east is the 'eye' (=Locanā) and love, with light the same as a blue cloud. In the south-west is compassion with the diamond of the Māmakī family.

In the north-west, there is the lotus, the unshaken face of sympathetic joy. The lotus of the north-east shines in blue fashion with impartiality.

As the eastern giving at the gate is a mallet lovely in appearance, so also pleasing words are a staff (in the south) appearing with diamond light.

Acts in accordance are the lotus in the western horse-neck, and exemplary conduct is the (viśva-)vajra of the vajrin of diamond winding (=ambrosia).

The characteristic of placing seals is what has been thus rightly explained. By contemplations of three kinds (arcane body, speech, and mind) there would be the worship according to the proper place. This mudrā preceded by greatness is said to be the maṇḍala.

Besides, there are varieties of maṇḍala. The *Guhyasamājatantra*, Chapter XVIII, verse 99, mentions three kinds : *bhaga-maṇḍala*, *bodhicitta-maṇḍala*, and *deha-maṇḍala*. Tsoṅ-kha-pa, in his independent *Don gsal ba* commentary on the Guhyasamāja devotes individual sections to the three *maṇḍalas*, keeping the terminology of 'body-maṇḍala' (*deha-maṇḍala*), while substituting other names for the two other maṇḍalas. In place of '*bhaga-maṇḍala*', he employs the term '*utsarga-maṇḍala*' (emission m.')from the *Pradīpoddyotana* on Chapter VII (equivalent to its terminology 'house-m.' *puraṃ maṇḍalaṃ*, Pradīpoddyotana MS., chapter one). Tsoṅ-kha-pa, following the *Pradīpoddyotana* on chapter VII, replaces the '*bodhicitta-m.*' with the expression *paramārtha-maṇḍala*. He makes it clear that the thirty-two Guhyasamāja deities are involved in all three of the above-mentioned maṇḍalas, which are evoked in the order *deha-maṇḍala*, *utsarga-maṇḍala*, and *paramārtha-maṇḍala*. The *deha-maṇḍala* is perfected in the phase of *yoga* called Atiyoga, and both the *utsarga-m.* and the *paramārtha-m.* belong to the phase of *yoga* called Mahāyoga, or Mahāsādhana; and are respectively equivalent to the two sub-phases of Mahāsādhana called 'Victorious Maṇḍala' (*vijaya-maṇḍala* and 'Victory of the Rite' (*karma-vijaya*). So much for the terminological side.

What is meant, is that the 'body-maṇḍala' of Atiyoga overflows into the *bhaga*, or mother-lotus, whereupon the latter becomes the *bhaga-maṇḍala*. This phase is called 'letter placement' (*akṣara-nyāsa*) in the discussion of the fourth *yoga* (cf. the section 'Four steps of yoga....'); and this is the position of the *Pradīpoddyotana* (Documents) when in its treatment of the fourth member it refers to the instigation of the *vajra* and *padma* and then to the mantras (32 in no.) Vajradṛg, etc. This is also the phase discussed in the section 'Title of the work and nidāna', where the quotation from the *Devendraparipṛcchā* refers to the placement of the gods in the goddess (the *karma-mudrā* or *jñāna-mudrā*). The difficulty is that this process has several explanations going respectively with the 'Stage of Generation' and the 'Stage of Completion'. The explanation that agrees with both Stages, is that this phase is the demonstration of the maṇḍala, the objective showing of the deity circle, either in its restricted form as in *Guhyasamājatantra*, chapter one, or in the full 32-deity group. Hence the *Pradīpoddyotana* ('Documents') refers to this fourth *yoga* as 'accomplishment of the great aim of others'.

The third maṇḍala, the *paramārtha-m.*, refers to the Guhyasamāja deities being drawn into *paramārtha*, or the absolute realm. Tsoṅ-kha-pa explains in his *Mchan ḥgrel* on Chapter VII that this means that the five personality aggregates (*skandha*), five elements (*dhātu*), five sense organs (*indriya*), five sense objects (*viṣaya*), and five knowledges (*jñāna*), a total of 25, are successively drawn into the Clear Light (where, according to the *Pradīpoddyotana* on Chapter eight, verse 7, they unite with the '25-year old girl').

## III. INTRODUCTION TO THE YOGA OF THE GUHYASAMĀJA SYSTEM

### A. *The chapters of the Guhyasamājatantra and yoga*

The Eighteen chapters are discussed here because, as will be soon demonstrated, chapters 2 to 17 are divided into four groups with titles almost identical with those of the four *sādhana* steps.

The word for 'chapter' employed by the *Guhyasamājatantra* is *paṭala*. The *Pradīpoddyotana*, at the end of its commentary on chapter one, explains this word in two senses, going with *paṭa-* ('cloth') and *-la* ('grasping'):

> / *paṭo yathā daṃśamaśakādyupadravaṃ nivārayati / tathāyaṃ tantrārthaḥ kleśakarma janmādyupadravaṃ nivāraṇāt paṭa iva paṭa(la)ḥ / taṃ lāti gṛhṇātīti taddhārako granthasamūhaḥ paṭalaḥ* /
>
> Just as a cloth covering (*paṭa*) wards off the attack of gnats, mosquitoes, etc., so also, by warding off the attack of defilement, *karma*, and rebirth, '*paṭala*' as the meaning of the Tantra, is like a cloth covering. Since it grasps and holds that (meaning), '*paṭala*' as the collection of compositions, is its receptacle.

Also, at the end of its commentary on chapter thirteen, the *Pradīpoddyotana* equates a *paṭala* with 'the collection of compositions which teach it' (*tatpratipādako granthasamūhaḥ*).

The following chapter titles as preserved in Sanskrit have varying relevance to the chapter contents. For example, of the two chapters translated in 'Documents', chapter six does adhere to indications of its title, while chapter twelve is scarcely described by its title.

1. "Blessing of the samādhi-maṇḍala of all the Tathā gatas" (sarvatathāgatasamādhimaṇḍalādhiṣṭhāna).
2. "The Mind of Enlightenment" (bodhicitta).

3. "Samādhi called 'Diamond Array' " (vajravyūho nāma samādhi).

4. "Secret maṇḍala of Body, Speech, and Mind" (guhyakāyavākcittamaṇḍala).

5. "Best of all praxis" (samantacaryāgra).

6. "Empowerment of the Body, Speech, and Mind" (kāyavākcittādhiṣṭhāna).

7. "Praxis of mantras" (mantracaryā).

8. "Pledge of consciousness" (cittasamaya).

9. "Pledge whose goal is the reality of the non-dual supreme entity" (paramārthādvayatattvārthasamaya).

10. 'Exhorting with the heart (mantras) of all the Tathāgatas " (sarvatathāgatahṛdayasañcodana).

11. "The highest vidyāpuruṣa who has the mantra-pledge and the reality-diamond of all the Tathāgatas" (sarvatathāgatamantrasamayatattvavajravidyāpuruṣottama).

12. "Instruction on the best evocation of the pledge (samayasādhanāgranirdeśa).

13. "Revelation contemplating the meaning of the reality of the array of pledges" (samayavyūhatattvārthabhāvanāsambodhi).

14. "Samādhi called 'King of sporting with attraction (of deities) by mantras' " (mantrākarṣaṇavijṛmbhitarājo nāma samādhi).

15. "Source of the diamond whose essence is the pledge of all sentient beings" (sarvasattvasamayasāravajrasaṃbhūtir nāma) (edited citta replaced by sattva).

16. "Revelation of the maṇḍala-diamond of all siddhis" (sarvasiddhimaṇḍalavajrābhisambodhir nāma).

17. "Blessing of the pledge—and—vow-diamonds of all the Tathāgatas" (sarvatathāgatasamayasambaravajrādhiṣṭhāna).

18. "Blessing of the diamond knowledge which explains all the secrets (sarvaguhyanirdeśavajrajñānādhiṣṭhāna).

The *Pradīpoddyotana* commentary covers only the first 17 chapters, although it cites the 18th chapter ('Documents') ; while the 18th chapter itself has some separate commentaries preserved in the Tibetan Tanjur. The reason is that there is a block of verses in the 18th chapter (verses 25-31 in S. Bagchi's numbering) which group the previous chapters 2-17 in four sets.

Consequently, the Guhyasamāja tradition generally labelled the 18th chapter a 'Continuation Tantra' (*uttara-tantra*). The fact that those sixteen intermediate chapters fall into four sets by authority of those verses is hardly noticed in the present edition of the text, because of corruptions which cannot be corrected without consultation of the Tibetan translation. Indeed, there are even two important lines missing from the current edition, which I have restored along with the other corrections, with the help of Nāgārjuna's commentary (*Aṣṭādaśa-paṭala-vistara-vyākhyā*, PTT, Vol.60, p. 4). The two lines were still part of the *Guhyasamāja-tantra* when Ratnākaraśānti composed his *Kusumañjali-guhyasamāja-nibandha-nāma* (PTT, Vol. 64), which explains how to pair the verses for translation purposes. What is presently numbered verse 30 is in fact the first line (hemistich) of one verse and the second line of another verse. I have made two new verses numbered 30' and 30'' in the following text of corrected Sanskrit. It can be speculated that factors in the gradual corruption of the lines are the original presence of 9-syllable *pādas* in some places, and the use of infrequent ordinal forms of numbers. The translation will follow the order in which the Sanskrit verse mentions the ordinal numbers, in the first-mentioned set, the fifth, ninth, seventeenth, and thirteenth (chapters).

*pañcamaṃ navamaṃ caiva daśasaptamaṃ trayodaśam* /
*buddhānāṃ bodhisattvānāṃ deśanāsādhanaṃ mahat* //25//
*caturthaṃ ṣoḍaśaṃ caiva aṣṭamaṃ dvādaśaṃ tathā* /
*ācāryakarmasāmānyaṃ siddhiś ca vratasambaram* //26//
*ṣaṣṭhaṃ caiva dvitīyaṃ ca daśaṃ caiva caturdaśam* /
*haṭham anurāgaṇaṃ ca upasādhanasambaram* //27//
*saptamaṃ ca tṛtīyaṃ ca ekādaśaṃ daśapañcamam* /
*siddhikṣetranimittaṃ ca sevāsādhanasambaram* //28//
*sarvatathāgatakarma nigrahānugrahātmanam* /
*dāntadaurdāntasaumyānāṃ sattvānām avatāraṇam* //29//
*utpattikramasambandhaṃ sevāvajravidhiś catuḥ* /
**sāmānyasiddhisambandham agrabhūtaṃ ca granthanam* //30'//
**maṇḍalavratasambandham ācāryasampattigranthanam* /
*gurūṇāṃ mantramārgeṇa śiṣyāṇāṃ paripācanam* // 30'' //
*suvratasyābhiṣiktasya svaśiṣyasya mahātmanaḥ* /
*buddhānāṃ bodhisattvānāṃ deśanāparimocanam* //31//

25, 31 : The fifth, ninth, seventeenth, thirteenth (chapters) have the great perfection of the teaching of the Buddhas and Bodhisattvas, to wit, liberating one's great-souled disciple who is goodly vowed and initiated, by means of the teaching of the Buddhas and Bodhisattvas.

26, 30" : The fourth, sixteenth, eighth, and twelfth have the common acts of the *ācārya*, occult powers (*siddhi*), and the Vratasambara, to wit, the compositions on the *ācārya's* perfection, associated with maṇḍala-rites, maturing the disciples by way of the guru's mantras.

27, 29 : The sixth, second, tenth, and fourteenth have the fierce act (*haṭha*), attraction (of deity), and vows of the Upasādhana, to wit, all the Tathāgata acts with the nature of taming and assisting, introducing the sentient beings whether tamed, obdurate, or mild.

28, 30': The seventh, third, eleventh, and fifteenth have the cause of the field of occult powers, and the Sevā-sādhana-sambara, to wit, the four diamond rites of Sevā, associated with the Stage of Generation; both the compositions associated with common siddhis and (those) which show the superior kind.

The tantric Nāgārjuna in that commentary on the 18th chapter (*op. cit.*, p. 4) briefly alludes to the contents of each chapter as he groups them by fours with titles :

Mahāsādhana chapters (5, 9, 13, 17):

Chap. 5 on the praxis (*caryā*)
Chap. 9 on the *yogasamādhi*
Chap. 17 on *samaya* and *saṃvara* (pledges and vows)
Chap. 13 on extensive treatment of rites (*karma*)

Vratasambara chapters (4, 8, 12, 16):

Chap. 4 on the *citta-maṇḍala*
Chap. 16 on the *kāya* and *vāg-maṇḍalas*
Chap. 8 on the *guhya-abhiṣeka*
Chap. 12 on the change into the *Mahāmudrā*

Upasādhana chapters (2, 6, 10, 14) :

Chap. 6 on the *adhiṣṭhāna* of body, speech, and mind
Chap. 2 on the *bodhicitta*
Chap. 10 on exhorting all the Tathāgatas by their heart-mantras
Chap. 14 principally devoted to mantras

Sevā chapters (3, 7, 11, 15):

Chap. 7 on special practices (*caryā*)

Chap. 3 on the gods

Chap. 11 on the series of *mantras* and the knowledge body

Chap. 15 on the illusory divine body

Ratnākaraśānti's commentary (*op. cit.*, PTT, Vol. 64, p. 98 and p. 201) mentions that chapter 1 is the goal-tantra (literally: 'the tantra of what is to be approached'. S. *upeya-tantra*, T. *thabs las byuṅ baḥi rgyud*), while the chapters 2-17 are the 'tantra of the approach' (S. *upāya-tantra*. T. *thabs kyi rgyud*), and that the chapter 18 is the 'continuation tantra' (*uttara-tantra*). Furthermore, each group of four chapters from 2-17 is also known by a numerical title. The Sevā chapters are 'Tretā'; Upasādhana, 'Dvāpara'; Vratasambara, 'Kṛta'; and Mahāsādhana, possibly* 'Nandin' (T. *dgaḥ ba can*). However, the words Sevā, and so on, appear to be employed as categories rather than as steps, in which meaning virtually the same set of terms is employed below (sub-section C). Candrakīrti's *Pradīpoddyotana* differs from Ratnākaraśānti, by treating the first chapter as a basis for the remaining sixteen; and so, for example, includes the forty nidāna verses in the commentary on Chapter 1.

There is a problem of how practical is that grouping by fours. There is some confirmation for the validity of the grouping in terms of the Mahāsādhana and Vratasambara (=Sādhana) sets when these terms are equated with the 'vajras', namely, Mahāyoga and Atiyoga. As was shown, the 'body maṇḍala' is associated with Atiyoga, and this is indicated by the Vratasambara chapters, namely, Chapter 16 (on the kāya-and vāg-maṇḍalas) and Chapter 12 (on the change into the Mahāmudrā). The samādhi 'Victory of the Rite', associated with Mahāsādhana, is the topic of Chapter 13 (on extensive treatment of rites), and the utsarga-and paramārtha-maṇḍalas, while not explicitly stated for the Mahāsādhana chapters, presumably go with Chapter 5 (on the praxis, caryā) and possibly with Chapter 9 (on the yogasamādhi), while the paramārtha-maṇḍala also goes with Chapter 13. Even clearer is the consistency of the Upasādhana chapters (2, 6, 10, 14) with the equivalent 'vajra' called Anuyoga (as shown later) because this involves depositing mantras (parts of the bodhicittta) in spots of the body. Also when *Guhyasamāja*, Chapter 18, associates 'the four diamond rites of Sevā' with the Sevā chapters (3, 7, 11, 15) this is consistent with my later grouping of the first six nidāna syllables (for Evaṃ mayā śrutam) with Yoga (=Sevā) because, as I later show, the four syllables E, VAM, MA, YĀ can indicate any four steps of yoga, and 'śrutam' means hearing or learning them. However, insofar as I have noticed cross-referencing in the *Pradīpoddyotana* and its *Mchan ḥgrel*, the associations appear to be independent of such grouping. For example, the important verses on the meditation on the tip of the nose are found in Chapters three and six, which belong to two different groups. Perhaps because there was a question of the viability of this grouping, Ratnākaraśānti composed his commentary (*op. cit.*) by first commenting on chapters 2-17 in the above grouping, and then commenting on each of the 17 chapters in their normal order.

Of those chapters, my researches indicate that the first twelve are the most important. This is indicated in part by the fact that the explanatory tantra *Saṃdhivyākaraṇa*, which expands the *Guhyasamājatantra* in chapter order, only goes up through chapter twelve. This set of chapters includes chapter 1, which is the 'goal' or 'basis' chapter; chapter 2, with the all-important topic of *bodhicitta*; chapters six and twelve with the steps of yoga; and chapter seven with the three kinds of praxis (*caryā*). Also, the theory that the chapters 2-17 are grouped by fours in the scheme given above, acknowledges that the later chapters expand on materials of the earlier chapters rather than start completely new topics.

### B. *The two stages, initiations and the Clear Light*

The *Guhyasamāja*, in common with other Tantras of the Anuttarayogatantra class, whether Mother or Father Tantras, is divided into two stages of application, the Stage of Generation (*utpatti-krama*) and the Stage of Completion (*sampanna-krama*) (or *utpanna-krama*). This is said in the *Guhyasamājatantra*, Chapter XVIII (p. 157) : /kramadvayam upāśritya vajriṇāṃ tatra deśanā / kramam autpattikaṃ caiva kramam autpannakaṃ tathā / "Taking recourse to two stages, the adamantine ones have therein the instruction, namely, the Stage of Generation and the Stage of Completion." Also, the *Pañcakrama*

(I, 2) states : /utpatti-kramasaṃsthānāṃ niṣpannakrama-kāṅkṣiṇām / upāyaś caiṣa sambuddhaiḥ sopānam iva nirmitaḥ/ "The Complete Buddhas have formulated like a ladder this means for those well standing in the Stage of Generation and desiring the Stage of Completion." In terms of yogins, Candrakīrti at the beginning of his commentary on Chap. XI, distinguishes them as the *kalita-yogin* ("imagining y.") and the *niṣpannayogin* ("completed y.").

In his *Sṅags rim chen mo* (f. 340a-5), Tsoṅ-kha-pa illustrates the necessity to have the Stage of Generation precede the Stage of Completion, by citing Vajragarbha's commentary on the *Hevajratantra*:

> /mi yi skye ba dag źiṅ la // dmigs med sñiṅ rjeḥi sa bon ni/ /btab pas gaṅ phyir de yi phyir // stoṅ ñid dpag bsam ljon śiṅ ḥbyuṅ / By reason of having cast the seed of aimless compassion into the pure field of human birth, there arises the 'wishing tree' of voidness.

Tsoṅ-kha-pa explains that the 'field' is 'purified' by the Stage of Generation; and that the 'seed' of aimless compassion attended with great ecstasy (*mahāsukha*) is cast therein by the Stage of Completion.

The Stage of Generation is conceptual, the Stage of Completion concrete. The reason the Stage of Generation must precede can be illustrated in terms of the theory of winds. In this first stage the candidate comes to understand the nature of the winds which are not visible to the ordinary senses, and in the course of the yoga proper to this stage recites in accordance with the natural cycle of the winds. In the Stage of Completion he proceeds to combine those winds in extraordinary ways. Of course one must understand a thing (first stage) before one can manipulate it (second stage). It follows that unless one believes that there are these mystic winds the Upaniṣads speak about and which are so prominent in the commentarial literature of the *Guhyasamājatantra*, he can see little point to having these two successive stages of yoga; and, in fact, there is little profit to his pursuing the system at any level of application.

Tsoṅ-kha-pa's remark, cited above, is clarified textually with such an expression as 'knowing the intrinsic nature' (*svabhāvajña*) (see also, *nidāna* verse 33), that is to say, knowing the natural cycle of the world in terms of the mystic forces, as the achievement of the Stage of Generation, prior to the 'great ecstasy' (*mahāsvkha*) of the Stage of Completion. Here there are two passages that show what is meant. The first is in Āryadeva's *Cittaviśuddhiprakaraṇa*, verse 20, where 'intrinsic nature' translates *svabhāva* :

*bālā rajyanti rūpeṣu vairāgyaṃ yānti madhyamāḥ |*
*svabhāvajñā vimucyante rūpasyottamabuddhayaḥ ||*

Children delight in forms; the middle-aged pass to aversion. Understanding the intrinsic nature of form, those with best intelligence are liberated (from it).

The second passage is from Saraha's *Dohā-koṣa*, verse 23 in Shahidullah's numbering, translated here from the Prakrit (given) and Tibetan text. While it does not have such a term as 'intrinsic nature', it seems to have the same message.

jallaī maraī ubajjaī [bajjhaī]
tallaī parama mahāsuha sijjahī.
[Sarahe gahaṇa guhira bhāsa kahia
pasu-loa nibboha jima rahia.]

Having taken which (jallaī), one dies,
is reborn, and is bound;
Taking that very thing (tallai) one achieves
the supreme 'great ecstasy'.
But Saraha speaks these inexplicable and
profound words so this beastly
world will not understand.

Interpreting Saraha's verse in the present context, in the Stage of Generation one contemplates those natural forces behind the cycles of birth, staying for a while, and dying, and the repetition of those three again and again, and then in the Stage of Completion, manipulates those same forces to achieve the 'great ecstasy'.

Both stages have their own forms of 'subtle yoga' (*sūkṣma-yoga*) of *prāṇāyāma*. The former stage is held to extend certain worldly magical powers (*siddhi*) to its successful candidates. The latter stage is held to confer the supreme achievement of Complete Enlightenment, which is the goal of non-tantric Buddhism as well. In the commentarial period, treatises were composed especially for one or other of the two stages. The most famous of such treatises, Nāgārjuna's *Pañcakrama*, is devoted to the Stage of Completion but is also helpful for the prior stage.

This is because the treatise is first to be read or heard with conviction, and this conceptual reading is an elementary form of the Stage of Generation which is the conceptual preparation for the second stage.

The commentators of the 'Ārya' tradition of the Guhyasamāja tried to combine this theory of stages with the well-known Bodhisattva stages of non-tantric Mahāyāna Buddhism, thereby clarifying the tantric version as the 'quick path'. These ten stages either fall into a 5-5 grouping or a 7-3 grouping. Both groupings are adopted in tantric literature, but the latter grouping was accepted for the correlation in this case, as is suggested by the *Pañcakrama*, 2d krama, verse 79:

*ādikarmikayogena cāṣṭamīṃ bhūmim āpnuyāt /*
*ālokatrayadarśī ca daśabhūmyāṃ pratiṣṭhitaḥ //*

By *yoga* of a beginner, he attains the Eighth Stage, and seeing the three Lights he is settled in the Tenth Stage.

Tsoṅ-kha-pa's *Pañcakrama* comm., Vol. 159, p. 4-4, 5, cites the view of *Spyod bsdus* (Āryadeva's *Caryāmelāpaka*) that one attains the Eighth Stage by the Stage of Generation. The implication is that the last three stages of the Bodhisattva Path constitute part of the Stage of Completion. Thereafter, the commentators differ along sectarian lines. Commentators of Yogācāra preference would combine this tantric theory with the terminology 'revolution of the basis' (*āśraya-parāvṛtti*) of the set of perceptions, especially the 'store consciousness' (*ālayavijñāna*) often associated in that Yogācāra literature with attainment of the Eighth Bodhisattva Stage. Mādhyamika-type commentators would avoid the term 'store consciousness' in this connection. However, no attempt is made in these tantric correlations to make a full-scale dovetailing with the theory of ten Bodhisattva Stages, in the manner as these are portrayed in great detail especially in the *Daśabhūmikā-sūtra*.

The old theory of ten Stages implies an eleventh (the Samantaprabhā), the stage of the complete Buddha. A further difficulty arose when three extra Stages (*bhūmi*), with varying names, were added to the traditional ten, with the previous name Samantaprabhā moved to the thirteenth. For example, Alaṃkakalaśa, PTT, Vol. 61, p. 182-2, explains the name 'Vajramālā' as the Stage called Samantaprabhā, and cites the verse (the original Sanskrit given under 'Bhageṣu vijahāra'), including: "The Stage resorted to by all the Buddhas is the Thirteenth, and it is called the 'lady'." The two systems of stages, the ten plus one, on the one hand, and thirteen on the other, relate to two ways of assigning the initiations (*abhiṣeka*) and mystical visions of the *Guhyasamājatantra*.

According to the notes to *Mkhas grub rje's Fundamentals of the Buddhist Tantras*, initiations are the means of attaining power over nature. There are two kinds, initiation simply in an honorary way, namely to the Buddhas; and initiation for the purpose of generating the power, namely to the Bodhisattvas. There are further varieties, such as those stated in the *Guhyasamāja*, Chap. XVIII, verses 111-112A:

> *abhiṣekaṃ tridhā bhedam asmin tantre prakalpitam /*
> *kalaśābhiṣekaṃ prathamaṃ dvitīyaṃ guhyābhiṣekataḥ //*
> *prajñājñānaṃ tṛtīyaṃ tu caturthaṃ tat punas tathā /*
>
> A distinction of three initiations is prepared in this Tantra, to wit : initiation of the flask as the first; the second, as the secret initiation; insight-knowledge, the third; and the fourth, precisely the same (as the third).

The first initiation, that of the flask, is laid in the Stage of Generation, and is usually divided into five initiations of the flask, going with the five Tathāgatas, and all accompanied by sprinkling rites. An initiation of the hierophant (*vajrācārya*) is laid in the transition to the Stage of Completion. The last three initiations, the 'secret', the 'insight-knowledge', and the 'fourth' are laid in the Stage of Completion. All those initiations are described at length in *Mkhas grub rje's Fundamentals of the Buddhist Tantras*; here some correlative materials are presented in order to clarify the role of the initiations in the Yoga of the *Guhyasamājatantra*.

Candrakīrti's *Guhyasamājābhisamayālaṃkāra-vṛtti* (PTT, Vol. 62, p. 26-5) mentions three kinds of 'flask initiation' : outer, inner, and 'pregnant' (phyi daṅ naṅ daṅ sbas paḥo). The outer kind uses a flask made of precious material for the five initiations of the flask. The inner kind also uses a precious flask for the five kinds of ambrosia, empowered by the Tathāgatas. The 'pregnant' kind also has two varieties, 'means' (*upāya*) and 'insight' (*prajñā*) flasks. The pregnant flask of means has the water from the mouth of the guru; the pregnant flask of insight has the water from the lotus of the prajñā lady.

The 'pregnant' kind of flask initiation appears to be the 'unshared kind' (*asādhāraṇa*) involved with the Hierophant's Initiation. In the latter initiation, the candidate is given the *vidyā* (goddess) called the 'seal pledge' (*mudrā-samaya*) and made to enter the union 'bliss-void' (*sukha-śūnya*) by embracing that *vidyā*.

Passing to the three initiations of the Stage of Completion, we note two ways of relating those initiations to the system as stages, as is set forth in Alaṃkakalaśa's commentary on the *Vajramālā* (PTT, Vol. 61, p. 180-2, 3) :

> / deḥi phyir las daṅ po paḥi rnal ḥbyor gyi ṅo bo slob dpon daṅ gsaṅ baḥi dbaṅ bskur ba dag ni sa brgyad pa źes bya ba rnam par bźad go / / śes rab ye śes kyi dgu paḥo / /bźi pa dpeḥi rnam pas ni bcu paḥo /. . . ./ yaṅ na slob dpon gyi dbaṅ ni sa brgyad paḥo / /gsaṅ baḥi dbaṅ gis ni rnam pa gaṅ gis rdo rje bzlas pa la brten nas dgu paḥo / / śes rab ye śes kyi dbaṅ gis sems rnam par dag paḥi ṅo bo ñid kyi bcu paḥo / raṅ byin gyis brlab pa yaṅ de ñid do / / bźi pa ñid kyi mṅon par byaṅ chub paḥi ṅo bo ñid kyis bcu gcig paḥo / /mos pa spyod paḥi sa daṅ bcas pa ni bcu gñis paḥo // zuṅ du ḥjug paḥi rim pas ni bcu gsum paḥo /
>
> Hence, the initiation of the hierophant (*vajrācārya*) who is a 'beginner *yogin*' and the Secret Initiation are laid in the Eighth (Bodhisattva) Stage; the Prajñā-jñāna initiation is on the Ninth; the Fourth Initiation, by form of example (i.e. taking the preceding initiation as example), on the Tenth. . . . In another way, the Hierophant's Initiation is on the Eighth Stage; the Secret Initiation for which one depends on Diamond Muttering (*vajra-jāpa*) on the Ninth; the Prajñā-jñāna Initiation whereby there is *cittaviśuddhi* is on the Tenth, as is also the *svādhiṣṭhāna*; the Fourth through *abhisaṃbodhi* is on the Eleventh; the Twelfth has the Adhimukti-caryā Stage; and with the Yuganaddha-krama there is the Thirteenth.

The second type of correlation involves the five *krama* titles of Nāgārjuna's *Pañcakrama* (Vajrajāpa, Cittaviśuddhi, Svādhiṣṭhāna, Abhisaṃbodhi, and Yuganaddha). The first type stems from Āryadeva's *Caryāmelāpaka*, in a passage cited in the notes to Mkhas grub rje's work, pp. 312-3: (Tibetan omitted):

> Moreover, Dbyaṅs-can-dgaḥ-baḥi-blo-gros, following the Ārya school of the *Guhyasamāja*, writes in his *Dpal gsaṅ ba ḥdus pa ḥphags lugs daṅ mthun paḥi sṅags kyis lam rnam gžag legs bśad skal bzaṅ ḥjug ṅogs*, folio 20b-1, f.: "The one who has arrived at the limit of the subtle and the coarse of the Steps of Production which conclude the maturation of the stream of consciousness, is associated with attainment of the eighth stage. Both the arcane body and arcane speech of the Steps of Completion are associated with the latter part of the eighth stage as well as with the ninth stage. Both the arcane mind and the illusory body are associated with the first part of the tenth stage. Both the Clear Light and the coupling in the realm of learning are associated with the latter part of the tenth stage. The coupling beyond learning is posited on the eleventh stage, Samantaprabhā. That is the purport of the *Caryāmelāpaka* (Toh. 1803.)"

Furthermore, there is a difference in where the initiations of the Stage of Completion are conferred. The notes to Mkhas grub rje's work show that the Secret Initiation is attained in the relative *bodhicitta-maṇḍala*, the Insight-Knowledge (*prajñā-jñāna*) one in the *bhaga-maṇḍala* of the vidyā, and the Fourth Initiation in the absolute *bodhicitta-maṇḍala*. Comparing this terminology with the previous discussion of the maṇḍala, it is easy to observe that the relative *bodhicitta-maṇḍala* is the 'body-maṇḍala' (*deha-maṇḍala*), and the other two, the *utsarga-maṇḍala* and the *paramārtha-maṇḍala*; while all three are understood in the present case with interpretations of the Stage of Completion.

Also, these initiations can be stated in terms of the consorts (*mudrā*). Following the exposition of the Kloṅ-rdol bla-ma as set forth in my "Female Energy..." article, the 'incantation-born female' is the yoginī at the final limit of the Stage of Generation; hence is involved in the Mahāsādhana phase of 'invariant (letter) placement' (in the *samādhi* 'Victorious Maṇḍala'), and presumably is the vidyā of the Preceptor's Initiation. The 'field-born female' enables one to attain the Symbolic Clear-Light with the arcane state of body, speech, and mind; and so is the vidyā of the 'Secret Initiation'. The 'together-born female' enables one to attain the Illusory Body and the Goal Clear-Light (or the Clear Light of the Absolute Entity): hence is the vidyā of the Prajñājñāna Initiation; and since the Fourth Initiation is said to be just the same as the third, she is also the vidyā or mudrā intended here.

Regarding the 'Secret Initiation', the *Pradīpoddyotana* in its chapter eight devoted to this initiation cites the Tantra catalogued as *Candraguhyatilaka* ("yathoktaṃ bhagavatā *guhye candratilake*"):

> *utsṛjya ratnojvala-*bodhicittaṃ saṃśuṣkamūrtiṃ sakalaṃ jinānāṃ* /
> *abhiṣiñcya mūrdhnāmalaratnavaśair viśuddhavajrodbhavajñāna-toyaiḥ* //
>
> Having drawn forth the *bodhicitta* jewel-blazing of the Jinas, he sprinkles all the arid body by way of the head with knowledge drops issuing from the pure *vajra*, (drops) with the power of the immaculate jewel.

The context shows that the expression 'by way of the head' means that the candidate imagines that the substance flows down from the crown of the head and first stimulates the 'little tongue' (the uvula). For a clear statement of its further progress through the body, see Śrī Lakṣmī's passage presented under nidāna verse 'KĀ' (No. 22). For the reference to the tongue, the *Pradīpoddyotana* on chapter seventeen quotes the '*Mūlatantra*' (in fact, the *Tattvasaṃgraha* of the Yoga-tantra class):

> *jihvāṃ talagatāṃ kṛtvā nāsikāgraṃ tu cintayet* /
> *sūkṣmavajrasukhasparśād bhavet cittaṃ samāhitam* //
>
> Having placed the tongue on the 'roof of the mouth', he should contemplate the tip of the nose (of the face). From blissful contact with the subtle *vajra* (the little tongue), the mind becomes stabilized.

In the same place the *Pradīpoddyotana* cites a clarifying passage from the '*Prajñāsūtra*' (which *Mchan ḥgrel* identifies only as 'Mother Tantra'):

> *dhārāmṛtamayī nityaṃ yā mūrdhni varṣate dhruvaṃ* /
> *pītvā hayayogīndreṇa jarāmṛtyuvināśakaḥ* //
> *yathotpalanālena (tu) toyam ākarṣate naraḥ* /
> *evam upajīvya jīved yogī mahābala iti* //
>
> What consists of streaming ambrosia continually and

> steadily rains in the head. Having drunk (that) with the 'yogi organ of a horse' (i.e. the stretched-out tongue curled back to the uvula) one destroys old age and death, (drinking) like a man sucks water through the stalk of an utpala-lotus. So having subsisted, the yogi lives with the name 'Mighty One'.

Furthermore, according to that work of Candrakīrti's, the *vṛtti* (*op. cit.*, p. 29-3), the place where the initiation is conferred is the disciple's tongue, of which there are three: in the throat, the heart, and the navel, the places where he enjoys the substance. This refers to the downward passage of the white-and-red bodhicitta drop.

In the case of the third initiation, this is the 'knowledge based on the insight' (Candrakīrti's explanation, the *vṛtti*, p. 30-3, 4) as a definition of *prajñā-jñāna* ('insight-knowledge'). According to Mkhas-grub-rje's work, the Insight-Knowledge Initiation is associated with the passage of winds in the 'central vein' arousing ecstasies in four *cakras*. Hence it is understandable that definitions of *mahāsukha* are given in connection with this Initiation. Thus, Tsoṅ-kha-pa's *Sṅags rim chen mo*, in the Prajñā-jñāna Initiation section, quotes Vitapāda's *Yogasapta-nāma-caturabhiṣekaprakaraṇa*: "The distinction of whether there is or is not the great ecstasy (*mahāsukha*) is accordingly the last of explanations. However, in the Prajñā-jñāna the characteristic of *mahāsukha* takes shape. . . . 'Because it is without place and without deception, it is explained as *mahāsukha*' " (sbyor ba bdun pa las kyaṅ // bde ba chen po yin ma yin gyi khyad par de bźin du bśad paḥi mthar / ḥo na kyaṅ śes rab ye śes la bde chen mtshan ñid gzugs su gnas / źes daṅ // mi gnas kyaṅ ni mi sluḥi phyir // bde ba chen po źes su bśad / ces dbaṅ gsum pa la. . . .). Also, Tsoṅ-kha-pa's commentary on the "Six Laws of Nāro-pa," (PTT Vol. 161, p. 8-2,3) states: "The main thing here is the requirement that the ecstasy of the Stage of Completion belong to the 'consubstantiality' (*sahaja*) arising from making the wind(s) enter, dwell, and dissolve in the 'central vein' " (/ ḥdiḥi yaṅ gtso bo ni rluṅ dbu mar źugs gnas thim gsum byas pa las byuṅ baḥi lhan skyes kyi rdzogs rim paḥi bde ba dgos so / ). In Candrakīrti's way of explaining (the *vṛtti*, p. 30-3, 4) the initiation is conferred in the three series of caves or in the padma. Since the *bodhicitta* proceeds downward in the 'central vein' through four *cakras*, we may understand Candrakīrti's remark as intending the upper three cakras as 'caves' and the lowest cakra as the 'padma', where the bodhicitta should not 'fall out' or be released.

The Fourth Initiation, also called 'Initiation of the Name', is said to be just like the Prajñā-jñāna one, meaning that the bodhicitta passes through the reverse order of the same *cakras*; and, according to the note in Mkhas grub rje's work, p. 36, upon reaching the forehead cakra, the small circle called *ūrṇā-kośa*, passes out into the ten directions like a lightning flash.

Furthermore, the theory of the Clear Light preceded or followed by three Lights, is related to the division into two stages. Now I shall present material from several works of Tsoṅ-kha-pa, leading up to a convenient table, after which some classifications in Tanjur works can be appreciated better. Tsoṅ-kha-pa, in his commentary on the *Caturdevīparipṛcchā* labelled '*Bźis źus*' (PTT, Vol. 159, p. 97-4) writes: "That is the concise *paramārtha-maṇḍala* as the 'Clear Light of conviction' in the phase of the Stage of Generation, and is comparable to the four voids of which the Clear Light belonging to the Stage of Completion is the chief one" ( / de ni bskyed rim gyi skabs su lhag mos ḥod gsal du bsdus paḥi don dam paḥi dkyil ḥkhor daṅ/ rdzogs rim gyi ḥod gsal gtso bor byas paḥi stoṅ pa bźi lta buḥo / ). Restricting ourselves to this 'Clear Light of conviction' concerned with imagining the 'basic time'—the cycle of life and death—we find that there are two kinds. There is a Clear Light of deep sleep which contrasts with dream, and a Clear Light of death which contrasts with the intermediate state, as in this passage of Tsoṅ-kha-pa's *Gsaṅ ba ḥdus paḥi źal śes yig chuṅ thor bu pa* (Vol. 159, p. 136-2): "Since the Clear Light of deep sleep, and dream are controlled by the power of wind, there is the invariable accompaniment that the Clear Light of death, and the intermediate state are controlled by the power of wind. In the same way, since the Clear Light of deep sleep, and dream are controlled by craving, there is the invariable accompaniment that the Clear Light of death, and the intermediate state are controlled by craving" ( / gñid kyi ḥod gsal daṅ / rmi lam rluṅ stobs kyis zin na / ḥchi baḥi ḥod gsal daṅ / bar do rluṅ stobs kyis zin pas khyab / de bźin du gñid kyi ḥod gsal daṅ / rmi lam ḥdun pas zin na / ḥchi baḥi ḥod gsal daṅ / bar do ḥduu paḥi zin pas khyab ciṅ /). According to this passage, the 'basic time' is controlled by wind and craving; deep sleep corresponds to death; dream corresponds to the intermediate state.

Turning to the 'time of the path' in the Stage of Completion, when the four voids are evoked concretely, there is also a terminology of two kinds of Clear Light, as in Tsoṅ-kha-pa's *Gsal baḥi sgron me* (Vol. 158, p. 194-1) : "Moreover, at the conclusion of the Clear Light of the (Supreme) Entity, he accomplishes the Yuganaddha-deha (pair-united body); and at the end of the Symbolic Clear Light, he accomplishes the Illusory Body" ( / de yaṅ don gyi ḥod gsal gyi mjug tu zuṅ ḥjug gi sku daṅ / dpeḥi ḥod gsal gyi mjug tu sgyu maḥi sku ḥgrub po /).

However, both the 'basic time' and the 'time of the path' are involved in the varieties of intermediate states and of births, as in that same work of Tsoṅ-kha-pa (his commentary on the *Pañcakrama*), first the intermediate states (*bar do*) (Vol. 159, p. 53-4): (1) bar-do of gestation (*srid pa bardo*), which agrees with (2) the bar-do of dream (*rmi lam gyi bardo*) according to the Mar-pa school—the two being the bar-do of the basic time (*gźiḥi bar do*); (3) bardo of the path (*lam gyi bardo*). Next the births (Vol. 159, p. 53-5): (1) birth in a womb through intermediate state of gestation; (2) birth through 'bar-do of dream' at the time of waking up to reoccupy the gross personality aggregates—the two being the 'birth' of the basic time (*gźiḥi skye ba*); (3) birth of apprehending the gross personality aggregates by the bar-do of the illusory body (*sgyu lus kyi bardo*).

The above data can be clarified in tabular form, where the Clear Lights of deep sleep and death of everyday life correspond respectively to the Symbolic Clear Light and the Clear Light of the Absolute Entity.

Now for the Tanjur classifications, of which a good start is Śākyamitra's *ṭīkā* on the *Caryāmelāpakapradīpa* (PTT, Vol. 62, p. 300-5) : "The varieties are Clear Light of (1) training (*śaikṣa*), (2) beyond training (*aśaikṣa*), (3) true mind (*cittatā*), and (4) entity (*artha*). Nos. 3 and 4 in his classification seem to be the two mentioned by Śrī Lakṣmī (Vol. 63, p. 29-4): "The Clear Light is of two kinds, Clear Light of consciousness and Clear Light of intrinsic nature. Among those, the Clear

## III. THE CLEAR LIGHTS

| | *Basic Time (in Stage of Generation)* | | *Time of the Path (in Stage of Completion)* | |
|---|---|---|---|---|
| Clear Light | Deep Sleep | Death | Symbolic | Supreme Entity (paramārtha) |
| Intermediate State | Dream | Gestation | Illusory Body (māyā-deha) | Yuganaddha-deha (pair-united body) |
| Birth | Waking up | Birth (exit from womb, or by some other means) | (apprehending the gross personality aggregates-vipāka-kāya) | (apprehending the world, in the Nirmāṇa-kāya) |

Light of consciousness is the (Yogācāra's) 'representation' (*vijñapti*) without aspect (*nirākāra*); and the Clear Light of intrinsic nature is universal void (*sarvaśūnya*) which is obtained at the fourth stage" (/ ḥod gsal ba ni rnam pa gñis te / sems kyi ḥod gsal ba daṅ / raṅ bźin gyis ḥod baḥo // de la sems kyi ḥod gsal ba ni rnam pa med paḥi rnam rig daṅ / raṅ bźin gyis ḥod gsal ba ni thams cad stoṅ pa ste / rim pa bźi pas thob par byaḥo/). That is to say, Śākyamitra's kind called 'true mind' would be the Yogācārin's 'representation without (external) aspect': and the one of 'entity' (short for 'supreme entity') would be the universal void.

Nos. 1 and 2 of Śākyamitra's classification are explained in Candrakīrti's *Guhyasamājābhisamayālaṃkāra-vṛtti* (PTT, Vol. 62, p. 35-3) in summary verses: "One should understand two Clear Lights by 'training' (*śaikṣa*) and 'beyond training' (*aśaikṣa*). The Clear Light of training is explained as (the *dhyānas* of) 'contraction' (*piṇḍagrāha*) and 'expansion' (*anubheda*). The one beyond training is non-discursive (*avikalpa*), not perceptively reached (*anupalabdha*), pure from the outset (*ādiśuddha*)." These two are respectively equivalent to the Symbolic Clear Light and to the Clear Light of the Absolute entity in the time of the path. Therefore, Śākyamitra's varieties (1) and (2) are respectively equivalent to his varieties (3) and (4). All of the above Tanjur classifications apply to "Time of the Path." The Clear Light of Deep Sleep appears mainly a matter of oral instruction.

Finally, there is the difficult but important topic of three *caryās* in relation to the two Stages. In his *Mthaḥ gcod*, Tsoṅ-kha-pa points out that Āryadeva's *Caryāmelāpaka* took account of the three *caryās* only for the Stage of Completion, but that the *Pradīpoddyotana* on Chapter X (in fact the initial sentence) implies that both Stages have their version of the three *caryās*. The three according to the *Pradīpoddyotana* manuscript on Chapter VII are *prapañca-caryā*, *niṣprapañca-caryā*, and *atyantaniṣprapañca-caryā*. Tsoṅ-kha-pa elaborately discusses these matters in his *Pañcakrama* commentary (PTT, Vol. 159, pp. 67 to 78), the section entitled "The *caryā* which is the means of issuing the profit in the two States" (*rim gñis la bogs ḥbyin paḥi thabs spyod pa*); and has a briefer, but also complicated discussion in his *Mthaḥ gcod* on Chapter VII (PTT, Vol. 156, pp. 42 to 45).

The discussion shows that in each case this is a *caryā* (advanced yoga technique) connected with the female element of the world. The word *prapañca* has here the special meaning, "involvement with the five sense objects". In ancient Buddhist texts, these five are called the *pañcakāmaguṇa* ("the five strands of desire"), and they promote development of the being, his taking a place in phenomenon (a more usual Indian meaning of the Sanskrit word *prapañca*). The addition of the word *caryā* serves for classifying the yoga techniques of this Tantric tradition. Candrakīrti's commentary on Chapter VII associates the three in the given order with three of the four ways of interpreting *Guhyasamājatantra* passages, namely with the "shared sense," and "pregnant sense," and the "ultimate sense" (see my section "Seven ornaments and subdivisions"). In illustration, when one contemplates the deities in their proper dress, hence in their corporeal form, this is a case of *prapañca*; however, properly speaking, the addition of the word *caryā* restricts this case to the five sense objects deified as goddesses (as in *nidāna* verse 21). Again, in relation to the three Lights, the *caryā* would be of the "non-*prapañca*" type; and in relation to the Clear Light, the *caryā* would be of the "extreme non-*prapañca*" type. Hereafter, the term *prapañca* will be left untranslated; '*caryā*' is either translated as 'praxis' or left untranslated.

Now that we have alluded to both superficial and profound aspects of the two stages, we should prepare for the separate discussion of the two stages by the verse cited in 'Documents' (*Pradīpoddyotana* on XII, 60-64) :

By the distinction of 'shared' and 'superior',
one posits two kinds of service :
The 'shared' one by the four *vajras*, the 'superior'
one by members six in number.

This verse shows that the word 'Service' (*sevā*) can be employed in generalized ways to indicate the entire praxis of the Guhyasamāja. Previously in section A, on the chapters, we have translated that there are four diamond rites of Sevā associated with the Stage of Generation. Then the superior service is the six members of yoga in the Stage of Completion. To anticipate, the four diamond rites are named 1. yoga, 2. anuyoga, 3. atiyoga, and 4. mahāyoga. The six members of yoga have already been defined in 'Documents' : 1. pratyāhāra, 2. dhyāna,

3. prāṇāyāma, 4. dhāraṇā, 5. anusmṛti, and 6. samādhi. What is meant by 'shared' service is that the terms 1. sevā 2. upasādhana, 3. sādhana, and 4. mahāsādhana, can be employed in one sense of the words as equivalent to the four vajras as named above, and can be employed in another sense as equivalent to the six members of yoga. In the latter case, sevā covers pratyāhāra, dhyāna, prāṇāyāma, and dhāraṇā; upasādhana equals anusmṛti; and both sādhana and mahāsādhana are included in samādhi. Moreover, as has been shown, sixteen chapters (2-17) of the *Guhyasamājatantra* are labelled by these four generalized terms of service. It may be the intention of such labelling to indicate the shared aspects of the two stages insofar as these aspects can be assigned in four groups by those four labels of the chapters.

However, the *Guhyasamājatantra* has itself briefly defined the common elements indicated by the four vajras in its chapter XVIII, verse 137 :

> *prathamaṃ śūnyatābodhiṃ dvitīyaṃ bījasaṃhṛtam /*
> *tṛtīyaṃ bimbaniṣpattiś caturthaṃ nyāsaṃ akṣaram //*
>
> The first is the revelation of voidness; the second is the drawing togethe of germ syllables; the third is the perfection of the image; the fourth is the invariant (=letter) placement.

In order to apply to both stages, those four have to be explained with utmost generality. The first indicates the yoga of reaching up through the void or light stages to the Clear Light. The second is a descent of divine elements. The third is the consummation of the candidate. The fourth is the saintly re-involvement with the world.

### C. *The four steps of yoga and the three samādhis in the Stage of Generation*

The four steps of yoga in the Stage of Generation are frequently referred to as the four steps of service (*sevā*) or of evocation (*sādhana*). They are presented this way in the *Guhyasamāja*, XVIII, p. 162:

> *yogatantreṣu sarveṣu śasyate yoginā sadā /*
> *sevāvidhānaṃ prathamaṃ dvitīyam upasādhanam /*
> *sādhanaṃ tu tṛtīyaṃ vai mahāsādhanaṃ caturthakam //*
>
> The yogin always praises in all Yogatantra—the rite of

service as first, the near-evocation as second, evocation as third, and great evocation as fourth.

These steps are stated somewhat more fully in *Ibid.*, XII, p. 58 (completely given in 'Documents') : "He should contemplate the samādhi-praxis of service (*sevā*) as the supreme revelation (*uttama-bodhi*)" (sevāsamādhisaṃyogaṃ bhāvayet bodhim uttamam). "....the deliberation on the 'base of vajra' (*vajra-āyatana*) when there is foremost success is the near-evocation (*upasādhana*)" (upasādhanasiddhyagre vajrāyatanavicāraṇam). "The contemplation of the lords of the mantras stated to be the exhortation at the time of evocation (*sādhana*)" (sādhane codanaṃ proktaṃ mantrādhipatibhāvanam). "At the time of great evocation (*mahāsādhana*), when he imagines the form of his own *mantra-vajrin* as the lord on the crown of the head, he is successful because of the *jñāna-vajrin*" (mahāsādhanakāleṣu bimbaṃ svamantravajriṇaḥ / mukuṭe 'dhipatiṃ dhyātvā siddhyate jñānavajriṇaḥ).

Tsoṅ-kha-pa further clarifies the four steps by identifying them with the four yogas of the *Kṛṣṇayamāri-tantra* (presumably Tohoku No. 467) in this passage (*Sṅags rim*, f. 364b) :

> */ rdo rje sems dpaḥ rdzogs pa ni // rnal ḥbyor yin par ḥdi ltar ḥdod / / de yi rgyu mthun lha yi sku / rjes kyi rnal ḥbyor yin par grags / / ḥkhor lo thams cad yoṅs rdzogs pa // śin tu rnal ḥbyoryin par ḥdod // sku daṅ gsuṅ daṅ thugs rnams daṅ // lha yi mig sogs byin brlab daṅ / / ye śes ḥkhor lo gźug pa daṅ // mchod daṅ bstod pa chen po ni / /rnal ḥbyor chen po źes byaḥo /*
> The perfection of Vajrasattva is thus held to be *yoga*. His affiliated divine body (**devatā-kāya*) is known as *anuyoga*. The perfecting of all the 'circles' (*cakra*) is held to be *atiyoga*. The blessing (*adhiṣṭhāna*) of *body*, speech, and mind, and of the divine eye (*divya-cakṣus*), etc.; the drawing in of the Jñāna-cakra (=knowledge beings, *jñānasattva*), the great offerings and praises—is called *mahāyoga*.

Nāgārjuna, in his *Piṇḍīkṛta-sādhana*, is consistent with his employment of this terminology of yogas, starting with verse 44 (in La Vallée Poussin's numbering). We learn that in *yoga* there is the rite involving the recitation of the celebrated mantras, Oṃ śūnyatājñānavajrasvabhāvātmako 'ham, and Oṃ dharmadhātusvabhāvātmako 'ham. With verse 51, he mentions the *anuyoga* and this culminates in the contemplation of the 'primeval lord' (*ādinātha*). Then the *atiyoga* develops vajrasattva (the 'diamond being') as the progressed self of the yogin with his body as a *maṇḍala* (the *deha-maṇḍala* mentioned earlier in our maṇḍala section). The *mahāyoga* starts with verse 70 and involves the blessing or empowerment of body, speech, and mind, using the mantras of *Guhyasamāja*, chapter 6 ('Documents').

Passing to some individual explanations for the four steps, especially as they apply to the Stage of Generation, we note that the *Pradīpoddyotana* ('Documents') is helpful for clarifying the 1st step. It is necessary to place consciousness in *samādhi*. The practitioner then reviews the evocation "from the spot of earth, etc. up to the maṇḍala circle." He then enters the realm of the void through contemplating the mantra, "Oṃ śūnyatājñānavajrasvabhāvātmako 'ham" (Oṃ. I am the intrinsic nature of the knowledge diamond of voidness). Hence in this step the officiant evokes the void maṇḍala-palace, also called the 'perfection of Vajrasattva'.

Commenting on the '*vajra-āyatana*' of the second step of sādhana, namely upasādhana, *Sṅags rim* says (f. 363a-6 to 363b-1): "Thugs-rje-źabs explains that *vajra* means the thirty-two deities from Vairocana down to Sumbharāja; while its base (*āyatana*) refers to the spots wherein are deposited the syllables of those (deities) in the aggregate of form all the way down to the soles of the feet." ( / rdo rje ni rnam snaṅ nas gnod mdzes kyi bar so gñis so // deḥi skye mched ni gzugs phuṅ nas rkaṅ mthil gyi bar yin te de dag gis yi ge ḥgod paḥi gnas bstan par thug rje źabs ḥchad do / ). This remark immediately shows the connection between the '*vajra-āyatana*' of the second sādhana step with the second vajra, the 'drawing together of germ syllables' (*bījasaṃhṛta*) (cf. preceding sub-section). This refers to the body-maṇḍala where thirty-two syllables representing the thirty-two deities are deposited in the appropriate spots of the body. But without this comment, the relation between the two second ones would not be clear. Also the comment clarifies the *Sṅags rim* remarks (362b-6, ff. through 363a-1, 2, 3) that on the Stage of Generation the second sādhana yields the 'incantation body' (*mantra-deha*) while the same sādhana, interpreted on the Stage of Completion, yields the 'knowledge body' (*jñāna-kāya*).

This evocation of a sanctified body, which the *Pradīpoddyo-*

*tana* calls the 'form of Mahāmudrā', is alluded to in Nāgārjuna's *Piṇḍīkṛtasādhana* (verses 51-52) :

> *....anuyogaṃ samācaret |*
> *tatas tryakṣarasambhūtaṃ sitakundendusannibham |*
> *ādināthaṃ vicintya....*
>
> ....He should engage upon the Anuyoga. Then, imagining the primeval lord (*ādinātha*) arisen from the three syllables like the white-Jasmine moon....

As to the three syllables, these can be either *ā*, *o*, and *ha*, or they can be Oṃ, Āḥ, and Hūṃ. Thus *Mchan ḥgrel*, PTT, Vol. 158, p. 14-3, states : "*ā*, *o*, and *ha* are the three basic syllables...; that means that from the thirty-two parts of the 'seminal drop' (*bindu-bodhicitta*) the three syllables become 32-fold and generate the gods on the lotus." This alludes to generation of the thirty-two Guhyasamāja gods from germ syllables. Furthermore, Tsoṅ-kha-pa's *Rnal ḥbyor dag paḥi rim pa* (PTT, Vol. 160, p. 91-1), shows the process of imagining a single *bindu* (of *bodhicitta*) as the syllable Bhrūṃ and from its transformation generating the 4-cornered, 4-doored, etc. palace along with thrones (Step No. 1); and continues :

> Then the single-part *bindu* becomes 32 parts upon the thrones, and from their transformation (there arise the syllables) Oṃ, Āh, Hūṃ. Then the incantation of each of the seed syllables Hūṃ, etc. gives rise to 32 Jñāna-adhiṣṭhānas of the three vajras. Therefrom there arise 32 hand symbols of thunderbolt (*vajra*), etc. (Step No. 2). Therefrom one generates sequentially the bodies of the deities (Step No. 3) :—the foregoing is the 'way of generating'.

In the case of the third step—generation of the bodies of the deities (especially within the practitioner's own body as a body-maṇḍala) is presumably what the *Kṛṣṇayamāritantra* (op. cit.) calls the perfecting of all the circles. The *Mchan ḥgrel* on chapter XII (Vol. 158, p. 92-2, 3) adds information for the third step that the perfection here comes from the five abhisaṃbodhis. In summary of Nāgārjuna's text, Ratnākaraśānti's *Piṇḍīkṛta-sādhanopāyikā vṛtti-ratnāvalī-nāma* (Vol. 62, p. 62) places here the blessing of the sense bases (*āyatana*), the personality aggregates (*skandha*), the elements, the major and minor limbs, by the various 32 deities; and (*ibid.*, p. 77) states that by divisions of the skandhas, there are Vairocana and the other Tathāgatas; and so on, down to Sumbharāja (in the feet). These are what the *Guhyasamāja* calls the 'lords of the mantras'. The *Pradīpoddyotana* ('Documents') alludes to verses XII, 70-71 to explain the blessing, but thereby disagrees with both the *Kṛṣṇayamāritantra* and Nāgārjuna's *Piṇḍīkṛta-sādhana* which place this blessing or empowerment of Body, Speech, and Mind in the fourth step.

The fourth step in the *Pradīpoddyotana* treatment involves imagining the lord on the crown of the officiant's head, and the five Tathāgatas on the heads of all the deities in their particular families. *Mchan ḥgrel* (PTT, Vol. 158, p. 92-2, 3) brings in the terminology of the fourth vajra, the 'invariant (=letter) placement', and states that this refers both to letter placement of the *samādhi-sattva* (*tiṅ ṅe ḥdzin sems dpaḥ*) and to letter placement in the body of the *vidyā* (rig maḥi lus la yi ge ḥgod pa), hence to letter placement of *vajra* and *padma* (rdo rje daṅ padmaḥi yi ge ḥgod pa ste), referring of course to the mention of *vajra* and *padma* in the *Pradīpoddyotana* comment ('Documents') on this step. This would then be the 'overflow maṇḍala' (*utsarga-maṇḍala*) spoken of in our maṇḍala section. As was mentioned, other sources place here the empowerment of Body, Speech, and Mind.

Furthermore, the *Pradīpoddyotana* ('Documents') clarifies that the Mahāsādhana, which is the fourth step, is the accomplishment of the aim of others. This agrees with the *Guhyasamājatantra's* explanation of Mahāsādhana as a title for chapters 5, 9. 17, and 13, that these chapters have the teaching that liberates one's great souled disciple. The *Pradīpoddyotana* mentions that the Mahāsādhana includes the 'best victorious maṇḍala' and the 'best victorious rite'. In fact, these are the second and third of a well-known set called the three samādhis.

The set of three samādhis constitute a terminology in common between the Yoga-tantra and the Anuttara-yoga-tantra classes of tantric literature. Even though there are some differences in explanation of those three, there are strong indications that the Stage of Generation of the Anuttarayoga-tantra is the portion of that kind of Tantra that has practices shared with the Yoga-tantra. The three samādhis are called 'preliminary praxis' (prathamaprayoga), 'triumphant maṇḍala' (vijaya-maṇḍala), and 'victory of the rite' (karma-vijaya). *Sṅags rim*, f. 364a-1, 2, mentions as the implication of those remarks of the *Pradīpoddyotana* that the first three steps of service are the 'preliminary praxis' and amount to steps that accomplish one's own aim. The employment of two samādhis to cover the 4th step of yoga helps to resolve the several ways of explaining the 4th step as not constituting rival methods of conducting the rite of that stage, but rather as suggesting the grouping into two phases. The 'victorious maṇḍala' is the initiation phase of the Stage of Generation, involving the five *vidyā* initiations, as they are called. The 'victory of the rite' includes those rather strange rites filling up a number of verses in both Chapter 6 and Chapter 12 ('Documents') about the ritual eating of different kinds of flesh, in fact the meditative eating of that flesh, credited with leading to supernormal powers (on which I once wrote an article, "Totemic beliefs in the Buddhist Tantras"). The apportionment of rites between the three samādhis can be seen rather clearly by placing in concordance with the four steps the maṇḍala rites of the Guhyasamāja which can also be arranged in four parts following the classification of *Mkhas grub rje's Fundamentals of the Buddhist Tantras*, which in turn is based on the *Sṅags rim*. These two works enabled me to group the rites in Nāgabodhi's *Śrī-guhyasamāja-maṇḍalopāyikāviṃśati-vidhi-nāma* (PTT, Vol. 62, pp. 12 to 18), where there are actually twenty-one rites despite the '*viṃśati*' of the title. Admittedly, this correlation demands more justification than here given, and a study of the Mkhas grub rje context will provide some of the missing links, for example, that the 'rite of the site' also requires contemplation of voidness (as we saw in the case of the first yoga step).

(A) Rites of the site:
1. Clearing the site (sa sbyoṅ ba)
2. Seizing the site (sa yoṅs su gzuṅ ba)
3. Elimination of the obstructing demons (bgegs ñe bar źi ba)

(B) Rites of preparatory acts :
4. Pitching the lines with chalk (thog le kor gyis thig gdab pa)
5. Preparing the flask (bum pa lhag par gnas pa)
6. Beseeching the gods (gsol gdab pa)
7. Preparation of the disciple (slob ma lhag par gnas pa)

(C) The main rite, beginning with construction of maṇḍala:

8. The five colored threads (tshon sna lṅa)
9. Putting in the colors (tshon dgyed pa)
10. Invitation of the gods (spyan draṅ ba)

(D) Initiations of the flask :

11. Drawing the disciple into the maṇḍala (slob ma gzug pa)
12. Diadem Initiation (cod pan gyi dbaṅ bskur)
13. Diamond Initiation (rdo rje dbaṅ bskur)
14. Mirror Initiation (me loṅ gi dbaṅ bskur) (=Water Initiation)
15. Name Initiation (miṅ gi dbaṅ bskur)
16. Emblem Initiation (phyag mtshan gyi dbaṅ bskur) (=Bell Initiation).

Offerings:

17. Offerings to the gods (lha la yon ḥbul ba)
18. Offerings to the guru (bla ma la yon ḥbul ba)

Permission and Unification :

19. Conferral of permission (*anujñā*) on the disciple (slob ma la rjes su gnaṅ ba sbyin pa)
20. Unification (of the Guhyasamāja deities that are in various spots of the body) (ñe bar bsdu ba)

Concluding Acts:

21. Release of the magic nail (phur bu dbyuṅ ba), i.e. dismissal of the deities, along with a burnt offering (*homa*).

In summary, one can establish the first samādhi of 'preliminary praxis' to cover the three parts. A. Rites of the site, B. Rites of the preparatory acts, and C. The main rite, where the three (as external ritual) are analogous to the first three steps of service (as internal ritual) which in both cases accomplish one's own aim. Then the second samādhi 'victorious maṇḍala' covers the initiations of the flask for the benefit of the disciple, but since in reality these initiations are conferred by the goddess, the female element enters at this point. The third samādhi 'victory of the rite' covers the offerings, permission to the disciple (to repeat the ritual himself) and re-unification of the 32 deities into Bodhicitta, as well as concluding acts. This helps to clarify the Mahāyoga as the second and third samādhi.

Also, it is becoming apparent that there are various ways of stating the four steps of service or yoga, and this may be the implication of the remark in *Sṅags rim*, f. 364a-1, 2 that for accomplishing the four steps there is a lesser, a middling, and a great (chuṅ ḥbriṅ chen po gsum ga dgos pas).

Besides, there is Tsoṅ-kha-pa's insistence on correlating tantric materials with the three phases, birth, death, and the intermediate state, which are referred to in nidāna verse 38, and those three with the three bodies of the Buddha. This is stressed among other places in his independent work *Don gsal ba* on the *Guhyasamājatantra* (PTT. Vol. 160, p. 128). In this way, Dharmakāya goes with death, Saṃbhogakāya with intermediate state, and Nirmāṇakāya with birth (cf. the table about the three phases in the preceding section). There Tsoṅ-kha-pa argues at length about the 'Ādinātha' (which according to Nāgārjuna is the germinal Vajradhara) to the conclusion that the generation of the 'ādinātha' agrees with the intermediate state. In the foregoing discussion of the four yogas, the generation of the ādinātha was placed in the second yoga called anuyoga. In my article, "The Five-fold Ritual Symbolism of Passion," I showed Tsoṅ-kha-pa's view that the contemplation of voidness is equivalent to death; and since this contemplation takes place in the first yoga, this step can be correlated with death. That leaves the third step to go with birth, which is reasonable since it is the culminating step for one's own sake. We therefore have the following line-up of the steps :

| | | | |
|---|---|---|---|
| 1. Yoga | — | symbolic death | — Dharmakāya |
| 2. Anuyoga | — | symbolic intermediate state | — Saṃbhogakāya |
| 3. Atiyoga | — | symbolic birth | — Nirmāṇakāya |

Of course, such concordances are not meant to suggest that the Yogin attains such bodies by following through with the several steps. Tsoṅ-kha-pa makes it plain that this correlation is meant to establish those steps as the causes in the 'Stage of Generation' for the subsequent attainment of those Buddha bodies in the 'Stage of Completion'.

### D. *The six members of yoga and the five kramas in the Stage of Completion*

The six members are stated in the *Guhyasamājatantra* for the first time in chapter 18, which is generally regarded in commentarial tradition as an Uttara-tantra 'continuation tantra' because it includes verses grouping the preceding chapters 2-17. However, Candrakīrti's *Pradīpoddyotana* on Chapter 12 (see 'Documents') insists that verse 64 has the implication of these members, especially by the words *sevājñānāmṛtena*; and accordingly wrote in comment upon that verse a fairly lengthy account of the six members. This account, curiously, is almost identical with the work *Ṣaḍaṅga-yoga* (extant in Tibetan), attributed to Nāgārjuna (in PTT Vol. 85). It may be that the comment was a traditional one for that block of verses in chapter 18. The same verse block that Candrakīrti quoted, plus some more, were later quoted by Nāro-pā in his *Sekoddeśaṭīkā*, a commentary on part of the *Kālacakra-tantra*. Nāro-pā devotes much of his subsequent commentary to aspects of those members, following the Kālacakra tradition. This shows that it was feasible to carry through the tantric praxis in terms of those six members; and the occurrence in the *Guhyasāmāja*, chapter 18, indicates that this formulation was once a viable procedure in this tantric cult.

Of course, the names of the six members of yoga are ancient. They are almost the same names as the members of yoga in the *Maitrī Upaniṣad*. However, over the centuries different interpretations have been made of the chief terms; and they do not always occur in the same order as in the *Guhyasamājatantra*. Also, the order of the members in this Tantra, while standard in the Anuttarayoga-tantra, has occasioned some sharp disputes. Of course, Nāgārjuna's commentary on the 18th chapter, where the six members are defined, was examined carefully by the commentators, but their silence regarding his commentary when they engage in disputes on these matters is due to Nāgārjuna's way of commenting, which we might call 'around' and not 'to' the point. However, it is interesting to observe how he did proceed in his commentary, the *Aṣṭādaśa-paṭala-vistara-vyākhyā*.

He found his first opportunity to go into the matter when commenting on chapter XVIII, verse 24 :

> *trividhaṃ kāyavākcittaṃ guhyam ity abhidhīyate* /
> *samājaṃ milanaṃ proktaṃ sarvabuddhābhidhānakam* //
>
> The three types, body, speech, and mind, are explained as the 'secret'.
>
> 'Samāja' is said to be union, the definition of all the Buddhas.

Using remarks based on those three, body, etc., he first explains the three samādhis, 'preliminary praxis,' etc.; then the Stage of Generation and the Stage of Completion; then his five kramas in order; the 'cause' (*hetu*), 'action' (*karma*), and 'fruit' (*phala*); then the six members of yoga in order. Then he starts over again, with somewhat different remarks based on those three, body, etc., with which he first explains the three samādhis, then the two stages, then the five kramas in order, then those three, 'cause', etc., and finally the six members in order. His next opportunity presented itself when commenting on the definition of Tantra (chapter XVIII, verse 33), in particular the expression '*asaṃhārya*' ('which cannot be led astray'). He says this means the Tantra of the Fruit, free from fear, wherein the achievement Vajradhara, and so on, is conferred by way of the yogin of subtle yoga in the Stage of Generation or the Stage of Completion, or of (the five krama) 'Diamond Muttering, etc., or of the six members. By this comment he clarifies that his five kramas and the six members are alternate ways of expressing the tantric path (in fact, the Stage of Completion). Then in verse 35, still devoted to definition of 'Tantra', the expressions 'pañcakaṃ trikulaṃ caiva....' gave him the opportunity to talk about five-fold sets, three-fold ones, and so on. His five kramas are such a five-fold set, so they are mentioned, along with the three samādhis again; and he cannot mention those without alluding to the six members, so now (PTT. Vol. 60, p. 6-3) he gives a brief definition of each of the six members. When he comes to the block of verses on which Candrakīrti commented ('Documents') he has a rather lengthy treatment of the six members (*op. cit.*, p. 14-3, 4, 5 and p.15-1) in a manner consistent with Candrakīrti's statement, although having some other materials, and in particular agrees on the disputed point that the *dhyāna* member has the five parts of non-tantric Buddhism and that these do reach up to the Spread-of-Light, Culmination-of-Light, and finally the Clear Light; while also placing the six members in the Stage of Completion. As though that were not enough, he continues (p. 15-1,2) with brief explanations of the benefit resulting from each member, for example, that dhyāna yields the five supernormal powers (the teaching of non-tantric Buddhism). There can be no doubt that Nāgārjuna gives the subject of the six members its proper due. He presents considerable information, all taken together. But since he introduced his five kramas into this commentary when they were not mentioned in the original text of chapter 18, he could have been helpful to show the relationship between his five kramas and the six members, which he avoided committing himself upon. And so subsequent centuries of commentators had to dispute over what was meant. In the Guhyasamāja cult, his *Pañcakrama* triumphed over the six-membered terminology, for which we are fortunate to have Candrakīrti's Sanskrit commentary.

As we consider Candrakīrti's comments, it seems that the first two members *pratyāhāra* and *dhyāna*, amount to a summary of non-tantric Buddhist meditation. In standard meditation, first there is withdrawal of the mind from the multiplicity of external objects, with focussing upon one properly chosen meditative object, which is contemplated in the mind. This is close to the *pratyāhāra* of Candrakīrti's explanation which, however, adds some tantric remarks. Then the five parts to Dhyāna are the traditional parts assigned to the dhyānas in non-tantric Buddhism which teaches that there are four Dhyāna levels or heavens constituting what is called the realm of form (*rūpa-dhātu*), below which is the realm of desire (*kāma-dhātu*) and beyond which is the formless realm (*arūpa-dhātu*). While it is true that the further explanations given by Candrakīrti for the five parts of *dhyāna* are not how those same words are explained in the Abhidharma treatises, it is intriguing to notice his remark that the fifth part "is engendered as light-only and the ultimate that is one with universal void." This claim that *dhyāna* reaches up to the Clear Light (of which 'universal void' is a synonym) practically admits that the Clear Light is an experience at the top of the realm of form, which is precisely where Mahāyāna Buddhism places the Complete Buddha in a heaven called Akaniṣṭha with a body called Saṃbhogakāya. But what sense is there to commenting that way, when *dhyāna* precedes the next member, 3. *prāṇāyāma*, in which there is no mention of experience of the Clear Light, but which is a necessary preliminary of the next member 4. *dhāraṇā* which covers the mystic experience of entering the Clear Light? It makes sense only if one takes into account the kinds of Clear Light as in the previous section that summarized the varieties in a table. That is to say, the

Clear Light reached by the *dhyāna* member is not the Clear Light of the 'Supreme Entity'; but, on the other hand, what is its Clear Light is not definite without further information about this member of yoga, especially since there was a controversy about the first two members.

Tsoṅ-kha-pa's commentary on *Pañcakrama*, PTT, Vol. 158, p. 196-4, says :

> / *sgroṅ ma rab gsal las sor bsam gñis sems dben daṅ* /
> *srog rtsol rdor bzlas daṅ* / *ḥdzin pa ḥod gsal daṅ* /
> *rjes dran daṅ tiṅ ṅe ḥdzin zuṅ ḥjug tu ḥdus par bśad de* /
> According to the *Pradīpoddyotana*, (among the six members) *pratyāhāra* and *dhyāna* are incorporated in secret state of mind (*citta-viveka*); *prāṇāyāma* in diamond muttering (*vajrajāpa*) (i.e. secret state of speech, *vāg-viveka*); *dhāraṇā* in Clear Light; *anusmṛti* and *samādhi* in pair-united (*yuga-naddha*).

This Tibetan tradition then proceeded to reject a portion of Candrakīrti's position, and by implication, Nāgārjuna's commentary on the 18th chapter. This is made clear in Tsoṅ-kha-pa's commentary *Mthaḥ gcod* (PTT. Vol. 156, pp. 50-52, 'Deciding among the alternatives' for chapter 12). He says (p. 51-2-4) : "According to the *Pradīpoddyotana*, both *pratyāhāra* and *dhyāna* are the arcane mind (*citta-viveka*) (*sor bsam gñis sems dben*)...." Later he says (p. 52-4-4): "In our school, if one treats the six members as six stages of the Stage of Completion, then we heartily endorse Sgra-dbyaṅs-bcu-gcig-pa (for his position) to treat both *pratyāhāra* and *dhyāna* as the arcane body (*kāyaviveka*)" (raṅ gi lugs kyis rdzogs rim gyi rim pa drug la yan lag drug sbyar na / sor bsam gñis lus dben la sbyor ba sgra dbyaṅs bcu gcig pa ltar legs so / ). The mentioned author (**Ekādaśasvara*) is the author of the *Mahāvajradharapathakramo-padeśāmṛtaguhya* (Tohoku catalog No. 1823). What Tsoṅ-kha-pa means by the words "if one treats" is that some authorities treated the first two members as part of the preceding Stage of Generation. Thus, there are three possibilities posited : 1. The first two members belong to the Stage of Completion as 'arcane mind'; 2. they belong there as 'arcane body'; 3. they belong to the Stage of Generation.

A part of the dispute is exposed in Bu-ston's commentary *Bśad sbyar* on the *Pradīpoddyotana* (Collected Works, Ta, f. 172 b, published in Part 9): "Here, the ācārya Abhayākaragupta held that *pratyāhāra* and *dhyāna* belonged to the Stage of Generation; that *prāṇāyāma* is Diamond Muttering, *dhāraṇā* is the Illusory Body and the Clear Light, and that *anusmṛti* and *samādhi* are Yuganaddha. And the author Kumāra claimed that *pratyāhāra* and *dhyāna* are the arcane mind, and that *anusmṛti* is the Illusory Body. Neither are correct" ( / ḥdir slob dpon a-bhyas/ sor sdud bsam gtan bskyed rim daṅ / srog rtsol rdo rje bzlas pa daṅ / ḥdzin pa sgyu lus ḥod gsal daṅ / rjes dran tiṅ ḥdzin zuṅ ḥjug bstan / źes pa daṅ / ku-mā-ras / sor sdud bsam gtan sems dben / rjes dran sgyu lus su byed pa mi ḥthad de /). In the case of Abhayākaragupta, Bu-ston gives the obvious reason that the position is in conflict with the Uttara-tantra (as cited in 'Documents') which places all six members in the superior category understood to be the Stage of Completion; but the reason Abhayākaragupta was forced into his position is that Nāgārjuna's *Pañcakrama* begins with Diamond Muttering (=*prāṇāyāma*, member No. 3). However, Bu-ston apparently believes that the refutation of Abhayākaragupta takes care of Kumāra's position as well—presumably on the grounds that *pratyāhāra* and *dhyāna* cannot be arcane mind except in the conceptual meaning proper to the Stage of Generation; but, as we saw, Candrakīrti may well have this position even though he places all six members in the Stage of Completion ('Documents'). Bu-ston continues by saying, "Some teach the *caryā* with *pratyāhāra* and the arcane body with *dhyāna*; that is most certainly wrong" ( / kha cig sor sdud kyis spyod pa bstan / bsam gtan gyis lus dben bstan / źes pa śin tu mi ḥthad de). By '*caryā*' Bu-ston refers to the technical use of this term, of which there are three kinds alluded to in Tsoṅ-kha-pa's annotation of *nidāna* verse 26 (which see).

Although Bu-ston denies 'arcane body' to *dhyāna*, he goes on to give his own position, "Hence, when one combines the six membered yoga with the five kramas, *pratyāhāra* and *dhyāna* are included in Illusory Body" ( / des na sbyor ba yan lag drug lam rim pa lṅar sdud na sor sdud bsam gtan sgyu lus su ḥdus te /). He also quotes approvingly that "one sees *saṃvṛti-satya* with *pratyāhāra*" (so sor sdud pas kun rdzob kyi bden pa mthoṅ baḥo). Although there may be a difference in usage of the term 'arcane body', it appears to me that Tsoṅ-kha-pa accepts Bu-ston's position; and Tsoṅ-kha-pa's annotation of nidāna verses 22-23 (on Kā-ya) seems indebted to Bu-ston's comment on this 'Kā' (*op. cit.*, f. 55b). The solution was to call these two members the 'saṃvṛti-māyā' stages.

My own solution of the nidāna grouping took account of the mention in verse 22 of the word niṣpanna-krama (Stage of Completion) and in verse 23 of the word niṣpanna-yoga (Yoga of Completion). Since these two verses go with the word 'Kā-ya', it is clear that the author of the nidāna verses of the *Vajramālā* explanatory tantra understood the Stage of Completion to begin with an emphasis on 'body'. To deny that this is 'arcane body' but then to affirm that it is Illusory Body—as Bu-ston did—seems an unnecessary quibbling over words. The nature of this 'body' will become clearer as we proceed.

Now, the *Guhyasamājatantra* has an earlier treatment of yoga that seems to belong to the Stage of Completion, namely in its chapter 6 (see 'Documents'). Verses 3-6 constitute the important block, and we present them here again with the Sanskrit corrected and translated with the help of the *Pradīpoddyotana*, Tsoṅ-kha-pa's *Mchan ḥgrel*, as well as with the *Saṃdhivyākaraṇa* (PTT, Vol. 3, p. 239-3-8) for verse 5:

*mantranidhyaptikāyena vācā manasi coditaḥ* |
*sādhayet pravarāṃ siddhim manaḥsantoṣaṇāṃ priyām* ||3||
*cittanidhyaptinairātmyaṃ vācākāyavibhāvanam* |
*niṣpādayet trisaṃyogam ākāśasamatālayam* || 4 ||
*kāyavākcittanidhyapteḥ svabhāvo nopalabhyate* |
*mantramūrtiprayogeṇa bodhir vinā ca bhāvanām* || 5 ||
*vicāryedaṃ samāsena kāyavākcittalakṣaṇam* |
*bhāvayed bodhisaṃyogaṃ samādhiṃ mantrakalpitam* || 6 ||

The one who has body as the mantra visualized should accomplish, exhorted by speech in the mind, the 'surpassing one', 'successful one', 'one satisfying the mind,' 'beloved one'.

He should accomplish the selflessness of *citta* being visualized, (then) the contemplation of speech (*vācā*) and body, (then) the triple conjunction, (finally) the abode equal to space.

The self-existence of body-, speech-, and mind-visualization is not reached by the praxis of mantra-body, nor is revelation in the absence of contemplation.

> Having pondered in brief this characteristic of body, speech, and mind, he should contemplate the samādhi 'Conjunction to revelation' as constructed by mantra.

Candrakīrti's comment on those verses implies a kind of six-membered yoga among them. 1. 'who has body as the mantra visualized'. 2. 'exhorted by speech in the mind'. 3. 'surpassing one'. 4. 'successful one'. 5. 'one satisfying the mind'. 6. 'beloved one'. There are four states (*avasthā*) to be achieved in the stream of consciousness of a yogin (*yogi-saṃtāna*) : 'surpassing one' because it outlasts diamond muttering (*vajrajāpād adhikatvāt*); 'successful one', i.e. the Svādhiṣṭhāna (=*mahāmudrā*); 'one satisfying the mind' because it is the purification of the *mahāmudrā* (*mahāmudrā-viśuddhikaratvāt*); 'beloved one', which generates the body of Mahāvajradhara. And these four successive states are respectively, 'the selflessness of citta being visualized'; 'the contemplation of speech and body'; 'the triple conjunction' as the divine body made of mind (*mano-maya-devatārūpaṃ*); and 'the abode equal to space'. Therefore, 'exhorted by speech in the mind' refers to the diamond muttering which is outlasted by the *citta* visualized. This diamond muttering is preceded by an achievement referred to as 'body as the mantra visualized'. The 'body as the mantra visualized' must be the achievement of the Stage of Generation kept over for the Stage of Completion, because having already achieved that much, the practitioner will naturally carry over that bodily attainment to the next stage, that of Completion.

The 'self-existence of body-, speech-, and mind-visualization' means the self-existence of the three lights, respectively prajñā, upāya, and upalabdhi, that is to say, 'the selflessness of citta being visualized'. That self-existence is not reached by the praxis of mantra-body, i.e. by having 'body as the mantra visualized', because, the foregoing members show that it is necessary to be 'exhorted by speech in the mind'. On the other hand, without contemplation ('body as the mantra visualized') neither is revelation reached. Having appreciated this point, 'he should contemplate the samādhi "Conjunction to revelation" as constructed by mantra.'

While there are definitely six stages in that formulation, there is no expressed indication that the *Guhyasamājatantra* (first 17 chapters) has in mind here such a division—as the Uttara-tantra imposes, of Stage of Generation and Stage of Completion. It may have implied the two in the *dvandva* of the title, *rahasyāti-rahasya*. But our foregoing materials make it quite clear that the 'body as the mantra visualized' is indeed the accomplishment of the Stage of Generation. If one leaves out that body, the remainder of the members in that passage of chapter 6 pertain to what became called the Stage of Completion. In such a case, the first member in this second series is the one called 'exhorted by speech in the mind', that is to say, diamond muttering attended with *prāṇāyāma*. Tsoṅ-kha-pa's commentary 'Deciding the alternatives' for the chapter 6 (op. cit., Vol. 156, pp. 25-5 to 26-1) cites in this connection the *Vajramālā* explanatory tantra (actually in chapter 68, the last chapter):

*| rdo rje bzlas par rab sbyor bas |*
*| rluṅ gi mtshan ñid śes nas ni |*
*| rnam rtog rluṅ rnams rnam par gcod |*
*| sems la dmigs pa thob par ḥgyur ||*
*| bdag la byin brlabs rim pas kyaṅ |*
*| dṅos grub brgyad ni thob par ḥgyur |*
*| snaṅ ba la sogs dbye ba śes |*
*| mṅon par byaṅ chub pa ni ḥthob |*
*| zuṅ ḥjug rim pa la gnas pa |*
*| dṅos grub thams cad bsdus pa ni |*
*| tshe ḥdi ñid la ḥgrub ḥgyur bar |*
*| rnal ḥbyor pa yis the tshom med ||*

> The one who by the praxis of diamond muttering understands the characteristic of the wind(s), destroys the *vikalpa*-winds and attains visualization of the *citta*. Then, by the Svādhiṣṭhāna-krama he wins the eight *siddhis*. Knowing (already) the distinctions of light (*āloka*), etc. he gains the Abhisaṃbodhi. Stationed on the Yuganaddha-krama, the yogin doubtless accomplishes in this very life the sum of all *siddhis*.

Immediately after this passage, Tsoṅ-kha-pa points out that this is the source of the five kramas. It cannot be doubted that Nāgārjuna based his *Pañcakrama* work especially upon the sixth chapter of the *Guhyasamāja* and the explanatory tantra *Vajramālā*. He has not altered the terminology in the names of the five kramas : 1. Diamond Muttering (Vajrajāpa), 2. Purification of consciousness (Cittaviśuddhi), 3. Personal Blessing (Svādhiṣṭhāna), 4. Revelation-Enlightenment (Abhisaṃbodhi). 5. Pair-wise united (Yuganaddha). Near the beginning of his first krama, he has this summary statement consistent with that sixth chapter and with the *Vajramālā* position :

4B. *mantranidhyaptim āgamya vajrajāpaḥ suśikṣyate*
5. *vajrajāpasthito mantrī cittanidhyaptim āpnuyāt*
*māyopamasamādhistho bhūtakoṭyāṃ samāviśet*
6. *bhūtakoṭeḥ samuttiṣṭhann advayajñānam āpnuyāt*
*yuganaddhasamādhistho na kiṃcic chiṣate punaḥ*

Having understood the mantra-visualization, he trains himself with diamond muttering. Firm in diamond muttering, the yogin achieves the citta-visualization. Stationed in the illusory samādhi, he enters the true limit. Emerging from the true limit, he achieves the non-dual knowledge. Stationed in the pair-wise united samādhi, there is nothing more for him to learn.

That is to say, after one has gained the mantra-body (in the Stage of Generation) he proceeds to the Stage of Completion with that kind of body prepared by yoga (which therefore may or may not be counted as the initial part of the Stage of Completion). If the mantra-body in its developed status as an "arcane body" is not counted in the numbering, then the first member is the diamond muttering. The yogin outlasts this with the state of visualizing the three Lights with their associated eighty *prakṛtis*. Stationed in the illusory samādhi, to wit, with the Illusory Body, he enters the Clear Light in this stage of Personal Blessing (*svādhiṣṭhāna*). In the stage of Abhisaṃbodhi, by the reverse order of the Lights, he achieves the non-dual knowledge. Finally, he attains the yuganaddha wherein there is nothing further to learn (*aśaikṣa-yuganaddha*).

Now returning to our considerations of the six-membered yoga on which Candrakīrti wrote his comments, it seems that the set of terms applies to the yoga praxis in a period prior to this terminology of two main Stages. When it was decided (per Nāgārjuna's system) to begin the Stage of Completion with the diamond muttering along with *prāṇāyāma*, the third member of the other terminological system, it became a problem of how to define the first two members 1. *pratyāhāra* and 2. *dhyāna* in a manner applicable to the Stage of Completion. Nāgārjuna evaded the issue in his commentary on the 18th chapter in which the six-membered yoga was presented. The solution adopted by Tsoṅ-kha-pa is that they represent the arcane body (*kāya-viveka*).

With the help of Candrakīrti's explanations ("Documents"), and availing ourselves of the preceding data, the rest of the correlation in terms of the Guhyasamāja cult can be set up as follows :

| *six-membered yoga* | | *five stages* |
|---|---|---|
| 3. Prāṇāyāma | — | 1. vajrajāpa |
| 4. dhāraṇā | — | 2. cittaviśuddhi<br>3. svādhiṣṭhāna |
| 5. anusmṛti | — | 4. abhisaṃbodhi |
| 6. samādhi | — | 5. yuganaddha |

It should be emphasized that such a correlation may help us to understand the stages of yoga in a terminological sense, and enable us to cross over from one system to the other one; and also that in practice authors settled on either set of terminology; and that either could be used by authority of the *Guhyasamāja-tantra*, which presents them in its Chapter VI and Chapter XVIII.

Finally, I wonder if this remarkable description of yoga is meant to duplicate the Buddha's feat in the celebrated account of the *Parinirvāṇa-sūtra*. Here the Buddha passed beyond the realm of desire up through the various divisions of the realm of form and then the divisions of the formless realm until he reached the cessation of ideas and feelings. He then reversed himself, going through the downward stages in order until he arrived at the lowest division of the realm of form. He then proceeded upwards again until he arrived at the top of the realm of form and then entered Parinirvāṇa. Later, in Mahāyāna Buddhism, for example in the *Laṇkāvatāra-sūtra*, the place where he had entered Parinirvāṇa was considered the place where one is initiated as a Complete Buddha.

### E. *Grouping the nidāna kārikās*

The reason for including this topic under the general discussion of yoga, is that repeated consideration of these forty verses with great labor of collecting commentarial materials for them, finally convinced me that they represent a sequence of yoga, and in that case the only yoga that can apply by authority of the *Guhyasamājatantra* toward any grouping is the four steps in the Stage of Generation and either the six-membered yoga or the five stages in the Stage of Completion.

But before we can take up this matter of grouping, it will be necessary to establish where to place what is called the "hundred lineages". This involves some disputed points about the "arcane body". Some authorities held that the "arcane body" was restricted to the Stage of Completion. In the course of Tsoṅ-kha-pa's lengthy discussion of this topic in his *Pañcakrama* commentary, he states (PTT, Vol. 158, p. 201-4,7,8) : "Since the *Caryāmelāpaka* has stated the arcane body of one hundred lineages to three lineages and then compressed into one lineage, with the Stage of Generation as the basis of inclusion, they should be included there, and so (in that case) it is not proper to include them in the Stage of Completion (rigs brgya nas gsum gyi bar gyi lus dben rnams rigs gcig gi lus dben du sdud par spyod bsdus las gsuṅs pas / bsdu rgyu bskyed rim der de rnams bsdus pa rdzogs rim du mi ruṅ baḥi phyir ro/). When we know that Tsoṅ-kha-pa held Āryadeva's *Caryāmelāpakapradīpa* in highest esteem and drew from that work the entire material on the "hundred lineages" after comparing three versions of Āryadeva's text then extent in Tibet, we must conclude that Tsoṅ-kha-pa gives his own position as far as the "hundred lineages" is concerned. Since Tsoṅ-kha-pa refers to those "hundred lineages" as "arcane body", it is clear to me that his "arcane body" annotations on *nidāna* verses, starting with verse 14 in my third group, is his way of placing those verses in the set describing the Stage of Generation. Although the "hundred lineages" stem ultimately from Āryadeva's work (in the Peking edition, PTT, Vol. 61, p. 295-5, line 7, to 297-5, line 8), I have taken them from the edited form in Tsoṅ-kha-pa's *Pañcakrama* commentary. Here, Tsoṅ-kha-pa (PTT, Vol. 158, p. 201-3-7) mentions that when the "arcane body" is included in the Stage of Generation, it is placed in the Atiyoga step, which is the third of the four steps. Ratnākaraśānti also implies that the "arcane body" is located in the third step by our information included from his book that the blessing is of the sense bases, personality aggregates, the elements and the major and minor limbs.

The "arcane body", which thus begins with yoga praxis in the third step, must continue through the fourth step for the simple reason that it is present at the outset of the next stage, that of Completion. We shall see that this observation agrees with the three kinds of *caryā* of the Stage of Generation, which are illustrated in the Tathāgata verses (*nidāna* verses 18-21). It thus becomes obvious that the *nidāna* verses which invite commentary of portions of the "hundred lineages" belong to the Stage of Generation, and also obvious that the *nidāna* verses beginning with verse 22, which speaks for the first time about the yoga of "completion", belong to the Stage of Completion. All my further collection of material confirmed this division and worked out with continual consistency.

Upon scanning the various commentaries on the *Pradīpoddyotana* in the Tanjur, I find only one commentator who attempts to group the *nidāna* verses. One reason for the general silence of the sub-commentators is that the commentarial flow is interrupted by stopping to comment in a completely different way, as would be necessary with arguments in the case of the *nidāna kārikās*, since Candrakīrti had cited them only in a block without individual remarks or grouping suggestions. Thus, even presuming that these commentators had their own thoughts about grouping, ordinarily it would be only such an independent commentary as the Dalai Lama referred to (cf. Preface) that would try to explain the verses from all possible angles including grouping. By the one commentator I mean the Kumāra whose *Pradīpoddyotana* commentary was noticed in a preceding section. He is probably the same Kumāra who is listed as a translator of Bhavyakīrti's long commentary on the same *Pradīpoddyotana*, so he may even have been a personal disciple of Bhavyakīrti. His commentary is rather brief; he calls it a *ṭippaṇī-hṛdayādarśa* ('Annotation which is the Mirror of the Heart'), and so he concerns himself with what he considers the most important elements of the work he is commenting on, rather than commenting on everything. It is worthwhile to present his solution, even though I do not accept it. He apparently followed this initial course of reasoning: At the end of the citation of the forty verses by the *Pradīpoddyotana*, there appears Candrakīrti's signal '*garbhyartha*' (T. *sbas pa* or *sbas don*). In a previous introduction, I have shown that Candrakīrti's '*garbhyartha*' has the three varieties of 'pregnant sense clarifying the doctrine of lust', 'pregnant sense revealing conventional truth' (=Illusory

Body), and 'pregnant sense considering the three *jñānas*'. Also Tsoṅ-kha-pa's *Mchan ḥgrel* mentions these three varieties when annotating that word '*sbas pa*' at the end of the forty verses, so it was quite reasonable for Kumāra to expect that the three varieties would be found presented among the forty verses. However, it is one thing to exemplify the three varieties somewhere or other; and another thing for the forty verses to fall into three groups, as Kumāra forces them (PTT, Vol. 60, p. 219-5). His first group amounts to verses 1 through 9 :

> */ E ni śes rab dam pa ñid ces bya ba nas / rnam śes ñid ni lṅa poḥo źes bya baḥi bar gyis ni sems rnam par dag paḥi rim pa yin no // ye śes gsum rnam par ḥbyed pa ni gcig tu sbas paḥi don no /.*
>
> From, ' "E" signifies the Noble Women Prajñā,' down to 'perception (*vijñāna*), the fifth', is the stage 'purification of the mind' (*citta-viśuddhi*). Analyzing the three gnoses (*jñānatraya*) is one kind of 'pregnant sense'.

The second group constitutes verses 10-18 :

> */ mñam ñid so sor rtog pa daṅ źes bya ba nas / de daṅ der rigs las ḥbyuṅ ba / lha daṅ lha mo tha dad pa de ni yod min de med kyaṅ / ḥgro baḥi don phyir ston pa yin źes bya baḥi bar gyis ni / lhaḥi sku rnam par dag pa mṅon tu ḥgro baḥi rdo rje bzlas paḥi rim pa bstan to / / deḥi naṅ nas phyag rgya bźi ni rgyas gdab ciṅ źes bya bas ni saṅs rgyas spyan la sogs pa ḥam dgug pa daṅ źugs pa la sogs pa ḥam / las kyi phyag rgya la sogs paḥo / / de ñid ḥdod chags kyi chos ston paḥi sbas paḥi don gñis paḥo /*
>
> From '(the knowledges) Equality, Discriminative....' down to 'Of the different gods and goddesses generated by him and his family, neither the gods nor the goddesses exist, but are displayed for the sake of sentient beings' —shows the stage 'Diamond Muttering' (*vajrajāpa*) which brings directly the pure body of a god. Among those (verses) the phrase 'sealed by four seals' (verse 16) implies either Buddhalocanā and the other goddesses; or attracting, drawing in, etc. (the four steps in bringing nonduality with the *jñāna*-being); or the *karma-mudrā*, etc. Exactly that is the other kind of 'pregnant sense' which teaches the doctrine of lust.

The third group includes verses 19-40 :

> */ ḥdi las gñis med mthoṅ baḥi źes bya ba nas / sbas paḥo źes*

*bya baḥi bar gyi ni sgyu ma lta buḥi tiṅ ṅe ḥdzin bstan pa ste / de kho na raṅ byin gyis brlab paḥi rim bstan paḥo / / kun rdzob kyi bden pa la de ma thag mṅon par byaṅ chub paḥi rim pa ni sbas paḥi don gsum paḥo /*

From 'Afterwards, who sees the non-duality' down to (the signal) 'pregnant sense'—teaches the illusory *samādhi* (*māyopama-samādhi*), and only that teaches the Svādhiṣṭhāna-krama. Immediately after that 'conventional truth', there is the Abhisaṃbodhi-krama. So the third 'pregnant sense'.

The weakness of Kumāra's solution can be judged from these viewpoints: (1) It was reasonable for him to impose stagesfrom Nāgārjuna's *Pañcakrama*, but he does not adhere to the order of the kramas, interchanging the first and second—Cittaviśuddhi and Vajrajāpa. By applying these stages throughout, which are prevalent on the 'Stage of Completion' he leaves no group of *nidāna* verses to depict the 'Stage of Generation', which belies Candrakīrti's verse to the effect that the forty verses explain the *Guhyasamājatantra*, which on the strength of Kumāra's divisions has no Stage of Generation at all. (2) It was reasonable for him to apply the terminology of three kinds of 'pregnant sense' but it is contrary to the obvious data of the verses to divide them into three consecutive groups on this basis. For example, the 'three knowledges (*jñānatraya*) kind of pregnant sense in fact covers the verses 1-7, 25-26, 30, 32, and 36-38. (3) His solution takes no account of the words of the *nidāna* sentence, because his second group (verses 10-18) goes down to the first *ta of tathāgata*. He evinces no indication that he tried to relate the subject matter of the verses to the words which furnish the forty syllables.

Having by those considerations eliminated the one classical attempt to group the verses, the way is clear to group them by appeal to the evidence of the verses themselves. The forty verses divide into sets on the basis of the Stage of Generation and the Stage of Completion, as previously discussed. Verse 22 employs the expression *niṣpanna-krama* ('Stage of Completion'). Therefore, the last nineteen verses are devoted to the Stage of Completion.

Then, within the two sets of verses some groups are obvious and others require further justification. The most difficult group in the first set is formed of the verses for Ekasmin Samaye, to which I assign the second vajra or step of service, *anuyoga*. The decision to make three groups out of the second set yields a solution compatible with the six-membered yoga, the five kramas, as well as with the four steps of service as shared with the Stage of Completion. The full picture in each case is provided in the respective groups. Now I present the final arrangement with some minimal remarks :

I. The Stage of Generation.
   - A. Evaṃ mayā śrutam. Yoga (= Sevā)
   - B. Ekasmin samaye. Anuyoga (= Upasādhana)
   - C. Bhagavān Sarva. Atiyoga (= Sādhana)
   - D. Tathāgata. Mahāyoga (= Mahāsādhana)

II. The Stage of Completion.
   - E. Kāyavākcitta. Pratyāhāra and Dhyāna (= kāyaviveka) Prāṇāyāma (= Vajrajāpa); Dhāraṇā (= Cittavisuddhi and Svādhiṣṭhāna) —Sevā
   - F. Hṛdaya-vajrayoṣid. Anusmṛti (= Abhisaṃbodhi) —Upasādhana
   - G. Bhageṣu vijahāra. Samādhi (= Yuganaddha) —Sādhana and Mahāsādhana

It might be objected that E-VAM applies to both Stage of Generation and Stage of Completion, and therefore it is improper to restrict it to the Stage of Generation, as in my solution. To this argument, one may respond that it is usual in the beginning of the path (e.g. the ten-staged Bodhisattva path, or the present Tantric path of two Stages) for the *guru* to tell the disciple the steps that lie ahead so that he may be realistic about the course he is to follow with its expected fruits. Accordingly, it is quite proper for E-VAM, which condenses the entire path, to appear first and to head the Stage of Generation. This would be the E-VAM of the path of attainment, among the three kinds of E-VAM to be explained later.

Here also a few remarks are in order regarding the correlation of the shared steps of service with parts of the Stage of Completion. Sevā in the Stage of Generation is the conceptual reach up to the Clear Light. In the second stage, the yogin is held to enter the Clear Light with a subtle body in the krama of Svādhiṣṭhāna. Therefore, all the members and kramas up to Svādhiṣṭhāna are the superior kind of Sevā. Upasādhana in the Stage of Generation evokes the 'primeval lord' (*ādinātha*) with a mantra-body (a kind of *mahāmudrā*). In the Stage of Completion, the Abhisaṃbodhi-krama represents the emergence from the Clear Light with the Saṃbhoga body, a knowledge-body (also a kind of *mahāmudrā*). Therefore Upasādhana is the superior step in this case. The remaining correlation is by reason of the distinction in this literature of 'coupling in the realm of learning' (*śaikṣa-yuganaddha*) and 'coupling beyond learning' (*aśaikṣa-yuganaddha*). While there is a beginning of this *śaikṣa-yuganaddha* in the Abhisaṃbodhi-krama, both kinds of *yuganaddha* are proper to Yuganaddha-krama. Sādhana in the Stage of Generation accomplishes the body-maṇḍala and one's own aim; therefore, in the Stage of Completion, it fulfills the *śaikṣa-yuganaddha* of being a Buddha 'in this life' as the lord 'with eight guṇas' (*nidāna* verse 34). Mahāsādhana in the Stage of Generation serves the aim of others; therefore, in the Stage of Completion it is the *aśaikṣa-yuganaddha*, equivalent to the 'Nirvāṇa of no-fixed abode', or the Complete Buddha (Saṃbuddha or Abhisaṃbuddha).

Besides, the basis laid in the Stage of Generation for the later accomplishment of the Stage of Completion can be treated in terms of Tsoṅ-kha-pa's correlation with the three Bodies of the Buddha.

The set "Thus by me it was heard" is associated with silence, death, and the Dharmakāya. For as Nāgārjuna pointed out in his commentary on chapter 18, when the Bodhisattvas were reduced to silence it was because they heard the teaching and entered one-pointed concentration. Thus they became affiliated with the Mind of the Buddha.

The set "Upon an Occasion" is correlated with magical Speech, the intermediate state, and the Sambhoga-kāya, by evocation of the primeval lord.

Then, the set "The Bhagavat—All" affiliates the yogin with the Buddha's Body, the Nirmāṇa-kāya, or birth, as the fulfilment of the microcosm.

The fourth set, "Tathāgata", involves all the previous three, by imagining the Acts of the Buddha in projection upon the external world, the macrocosm.

Then, in the direct order of the three 'doors', the yogin experiences the Body, the Speech, and the Mind, arriving at the supreme plane, the Clear Light. The Diamond Ladies of the Heart draw the yogin from the Clear Light. In the pregnant 'bhaga' they train him in the great attainment of the three mysteries of Body, Speech, and Mind, through which he can dwell, beyond training, to inspire the later candidates.

Also there are technical and scholarly aspects. The principal authorities for that grouping and the consequent annotation of the forty verses are : *Guhyasamājatantra*, especially chapters 6, 12, and 18; its explanatory tantras *Vajramālā* and *Saṃdhivyākaraṇa*; Nāgārjuna's commentary on chapter 18, his *Piṇḍīkṛtasādhana*, his *Pañcakrama* and its commentary by Śri Lakṣmī; Āryadeva's *Caryāmelāpakapradīpa*; Candrakīrti's *Pradīpoddyotana*, especially on chapters 1, 6, and 12; and among native Tibetan works, Tsoṅ-kha-pa's *Mchan ḥgrel* on the *Pradīpoddyotana*, his *Gsal baḥi sgron me* on the *Pañcakrama*, and his *Sṅags rim chen mo.*

PART THREE

# COMMENTARY ON THE FORTY NIDĀNA VERSES

## I. STAGE OF GENERATION

A. *Evaṃ mayā śrutam* (Thus by me it was heard).

Those initial words of the Tantra can be treated in several different ways: (1) separate treatment of the expression 'Evaṃ', (2) separate treatment of the expression 'Evaṃ mayā', and (3) treatment in terms of the six verses going with the words 'Evaṃ mayā śrutam'.

(1) For separate treatment of Evaṃ, there is the *Pradīpoddyotana* (*Mchan ḥgrel*, p. 13) citation of the *Devendraparipṛcchā*. This appears to be the only original passage extant from this Tantra; the selection found in *Subhāṣita-saṃgraha* is included within this longer selection.

*| uktaṃ bhagavatā | devendraparipṛcchāyāṃ | śakras āha |*
*kim artham evam ity etat kasmād ādau prayujyate |*
*kim idaṃ saugataṃ vākyaṃ kiṃ vā śrāvakabhāṣitam |*
*etan me saṃśayaṃ sarvam apanetu bhavāntakaḥ ||*
*śrutvā vākyaṃ surapates saddharmaguṇabhāṣitam |*
*sādhukāraṃ tato datvā bhagavān idam abravīt ||*
*ādav evam iti proktaṃ yad arthaṃ sarvadarśinā |*
*tat śṛṇu tvaṃ surapate yathāvad anupūrvaśaḥ ||*
*dharmaskandhasahasrāṇāṃ caturaśītisaṃkhyayā |*
*sarvāśrayaṃ pitāmātā dvyakṣaraṃ kathitaṃ tathā ||*
*ekāras tu bhaven mātā vakāras tu pitā smṛtaḥ |*
*bindus tatra bhaven yogaḥ sa yogaḥ paramādbhutaḥ ||*
*ekāraḥ padmam ity uktaṃ vakāre vajram eva ca |*
*bindus tatra bhaved bījaṃ taḥ prasūtaṃ jagat trayam ||*
*ekāras tu bhavet prajñā vakāraḥ suratādhipaḥ |*
*binduś cānāhataṃ tattvaṃ taj-jātāny akṣarāṇi ca ||*
*yo vijānāti tattvajño dharmamudrākṣaradvayam |*
*sa bhavet sarvasattvānāṃ dharmacakrapravartakaḥ ||*
*yo 'viditvā paṭhen nityam akṣaradvitayaṃ janaḥ |*
*sa bāhyo buddhadharāṇāṃ dhanivad bhogavarjitaḥ ||*
*evaṃ dvir akṣaraṃ māyā sarvajño 'tra by avasthitaḥ |*
*ādau saddharmaśāstrāṇāṃ tad evaṃ pratigīyate ||*
*tasmāt surādhipa śakra yadi cet śāśvataṃ padam |*
*saddharmo guru kartavyaḥ smara māyā dvir akṣaram ||iti|*

It was said by the Lord in the *Devendraparipṛcchā* : Indra asked :

> Why the term 'evam'? Why is it placed first? Is this an expression coming from the Lord, or is it a comment by a disciple? May the destroyer of phenomenal life remove from me all this uncertainty !
>
> Having heard this discourse of the master of the gods, concerning a merit of the Illustrious Doctrine, the Lord then conferred a 'Sādhu' ('Excellent !') and spoke as follows :
>
> For the purpose of seeing everything, the term 'evam' is stated first. Master of the gods, listen to that which, in regular order according to its full extent, has the count of 84,000 dharmaskandhas, namely, the two syllables, father-mother, the universal receptacle, which express the same.
>
> E is the mother; VA the father, the bindu (ṃ) there the union, and that union a marvel. E is said to be the lotus; diamond the meaning of VA; the bindu there the seed, and this engenders the three degrees of living beings. E is insight (prajñā); VA the lord of pleasure; the bindu is the inviolable reality, and from that arise the letters (of the alphabet).
>
> Whatever knower of the reality recognizes the two syllables as the 'seal of the doctrine', he becomes the setter into motion of the Wheel of the Law among all the sentient beings. Whatever person not knowing (the reality) would constantly recite the two syllables he, outside the Buddha-dharmas, would be like a rich man missing the enjoyment. The two-syllabled 'Evam' is illusion (*māyā*); since omniscience is located therein, that 'Evam' is rehearsed at the outset of treatises of the Illustrious Doctrine. Therefore, Indra, master of the gods, if you would have (your) rank be perpetual, let the Illustrious Doctrine be your master (*guru*). Remember that the two syllables are the *māyā* !

Vajrayāna ('the Diamond Vehicle') is summarized by the three meanings of E-vaṃ—(1) the fruit to be attained, (2) the path of attainment, and (3) the 'signs' guiding that path, for which there is Tsoṅ-kha-pa's summary from his *Mthaḥ gcod*, as presented in my "Female Energy and Symbolism in the Buddhist Tantras," p. 82 :

1. E is the secret place for teaching the doctrine (*dharma*), such as the sky, the *bhaga* ('female organ,' metaphorical), the *dharmodaya* ('source of natures'), the lotus, and the lion's seat. VAM is whoever the Tantra sets forth as the Teacher, be he Vajradhara, Heruka, and so on, who dwells in the *bhaga*, lion's seat, and so on. (These deities symbolize the inseparable union of the void and compassion).
2. E. is 'insight' (*prajñā*), 'voidness' (*śūnyatā*). VAM is 'means' (*upāya*), 'great compassion' (*mahākaruṇā*). Together they constitute the *bindu* (T. *thig le*).
3. E is the mother's *bhaga* place (*ādhāra*) (*yum gyi bhaga rten*). VAM is the father's *vajra* ('male organ,' metaphorical) placed (*ādheya*) therein (*de la brten paḥi yab kyi rdo rje*). This again is of two kinds : (*a*) the external E-vaṃ as 'signs,' the union with the 'seal' (*mudrā*); (b) the internal E-vaṃ as 'signs,' the guiding agent for the path of piercing the vital centers of the *cakras* (the 'wheels' imagined along the spinal column). "Here, 'signs' means signs of the genitals in the sense of shape." These shapes associated with the *cakras* are the triangle and the circle (in other texts, the four geometrical shapes associated with the four elements).

These three meanings of E-vaṃ are especially explained in certain verses. The E-vaṃ of the fruit to be obtained is in verses 30-36 (Vajrayoṣidbhageṣu). The E-vaṃ of the path of attainment is in verses 1 and 2 of the first group of verses. The E-vaṃ of the signs guiding that path is in verses 37 and 38 of the last group of verses.

(2) The separate treatment of Evaṃ mayā is to indicate any four steps of yoga. The four syllables are given symbolic values in Nāgārjuna's *Seka-catuḥ-prakaraṇa* (PTT. Vol. 61, p. 284-5), where the four are said to summarize the meaning of all the Tantras. For example, he says, "E is the voidness-Light; VAM the further voidness-Spread-of-Light; MA great voidness-Culmination-of-Light; and YĀ universal voidness-the single taste (*samarasa*)"/ E ni snaṅ ba stoṅ pas ste/ /VAM ni mched pa śin tu stoṅ/ /MA ni ñer thob chen po stoṅ/ /YĀ ni ro mñam thams cad stoṅ/ These values are immediately

applicable to the first four *nidāna* verses since these serially introduce the four voids or four lights, the fourth light being called the 'Clear Light' (*prabhāsvara*) in the verses, but called 'single taste' by Nāgārjuna at this point. Another set he gives suggests the four steps of *sādhana* in the shared sense : "E achieves the unachieved; VAM reveals the achievement; MA is the going successively higher; YĀ is the becoming of a Complete Buddha in this life"/ E ni ma thob thob par byed/ /VAM ni thob pa bstan par byed/ /MA ni goṅ nas goṅ du ḥgro / / YA ni tshe ḥdir rdsogs saṅs rgyas/. We can associate the four steps of *sādhana* (generalised) with Nāgārjuna's four values:

| *Syllable* | | | |
|---|---|---|---|
| E | 1. | The void palace | Achieving the unachieved |
| VAM | 2. | Residents in the palace | Reveals the achievement |
| MA | 3. | Perfection of the circles | Going successively higher |
| YĀ | 4. | Entrance of the knowledge being | Buddhahood in this life |

(3) When we treat the words Evaṃ mayā śrutam in accordance with the *nidāna* verses, they refer to Yoga, the first of the four parts of sādhana in the sense of the Stage of Generation. As this part is discussed in my sub-section 'The Yoga of the Guhyasamāja', the performer must first make his consciousness soar to the realm of the void. According to Candrakīrti's comment ('Documents') this is done with the help of mantras, of which the most popular one is: /Oṃ śūnyatājñānavajrasvabhāvātmako 'ham/ "Oṃ. I am the intrinsic nature of the knowledge diamond of voidness !" The occupation with the four voids corresponds conceptually to the maṇḍala ritual Rites of the Site'. To prepare the candidate for the later praxis in which the yogin learns to live in those void realms, now he merely imagines in conformity. Since the subsequent praxis involves the ascent into the void stages called Light, Spread-of-Light, and Culmination-of-Light, followed by the Clear Light, the candidate engages his mind with those same mystical states, principally along intellectual lines, but making a break with his previous habits of thought. He divides up the elements of consciousness into three groups. There are 33 female ideas, obscuring the moonlight; 40 male ideas obscuring the sunlight; and 7 androgyne ideas obscuring the dark

light. He contemplates the flow of those 80 ideas in day and night, making a total of 160. Verse E introduces the female, VAM the male, and MA the androgyne. Then verse YĀ, names the Clear Light, the fourth light, the negation of the 160 ideas. Those groupings of female, male, and androgyne ideas may first give the impression that the discussion devolves about our ordinary consciousness. On the contrary, they establish a kind of archetypal world, because those ideas are deemed not to belong to us: they enter our minds. Then the verses ŚRU and TAM turn to the phenomenalization of that anterior world, as indicated by the phrases "The *vijñāna* heard here" and "the wind... operates in the world of living beings".

> //E// *ekāro 'pi satī prajñā virāmādikṣaṇātmikā* /
> *etan mūlaṃ vinirdiṣṭaṃ parijñānaṃ bhavatraye* //1//
> "E" is the Noble Woman (*satī*) Prajñā, the moments of aversion, and so on. This root is designated as the experience in the three worlds.

*Mchan ḥgrel* (hereafter '*Mchan*' when on the verses in their regular order): 'Aversion, and so on'—'the thirty-three ideas, from aversion down to jealousy.' 'Moments'—'the wink of an eye, etc.' 'Designated'—in the Tantras. 'The three worlds'—'of desire, etc.', i.e. realm of desire (*kāma-dhātu*), realm of form (*rūpa-dhātu*), and formless realm (*arūpa-dhātu*).

*Pañcakrama*, II, 8-13: The thirty-three natures (*prakṛti*) are night-time signs (*niśā-saṃjñā*) and female ideas (*strī-saṃjñā*), 'with full-blown form of the covering process' (*saṃvṛtisphuṭarūpeṇa*), as follows (*Pañcakrama* order and my own grouping):

1-3. (incipient) aversion, medium aversion, intense aversion (*virāga*, madhyama-virāga, adhimātra-virāga).

4-9. (thinking of) future, (thinking of) past (anāgata, āgata); sorrow, of three degrees (śoka, madhyama-ś, adhimātra-ś); calmness (saumyam).

10-22. mental wandering (state of being scatter-brained) (vikalpa); fear, of three degrees (bhīta, madhyabhīta, atibhīta); craving, of three degrees (tṛṣṇā, madhya-t, ati-t); indulgence (upādāna); inauspiciousness (niḥśubham); hunger and thirst (kṣut-tṛṣā); feelings, of three degrees (vedanā, sama-v, ati-v).

23-30. intuition (vettivit); memory (dhāraṇāpadam); discrimination (pratyavekṣaṇam); shame of (lajjā); compassion (kāruṇyam); affection in three degrees (snehatas trayam), to wit: (a) protection of the object, (b) adoration of it, (c) over-possession of it (as of a son). 31-33. worry (cakitam); collecting (*saṃcaya*), of utensils, etc.; jealousy (mātsarya).

The annotations of this *nidāna* verse did not clarify the claim that this root is the experience in the three worlds. It may be intended that knowledge through experience is made possible by the degrees of aversion, which seems to be the psychological premise of the Apoha doctrine of Buddhist logic. In this doctrine a thing is defined by exclusion of what it is not. A 'cow' is the not not-cow. What might well be the explanation is that to have the concept cow in the mind requires that a distinct idea of cow be formed, the very clarity and determination of which invloves the removal (*apoha*) of all other non-cow entities. In this way, experiential knowledge (*parijñāna*) occurs with the 'aversion' to everything inconsistent with and contrary to that knowledge. Understanding begins with a kind of retreat. One must neglect the rest in order to appreciate something; and that thing understood means that a faculty of *prajñā* has arisen which understands the rest.

*Pañcakrama*, II, 29:

> */ āśvāsasas tu muhūrtaṃ syān nimeṣo 'kṣinimeṣaṇam/.*
> */ mātrā tu hastatālaṃ syāt kṣaṇādīnāṃ tu lakṣaṇam //*
>
> The characteristic of 'moments' etc. is the short time of an inhalation, the wink of the twinkling eye, the brevity in a clap of hands.

In the *Vajrajñānasamuccaya* (PTT, Vol. 3, p. 252-5), consciousness (*citta*), which is like a bright moon in the water, has the *prakṛtis*, aversion, etc. "In convention (*saṃvṛti*), it is symbolized by the directly manifested woman, the *bhaga*, the *padma*, and the host of goddesses." (kun rdzob tu ni mṅon sum kyi bu med daṅ bha-ga daṅ pad-ma daṅ lha moḥi tshogs kyi brdaḥo/).

> *//VAM// vaṃśas tad bhavad ābhāti rāgādiprasavānvitam/*
> *ālokābhāsa-vijñānam upāya iti saṃjñitam //2//*
>
> That Spread-of-Light *vijñāna* called 'means' (*upāya*),

attended with begetting of desire, and so on, appears like an emerging bamboo.

*Mchan*: 'Desire and so on'—'the forty conceptions from desire down to dishonesty'.

*Pañcakrama*, II, 16-21: The forty natures are daytime and male ideas or signs (*divā-puruṣa-saṃjñā*), as follows (*Pañcakrama* order and my own grouping):

1-7. desire (rāga); attachment (raktam); joy, medium joy, intense joy (tuṣṭam, madhya-t, ati-t); thrill (harṣaṇam); bliss (pramodyam).

8-13. surprise (vismaya); laughter (hasitam); refreshment (hlādana); embracing (āliṅganam); kissing (cumbana); sucking (cūṣaṇam).

14-26. firmness (dhairyam); striving (vīryam); pride (māna); getting things done (kartṛ); theft (hartṛ); strength (bala); enthusiasm (utsāha); daring, medium daring, super-daring (sāhasam, madhyama-s, uttama-s); aggression (raudra); coquetry (vilāsa); animosity (vairam).

27-34. auspiciousness (*śubha; text reads 'lābha') clarity of speech (vāk sphuṭā); truth (satyam); untruth (asatyam) certainty (niścaya); non-indulgence (nirupādāna); giving (dātṛtva); exhortation (codanam).

35-40. heroism (śūratā); lack of shame (alajjā); deception (dhūrta); wickedness (duṣṭa); oppression (haṭha); dishonesty (kuṭila).

The 'Spread-of-Light' *vijñāna* or means (*upāya*), is symbolized by the form of the male.

//MA// *mahāvidyā svayaṃ mūlam avidyayā vilomataḥ/*
*avidyayā bhavec caitat tasmād ālokasaṃbhavaḥ* //3//

In the reverse order, the great Science (=Wisdom) is itself the root of nescience. And the ('Spread-of-Light') arises from nescience (*avidyā*) while from that ('Spread-of-Light') arises Light.

*Mchan*: 'the great Science'—'the Clear Light' (*prabhāsvara*, *ḥod gsal*) (to be specifically mentioned in verse 4). 'nescience'—'the mixture of *prajñā* and *upāya*, thus of *citta* and *caitta*, and generates the seven conceptions of *prakṛtis*, indifference, etc.' (which are therefore androgynous ideas). *Prakāśikā* (by Bhavyakīrti) on MA, p. 292-5; "The great science (*mahā-*

*vidyā*) is the Dharmadhātu-nature, the Clear Light; and why ? As the verse says, it is the reverse of nescience (*avidyā*)" (rigs chen ṅi chos kyi dbyiṅs kyi ṅo bo ste ḥod gsal baḥo / / gaṅ gi phyir źe na / ma rig pa ni bzlog pa yin źes smos te).

*Pañcakrama*, II 24-25: The seven *prakṛtis* are as follows (*Pañcakrama* order and my own grouping):

1-4, indifference (madhyarāga); forgetfulness (vismṛti); illusion (bhrānti); speechlessness (tūṣṇīṁbhāva).

5-7. weariness (kheda); indolence (ālasya); ambivalence (dandhatā).

*Vajrajñāna-samuccaya* (PTT, Vol. 3, 252-4): "Here, the Clear Light is without location, without cessation or orgination, is Supreme Truth (*paramārtha-satya*), and True End (*bhūtakoṭi*). The dark light arisen therefrom is nescience (*avidyā*)"/ de la ḥod gsal ba gnas pa med pa / ḥgag pa med pa / skye ba med pa / don dam paḥi bden pa / yaṅ dag paḥi mthaḥ ste /d e las byuṅ baḥi mun paḥi snaṅ ba ni ma rig paḥo /.

*Guhyasamājatantra* (VII, verse 35):

*|tatra katham anutpādānusmṛtibhāvanā|*
*prakṛtiprabhāsvaraṃ sarvaṃ nirnimittaṃ nirakṣaram|*
*na dvayaṃ nādvayaṃ śāntaṃ khasadṛśaṃ sunirmalam ||*

Here, what is the contemplation, recollection of non-origination ?

The Clear Light with the intrinsic nature is completely signless, unlettered, neither dual nor non-dual, quiescent, spotless like the sky.

*Pañcakrama*, II, 53:

*śūnyatrayaviśuddhir yā prabhāsvaram ihocyate|*
*sarvaśūnyapadaṃ tac ca jñānatrayaviśuddhitaḥ ||*

That purity of the triple void is here called Clear Light. And that is the plane of universal void through purity of the triple knowledge.

*Pañcakrama*, II, 57-62:

57. *tathā coktaṃ mahāyānasūtre lalitavistare /*
*abhisambodhikāmo 'yaṃ śākyasiṃhas tathāgataḥ ||*
58. *mahāśūnyena buddhatvaṃ prāpsyāmīty abhimānataḥ /*
*nirañjanānadītīre niṣpādyāsphānakaṃ gataḥ ||*

59. *tilabimbīva sampūrṇaḥ khavajrasthā jinās tadā* /
*ekasvareṇa taṃ prāhur acchaṭena jinaurasam* //
60. *aviśuddham idaṃ dhyānaṃ na caitad iṣṭakāvaham* /
*prabhāsvaraṃ tu ālambyam ākāśatalavat param* //
61. *prabhāsvarapade prāpte svecchārūpas tu jāyase* /
*sarvaiśvaryaṃ tathā prāpya vajrakāye pramodase* //
62. *evaṃ śrutvā tu taṃ śabdaṃ visṛjyāsphānakaṃ tataḥ* /
*niśārdhasamaye tattvam ālambyaiva jinaurasaḥ* //

So it was said in the Mahāyānasūtra *Lalitavistara*:

The Lion of the Śākyas, the Tathāgata, thought, "I shall attain Buddhahood through the great void;" and seated on the Nairañjanā river bank, went into the Āsphānaka-samādhi (the breath-holding concentration). Thereupon the Victorious Ones dwelling in the diamond of the sky and fulfilled like the sesame fruit, spoke to the Son of the Victorious Ones with a single sound by the snap of fingers. 'Impure is this meditation and non-conducive to the desired goal. Take as meditative object the Clear Light, beyond like the dome of the sky. When you have attained the plane of the Clear Light, you shall emerge with a gratifying form, in that way acquiring universal sovereignty in a delightful diamond body.' Having thus heard that sound, he abandoned the breath-holding concentration, and at midnight visualized reality—did the Son of the Victorious Ones.

Of course, the account as the tantric Nāgārjuna states it, is not actually found in the *Lalitavistara* in those words. It appears to be one tantric interpretation of the purport of the *Lalitavistara*, the Mahāyāna biography of the Buddha. Tsoṅ-kha-pa, when citing the same passage in his *Pañcakrama* commentary (PTT, Vol. 159, p. 59) states (ibid., p. 59-2) that the passage maintains that after coming to the limit of the Mahāyāna path of the Pāramitā, one becomes a Buddha by the supreme path (*anuttara-mārga*) (which of course is the *Anuttara-tantra*) (ces pha rol tu phyin paḥi thegchen paḥi lam gyi mthar bla med kyi lam gyis ḥtshaṅ rgya tshul gsuṅs so /). Tsoṅ-kha-pa goes on to point out that while the part about dwelling in the 'Motionless Samādhi' (*āniñjya-samādhi*) (apparently equivalent to the 'breath-holding, concentration') on the Nairañjanā river bank is indeed in that scripture, the rest of the account is not expressly stated in the *Lalitavistara*. *Mkhas grub rje's Fundamentals of the Buddhist Tantras* devotes its first chapter to the various theories of how Gautama become a Complete Buddha; and in the Tantras the main theories diverge between the Yoga-tantra and the Anuttarayoga-tantra specialists.

Śrī Lakṣmī's discussion in her *Pañcakrama* commentary (PTT, Vol. 63, p. 29) mentions that the 'single sound' (*ekasvara*) refers to 'Thus' (*evaṃ*) 'on an occasion' (*ekasmin samaye*) by purport of single meaning (/de la dbyaṅs gcig ni don gcig la dgoṅs nas dus gcig tu ḥdi skad gsuṅs so /). She goes on to the two varieties of the Clear Light discussed previously in my introduction on this topic, and claims that the 'Clear Light of consciousness' is meant in the present account: "Here, according to what I heard from my venerable teacher, we maintain it is only *citta-prabhāsvara*" ( / ḥdir rje btsun gyi źal sṅa nas kyis/sems kyi ḥod gsal ba kho no bźed pa yin te/). Her statement implies the word '*prabhāsvara*' qualifying the word '*citta*' in the Abhisaṃbodhana chapter of the *Lalitavistara*, where the word is employed three times for each of the three watches of the night (an old division of time) during which Gautama attained Complete Enlightenment.' According to my introduction, the 'Clear Light of consciousness' is equivalent to the Clear Light of deep or dreamless sleep.

> //YĀ// *yāti vijñānam ādau tad ālokābhāsa-saṃjñitam/*
> *tan mahāśūnyatāṃ yāti sā ca yāti prabhāsvaram* //4//
>
> At first, that *vijñāna* (i.e. Light) passes to what is called 'Spread-of-Light'. That passes to the Great Void and the latter passes to the Clear Light.

*Mchan*: 'Passes to' in each case means 'dissolves in'.

This is the direct order, *anuloma*, of the three Lights leading into the fourth or Clear Light, the latter being mentioned in the *nidāna* verses for the first time along with the terminology of voidness. For the sequence, cf. *Pañcakrama*, II, 4: "Void, further void, and great void, the third, as well as universal void, the fourth—by distinction of fruit (the succeeding one) and cause (the preceding one)" (/śūnyaṃ ca atiśūnyaṃ ca mahāśūnyaṃ tṛtīyakam/ caturthaṃ sarvaśūnyaṃ ca phalahetuprabhedataḥ//).

Besides the direct and the reverse order, there is the recitation order, frequently indicated by the Sanskrit words rāga, dveṣa, moha, as in *Guhyasamāja* (Chap. VIII, p. 32):

*rāgadveṣamohavara vajrayānapradeśika/*
*ākāśadhātukalpāgra ghoṣa pūjāṃ jinālaya//*
"O, the best of lust, hatred, and delusion, explaining the Vajrayāna;
O, the best like the plane of the sky, the womb of the Victorious Ones,
Pray announce the *pūjā* !"

*Pradīpoddyotana* on the preceding: 'best of lust, hatred, and delusion', because the Vajrayāna purifies lust, hatred, and delusion.' *Mchan ḥgrel* on Chap. VIII (PTT, Vol. 158, p. 62-2): The three 'poisons' or basic defilements—lust, hatred, and delusion are associated with the three lights. 'Lust' stands for the 40 prakṛtis covering 'Spread-of-Light'; 'hatred' for the 33 prakṛtis covering 'Light'; 'delusion' for the 7 prakṛtis covering 'Culmination-of-Light'. (The three terms 'lust', 'hatred' and 'delusion' are apparently to be understood in generalized senses, to wit, 'lust'—all attraction towards, desire, 'hatred'-all repulsion, aversion; 'delusion'—all intermediate and indecisive states, indifference).

The following passages give further information on the direct order.

*Pañcakrama*, II, verse 5:

*prajñopāyasamāyogān niṣpannam upalabdhakam /*
*upalabdhāc ca niṣpannāt sarvaśūnyaṃ prabhāsvaram //*
Through union of *prajñā* and *upāya*, the Culmination (of Light) is perfected; and through Culmination perfected, there is universal void, the Clear Light.

Śrī-Lakṣmī comments (Vol. 63, p. 23-3-4):

/daṅ po śes rab kyi ye śes skye ba daṅ/ de nas gñis pa thabs kyi ye śes daṅ po las lhag pa skye ba ste / de gñis ga sbyor ba las ñe bar thob pa ni ye śes gsum pa rdzogs par ḥgyur ro / / de nas ñe bar thob pa rdzogs nas thams cad stoṅ paḥi ḥod gsal ba ni ye śes bźi paḥi ḥog nas bśad par ḥgyur baḥi sṅags daṅ/ phyag rgyaḥi rim pas rnal ḥbyor pa la snaṅ bar ḥgyur ro/

First arises the Prajñā knowledge; then, second, arises over the first the Upāya knowledge; from the union the third knowledge, which is Culmination (of Light), is completed. Then, through the completion of the Culmination, the Clear Light, the fourth knowledge, which is universal void, manifests to the yogin by a sequence of *mantra* and *mudrā*, as will be explained below (cf. *Pañcakrama*, II, 48-50, cited later).

Nāgārjuna's *Piṇḍīkṛta-sādhana*, 43-44A (some additions from Ratnākaraśānti's commentary, PTT, Vol. 62, p. 75-5) refers to the direct order with consideration of the body-maṇḍala:

*ūrdhvādhaḥkrodhasaṃyuktaṃ prakṛtyābhāsam eva ca* /
*vijñānaskandham āyāti vijñānaṃ ca prabhāsvaram* //
*sanirvāṇaṃ sarvaśūnyaṃ* (*ca*) *dharmakāyaś ca gadyate* /

Precisely the Light (triad) with its (160) prakṛtis, associated with the upper (i.e. Uṣṇīṣacakravartin at the Brahmarandhra, the orifice at crown of head) and the lower (i.e. Sumbharāja at sole of feet) Wrathful (Kings; cf. *nidāna* verse 17), passes to the aggregate of perceptions (*vijñāna-skandha*) (Akṣobhya and Māmakī); and perception (passes) to the Clear Light, also called 'universal void with *nirvāṇa*' and 'Dharmakāya'.

//ŚRU// *śrutaṃ yad iha vijñānam ābhāsatrayalakṣaṇam*/
*prakṛtīnām idaṃ mūlaṃ sattvadhātor aśeṣataḥ* //5//

The *vijñāna* heard here has the characteristics of the three lights. This is entirely the root of the *prakṛtis* (natures) of the sentient-being realm.

*Mchan*: "Heard here are both the essential nature (*ṅo bo*) and the sequence (*go rims*), meaning both the path and the four states (*avasthā*). First (the disciple) is taught how to dwell in the four, and then taught how to generate the path consistent therewith."

Tsoṅ-kha-pa's *Mchan* note about four states undoubtedly refers to the three lights and the Clear Light. The path doubles the (80) prakṛtis by contemplation in both day and night, per *Pañcakrama*. II, 27: "Those subtle prakṛtis proceed in both day and night, thus to total 160, by cause of wind-conveyance" (etāḥ prakṛtayaḥ sūkṣmāḥ śataṃ ṣaṣṭyuttaraṃ divā/ rātrau cāpi pravartante vāyuvāhanahetunā//).

But how should we understand the word '*vijñāna*' of *nidāna* verse 5? *Vajrajñānasamuccaya* (PTT, Vol. 3, 252-4): ',That *vijñāna* arisen from the Clear Light is called 'consciousness' (*citta*), 'mind' (*manas*), and 'perception' (*vijñāna*); and that is entirely the root (*mūla*, *rtsa ba*) of *dharmas*. Therefrom defilement and purification give rise to two false conceptions, that of 'oneself' and that of the 'other'." (/gaṅ ḥod gsal las byuṅ ba rnam par śes pa de ñid sems daṅ yid daṅ rnam par śes pa źes bya la / de ni chos thams cad kyi rtsa ba ste / kun nas ñon moṅs ba daṅ rnam par byaṅ baḥi bdag ñid de las rtog pa gñis su gyur te bdag daṅ gźan dag tuḥo/). Bu-ston (*Bśad sbyar* on ŚRU, f. 50a) says, "From the wind arises fire, from that water, from that earth; from that the personality aggregates, the elements, and the sense bases; (that is the meaning of the passage, to wit) 'from that, arise the three lights, and from that arise the 160 prakṛtis.' From that arise the 98 defilements, the 62 false views, and so on. Because sentient beings arise with a birthplace by dint of the so-amassed *karma*, the text says 'this is the inexhaustible root of the sentient-being realm'." (/ rluṅ las me / de las chu / de las sa / de las phuṅ po khams daṅ skye mched ḥbyuṅ / de las snaṅ ba gsum ḥbyuṅ / de las raṅ bźin brgya drug cu ḥbyuṅ ṅo / de las ñon moṅs pa dgu bcu rtsa brgyad daṅ lta ba drug cu rtsa gñis la sogs pa ḥbyuṅ / des las bsags paḥi dbaṅ gis skye gnas gźiḥi sems can ḥbyuṅ bas sems can gyi khams ma lus paḥi rtsa ba ḥdi yin no /). Besides, Tsoṅ-kha-pa, commentary on the *Vajrajñānasamuccaya* (PTT, Vol. 160, 154-3, 4), following the Mādhyamika point of view, insists that the *vijñāna* meant by the three lights is *manovijñāna*. Also, in his commentary on the *Caturdevīparipṛcchā* (Lhasa Coll. Works, Vol. Ca, f. 37b-6 to 38a-1): "The three *vijñānas* proceed from the 18-fold *dharmadhātu* which is the Clear Light of Death. They (the three) are *bodhicitta*—the Bodhisattva Samantabhadra." *Ibid.* f. 37b-3: "The *dharmadhātu* is the source of the six outer sense bases, the six personal sense bases, and the six perceptions (*vijñāna*), 18 in all." (The sixth perception is the *manovijñāna*, the other five being based on the five outer senses). This use of the Bodhisattva name 'Samantabhadra' presumably stems from the *Guhyasamāja*, Chap. IV. p. 17 (*Mchan ḥgrel*, p. 38):

> *śāntadharmāgrasambhūtaṃ jñānacaryāviśodhakam* /
> *samantabhadravācāgryaṃ bhāṣa maṇḍalam uttamam* //

"Pray explain the supreme maṇḍala having the best speech of Samantabhadra, arising from the summit of quiescent *dharmas* (=*paramārtha-satya*) and purifying (the 80 prakṛtis) by the praxis of the gnoses (=the three lights)."

My "Notes on the Sanskrit term Jñāna," p. 260, quotes from Tsoṅ-kha-pa's commentary on the *Vajrajñānasamuccaya* (Lhasa ed., Vol. Ca) to the effect that the *vijñāna* ('perception') arising from the Clear Light of dying from the Intermediate State (*bar do*) is the Culmination of Light; the *manas* ('mind') arising from that, is the Spread-of-Light; the *citta* ('consciousness') arising from that, is Light. Observe that the order: 1. delusion (=vijñāna), 2. lust (=manas), 3. hatred (=citta) is consistent with the order of appearance of the three 'poisons' in the Buddhist genesis legend, as discussed in my article "Buddhist Genesis and the Tantric Tradition."

But the tantric Nāgārjuna, Śrī Lakṣmī, Bhavyakīrti, and some other Tanjur commentators, employ a Yogācāra-type vocabulary, to wit: *ālaya-vijñāna*, *kliṣṭa-manas*, and *pravṛtti-vijñāna*. The following tabulation should make the difference clear:

| Lights=Voids | The Covering=80 Prakṛtis | | |
|---|---|---|---|
| | Mādhyamika terminology | Yogācāra terminology | Terminology in common |
| The Clear Light=Universal Void | | | |
| Culmination-of-Light=Great Void | Perception (vijñāna) | Basic perception (ālaya-vijñāna) | Nescience (avidyā) |
| Spread-of-light =Further Void | Mind (manas) | Defiled Mind (kliṣṭa-manas) | Mentals (caitta) |
| Light=Void | Consciousness (citta) | Evolving Perception (pravṛtti-vijñāna) | Consciousness (citta) |

Therefore, when Bhavyakīrti in his '*Prakāśikā*' (PTT, Vol. 60,

p. 293-1) comments on *nidāna* verse 5, he first states '*vijñāna*' to be the three as previously explained, meaning the three Yogācārā terms he has been employing for explaining the preceding *nidāna* verses; and states these *vijñānas* to have the characteristic (*lakṣaṇa*), i.e. the prakṛtis of (covering) the three lights; and so those lights appear when those *vijñānas* cease. Then Bhavyakīrti quotes two texts without naming their sources. The first is the celebrated verse of the *Saṃdhinirmocana-sūtra* (which was translated by Etienne Lamotte into French; and the verse is in Louis de la Vallèe Poussin, *Vijñaptimātratāsiddhi*, I, p. 173): "The *ādānavijñāna*, profound and subtle, like a violent current, proceeds with all its seeds (*bīja*). Deeming it improper for them to imagine it as a self, I have not taught it to the immature auditors" (/ ji skad du / len paḥi rnam par śes pa zab ciṅ phra / sa bon thams cad chu boḥi rgyun bźin ḥbab / bdag tu rtog par gyur na mi ruṅ źes / ñan thos byis pa rnams la ṅas ma bstan / źes ḥbyuṅ ba). The next one he quotes, is a well-known line from the *Madhyānta-vibhāga* (I, 8A; 20 in Gadjin M. Nagao's edition of the *Bhāṣya*): "And the imagination of unreality (*abhūtaparikalpa*) is the three worlds with their *citta* and caitta" (/ de bźin du yaṅ / yaṅ dag ma yin kun brtags ni / sems daṅ sems byuṅ khams gsum pa / źes ḥbyuṅ ṅo /). These quotations do not necessarily mean that Bhavyakīrti makes the usual identification of *ādānavijñāna* with *ālayavijñāna*, which he equates with the *avidyā* having seven prakṛtis; but it certainly means that he considers the '*vijñāna*' of *nidāna* verse 5 to be this *ādānavijñāna* as well as *abhūtaparikalpa*; and so he may understand by '*ādānavijñāna*' all three *vijñānas* rather than simply *ālayavijñāna*. Since his *ālayavijñāna* is equivalent to verse 3's '*avidyā*', it is unacceptable to Tsoṅ-kha-pa, who rejects the equation in PTT, Vol, 159, p. 31-3. In fact, both Bu-ston and Tsoṅ-kha-pa in their annotation of the *nidāna* verses agree in ignoring Bhavyakīrti's commentary. This subject is resumed under *nidāna* verse 7.

//TAM// *tam ekaikam arthābhāsaṃ vāyus saṃgṛhya dhārayet/*
*vāyuyuktaṃ ca vijñānaṃ śaśvaj jagati vartate* //6//

The wind seizing, takes hold of that entity-light in each case, and *vijñāna* joined with *vāyu* (wind) continually operates in the world of living beings.

*Mchan*: " 'Entity-light in each case' means the five sense objects as manifested. They arise by the 'reverse order' of the three lights (vijñāna-manas-citta) and dissolve by the 'direct order' (citta-manas-vijñāna). Vijñāna (=the three lights or vijñāna, manas, citta) rides on the winds which seize their respective sense objects."

*Pañcakrama*, II, 32-34:

*vayunā sūkṣmarūpeṇa jñānaṃ sammiśratāṃ gatam /*
*niḥsṛtyendriyamārgebhyo viṣayān avalambate //*
*ābhāsena yadā yukto vāyur vāhantāṃ gataḥ /*
*tadā tatprakṛtāḥ sarvā astavyastāḥ pravartayet //*
*yatra yatra sthito vāyus tāṃ prakṛtim udvahet/*
*yāvat samīraṇotpādo nābhāso niścalo bhavet //*

When 'knowledge' (jñāna = the three lights) becomes associated with subtle-formed wind, then issuing forth from the paths of sense organs it grasps ('hangs on to') the sense objects.

At whatever time the wind, having become a vehicle (for vijñāna), is yoked by the 'light', at that time all those prakṛtis are completely dissipated.

At whatever (vein, *nāḍī*) the wind stops, at that one it sustains some prakṛti (among the 80 prakṛtis). As long as (the wind) stirs up, the 'light' is not steady.

Verses 33-34 mention the alternate conditions of the three gnostic lights (Light, Spread-of-Light, and Culmination-of-Light), namely (II, 33) when those lights are free from the eighty prakṛtis, and (II, 34) when they are subjected to the eighty prakṛtis in which event their 'light' is not steady. The *Maṇimālā* commentary on the *Pañcakrama* (PTT, Vol. 62, p. 188-3, 4) explains the second verse:

/ re źig rluṅ gi rnam lṅa daṅ rnam pa bcu yin par sṅar bśad ciṅ deḥi gnas sñiṅ ga la sogs paḥi gnas rnams daṅ las kyi bye brag kyaṅ bstan mod kyi ḥon kyaṅ raṅgi ṅo bo dpyad na chos kyi dbyiṅs kyi ḥkhor lo ḥod gsal ba las rluṅ byuṅ ste / dehī phyir gYon daṅ gYas daṅ bar maḥi rtsa gsum ni lam yin no / de bas na gaṅ daṅ gaṅ du ste gYon nam gYas sam dbus su rluṅ gnas pa ni raṅ bźin de daṅ de ste sems las byuṅ baḥi chos de lta bu daṅ de lta bu skyed par byed ciṅ ḥbyuṅ bar byed do / / de bźin du yaṅ rtsa gVon paḥi lam nas byuṅ baḥi rluṅ gi śes rab kyi ṅo bo raṅ bźin rnams skyed par byed do / / gYas na gnas pas ni thabs kyi ṅo bo rnams so / / dbus na gnas pa ni ma rig paḥi ṅo bo rnams skyed par byed mod kyi ḥon kyaṅ dmigs pa la bltos dgos te /....../ de ltar rtsaḥi bye brag daṅ rjes su mthun paḥi yul ḥdzin pa las raṅ bźin rnams ḥbyuṅ ṅo /

Now the topic is the five kinds and the ten kinds of wind, as previously set forth, which are located in the heart and in the other places. While they are taught as the multitude of deeds ('perform all deeds'), if one ponders their intrinsic nature, they are the wind which arises from the Clear Light of the Dharmadhātu circle. Therefore their path is the three *nāḍis*, left, right, and middle. Hence, 'at whatever one,' left, or right, or middle, 'the wind stops', it generates while arising there the comparable prakṛti or sort of *caitasika-dharma*. Accordingly, the wind arising in the path of the left *nāḍi* generates the (thirty-three) prakṛtis which have *prajñā* nature; the one of the right, the (forty) prakṛtis of *upāya*; and the one in the middle generates the (seven) prakṛtis of *avidyā*. However, that needs dependence on a support of consciousness (*ālambana*)....Thus, the prakṛtis arise from apprehending a sensory object consistent with the basic multitude (of deeds).

The implication of the *Maṇimālā* commentary is that as long as the winds are correlated with external objects, the lights of the three *nāḍis* are unsteady. Hence the *yogin* must close the sensory doors to dissipate the prakṛtis associated with those *nāḍis*.

*Saṃdhivyākaraṇa* (PTT. Vol. 3, p. 236-2):

*/ byaṅ chub sems ni rluṅ gyur ciṅ /*
*/ nam mkhaḥ la ni rnam gnas pa /*
*/ sems can kun gyi srog gyur gaṅ /*
*/ lṅa yi bdag ñid bcu miṅ can //*
*/ rten ḥbrel bcu gñis źes grags pa /*
*/ ṅo bo ñid rnam gsum du gyur /*
*/ rluṅ źes bya baḥi byaṅ chub sems /*
*/ dbaṅ po kun gyi gtso ḥdi yin //*

> The *bodhicitta* which being wind and dwelling in space, then becomes the life wind of all sentient beings, is five and called ten.
> The *bodhicitta* called 'Twelvefold Dependent Origination' is the three natures; and called 'wind', governs all the sense organs.

*Pañcakrama*, I, 3 (and *Sṅags rim*, 408b-5 and 440a-4, etc.):

> *prāṇabhūtaś ca sattvānāṃ vāyv-ākhyaḥ sarvakarmakṛt |*
> *vijñānavāhanaś caiva pañcātmā daśadhā punaḥ ||*
> Being the life force of sentient beings, what is called 'wind' performs all deeds; and as the vehicle of *vijñāna* is five, besides is tenfold.

In the case of 'wind' as the vehicle of *vijñāna* it is the five secondary winds, to wit:—

1. nāga reveals forms through eye
2. kūrma reveals sounds through ear
3. kṛkila reveals odors through nose
4. devadatta reveals tastes through tongue
5. dhanañjaya reveals tangibles through torso

In the case of 'wind' identified with *prāṇa* itself, it is tenfold, i.e. the five basic winds as well as the five secondary winds. Cooperating with *vijñāna* the five basic winds perform all deeds and the five secondary winds perceive all things. Notice the respective approximation to the classical Sāṃkhya karmendriyas ('perform all deeds') and buddhīndriyas ('perceive all things').

Regarding the 'all deeds' performed by the five basic winds, *Sṅags rim* (f. 439b-2) draws upon a citation in *Caryāmelāpaka* about the function of those winds:

1. Prāṇa has the nature of streaming through the sense doors, coursing as the breathing and extending far (*prāṇa* and *āyāma*), and continually coursing.
2. The yogin will always understand *apāna* as (breaking) wind, expelling urine, excrement, and semen, and conveying downward.
3. Samāna is so called because it is what is always concomitant with tasting, eating, licking, drinking and sucking.
4. One understands udāna to have the action of drawing upwards, eating food and enjoying it, associating with awareness.

5. Vyāna has the function of filling, holding, (enabling) walking and returning, and of pervading all the joints.

*Pañcakrama*, III, 19:

*tad eva vāyusaṃyuktaṃ vijñānatritayaṃ punaḥ |*
*jāyate yoginā mūrtir māyādehas tad ucyate ||*

Besides, precisely that vijñāna-triad joined to the winds is engendered as a body by the yogin. That is called 'Illusory Body'.

The conception of these winds is a topic in the Stage of Generation. Later, in the Stage of Completion, the yogin learns to control them to engender a body called 'Illusory Body'.

### B. *Ekasmin samaye* (*Upon an Occasion*)

This group of verses represents the meaning of the Stage of Generation (*utpattikrama*) as ordinary generation, but with the 'climactic times' of birth, death, and intermediate state, which a theory (see verse 38 and annotation) correlates to the Bodies of the Buddha. The meaning of this group of verses is frequently referred to in Tibetan literature such as Tsoṅ-kha-pa's writings as 'the basic time' (*gźiḥi dus*) to contrast with 'time of the path' (*lam gyi dus*). In the path, the yogin seeks to evoke the entire cycle, passing through the portals of death as an experience of yoga and then returning to normal consciousness. In preparation for the separation from the coarse body of a subtle body called the Illusory Body that takes place in the Stage of Completion, in the present phase the practitioner develops a body which is called the Mantra body. This takes place in the second *sādhana* called Anuyoga with depositing of germ syllables in spots of the body. It corresponds in external maṇḍala ritual to the second part 'Rites of preparatory acts,' such as pitching the lines with chalk and beseeching the gods. A similar result is obtained in the present instance if the practitioner, following through the suggestions of this set of verses, goes through the imaginative procedure of analyzing his make-up and then of identifying his personality aggregates with the five winds and so on. In short, the verses can be interpreted as doctrinal assertions, but above all they are directions for praxis in the form of imaginative identifications.

Concerning the present and the anterior conditions of 'ordinary generation', Kluḥi-blo's (Nāgabuddhi's) *Samāja-sādhana-vyavasthāli* (PTT, Vol. 62, p. 7-5, ff.) mentions the standard four birthplaces, to wit, birth from eggs, birth from a womb, birth from warmth and moisture, and birth through transformation; and then gives standard examples, as birds, etc. from eggs; cows, etc. from a womb; worms, etc. from warmth and moisture; and the gods, hell beings, intermediate state beings, and men of the first aeon, through transformation. All those beings are called *sattva* ('sentient being'). This work also gives the tantric version of Buddhist genesis that was introduced into Tibetan literature such as Tsoṅ-kha-pa's writings. Kluḥi-blo mentions, p. 8-4, that after the men of the first aeon tasted the *amṛta*, and so on down to their partaking of the primeval grain, whereupon their bodies became heavy—the light disappeared, and a darkness ensued; and then the sun and moon appeared in the world. At this time, through the separation of *prajñā* and *upāya*, the beings became distinguished with the male and female organs. Gradually, mutual craving was aroused, whereupon these beings, known as *gandharvas*, experienced the three states (*avasthā*), and entered into the wombs of 'mothers'. Then the women, without illness, began to have menses; and a 'father' and 'mother' through desire for each other, engaged in various sexual techniques. Seeing this, for the sake of 'indulgence-in-desire', a *vijñāna-pati*, as though riding on a horse (=the wind), left the intermediate state and entered (the mother) through the Vairocana-portal (i.e. the crown of the head) (and then merged with the agglomeration in the womb). As to the reason these beings fell from the Clear Light (p. 8-2): "Although they possessed the gnosis body (*jñāna-deha*), they did not know the Illusory Samādhi, ...." (ye śes kyi lus can yin yaṅ de rnams kyis sgyu ma lta buḥi tiṅ ṅe ḥdzin mi śes śiṅ....).

Of course, that account has profound implications for the whole *Guhyasamāja* praxis. Tsoṅ-kha-pa's *Don gsal ba* commentary on the *Guhyasamājatantra* combines Kluḥi-blo's account with the *abhidharma* teaching of 'sentient-being worlds' (*sattva-loka*) and 'receptacle worlds' (*bhājana-loka*) as well as with the tantric idea of the 'primeval lord' (*ādinātha*). The whole idea of transmuting the body into a palace containing the thirty-two deities is to replace the impure receptacle worlds with a pure world, and this is founded on the evocation of the 'primeval lord' in the present (Anuyoga) phase. While most of the *nidāna* verses in this group do not obviously show themselves as a phase of yoga, the last one, *nidāna* verse 12, sets forth the praxis of *prāṇāyāma*, and *prāṇāyāma* is generally described as 'subtle yoga' (*sūkṣma-yoga*). *Prāṇāyāma* is accompanied by mantra-praxis, hence in this phase the yogin gains the 'mantra-deha'.

The school of Buddhajñānapāda, especially in Buddhaśrījñāna's *Mukti-tilaka-nāma*, and its commentary Vitapāda's *Muktitilaka-nāma-vyākhyāna*, discusses this situation using the terms 'the Profound (zab mo)' and 'the Bright' (gsal ba)'. Thus, in Vitapāda's commentary (PTT, Vol. 65, p. 136), we read that the meaning of 'the Profound' and 'the Bright' has been obscured for time immemorial by dint of habit forces (*vāsanā*), and because the ordinary persons do not understand those two, they are plagued by the sufferings of the three realms. "What is the 'Profound'?" In this regard, (Buddhaśrījñāna) states (the obscuration), 'discursive thought (*vikalpa*)....' That is to say, (the 'Profound') rightly and from the outset surpasses all forms of speech and conception because it is free from all forms of error (*bhrānti*)....What is the 'Bright'? (He) states, 'the Mahāmudrā....' That is to say,... the unborn body which is like an illusion and shines like a rainbow....The self-existence of the non-duality of the Profound and the Bright has the nature of pervading all states (*bhāva*) and is not included in the *dharmas* of *saṃsāra*; it is called Dharmadhātu." Combining this terminology with the previous account, the sentient beings did not know the 'Profound' because they lacked the Illusory Samādhi. Therefore they gradually lost the 'Bright', the Illusory Body.

> //E// *eṣo vāyur mahādhātur vijñānatrayavāhanaḥ* /
> *tebhyaḥ prakṛtayaḥ śaśvan nirgacchanti yathā yathā* //7//
> This wind, the great element, is the mount of the three *vijñānas*. By means of it, the *prakṛtis* always proceed accordingly.

*Mchan*: 'This wind' means the wind of action (cf. *Pañcakrama* verse cited under verse 6, wherein the wind is said to 'perform all deeds'), and therefore is called 'great element'.... It is written in the *Vajrajñāna-samuccaya*, "The wind is the mount of that *vijñāna*. From the wind arises fire; from fire, water; from water, earth. From those, the five personality aggregates (*skandha*), the six sense bases (*ṣaḍāyatana*), and the five sense objects;... and the *prakṛtis* are generated by reason of the manifestation." In that Tantra, the three lights are explained to arise from the Clear Light, and subsequently the wind, etc. arises. The mount of *vijñāna* as imagination (*parikalpa*) arises from the ordinary 'lights' of the reverse order, which are the phase of rebirth by transmigration into the womb.

The explanatory tantra *Vajramālā* states further how that wind is responsible for generation. This passage inaugurating its chapter 32 is involved with Yogācāra vocabulary; it is here translated with the help of Alaṃkakalaśa's commentary (PTT Vol. 61, p. 251-4,5 to p. 252-1, 2):

1. Now listen to a further explanation and rightly understand concretely how the wind has the characteristic of generation and seeks the temporal opportunity.

*| de nas gźan yaṅ bśad kyis ñon |*
*| rluṅ skye ba yi mtshan ñid ni |*
*| dus kyi glags ni brtsal ba ni |*
*| ji ltar dṅos su yaṅ dag śes ||*

2. The mind defiled (*kliṣṭamanas*) by habit-energy (*vāsanā*) sees its own (wind) nature as (though it were) another form. Not knowing the real state of affairs (the *prāṇa* and *apāna* winds), it is deluded by just wind alone.

*| bag chags ñon moṅs can gyi yid |*
*| raṅ gi ṅo bo gzugs gźan mthoṅ |*
*| don ni yod par mi śes śiṅ |*
*| rluṅ tṣam gcig pus rmoṅs paḥo ||*

3. Conjured up by *ālayavijñāna*, the habit-energies roam around within. *Vijñāna* is controlled by habit-energy through (death's) sequence of admixture with habit energy.

*| kun gźi rnam śes bkug nas ni |*
*| bag chags naṅ du rnam par spyod |*
*| bag chags kyis ni rnam śes bzuṅ |*
*| bag chags daṅ ḥdres rim pa las ||*

4. Then, by the infusion of inner habit-energy, at the time of (welling up) menses, it evolves in the mother's

channel as a diamond *bindu* of the melted semen and blood.

*| naṅ gi bag chags bsgos pa yis |*
*| de nas zla mtshan dus su ni |*
*| mṅal gyi rtsa la ḥjug pa ni |*
*| rdo rje khu khrag źu thig le ||*

5. It develops according to the admixture; *vijñāna* is aroused by the *ālaya* as though intoxicated by wine: from the habit-energies of *ālayavijñāna* the stream of *vijñāna* arises.

*| ḥdrespa ru ni gyur pa daṅ |*
*| kun gźi las ni rnam śes skye |*
*| ji ltar chaṅ ros myos pa bźin |*
*| kun gźi rnam śes bag chags las ||*

The verses 3-5 are the portion quoted by Tsoṅ-kha-pa in his commentary on the *Vajrajñānasamuccaya* (PTT, Vol. 160, p. 154-4, 5) with the remark, "The '*ālaya*' and '*kliṣṭamanas*' mentioned in this Tantra (the *Vajramālā*) are the same terms explained in other texts but have different meanings" (/rgyud ḥdir kun gźi daṅ ñon yid ces gsuṅs pa ni gźuṅ gźan nas bśad pa daṅ miṅ ḥdra yaṅ don mi ḥdra ste). I have come to understand that by 'other texts' he means the commentaries by the tantric Nāgārjuna and Bhavyakīrti, as well as Śrī Lakṣmī among others, that insist on assigning the terms *ālayavijñāna*, *kliṣṭamanas*, and *pravṛtti-vijñāna* to the three sets of *prakṛtis*, adding up to eighty, thereby equating *ālayavijñāna* with the 'nescience' (*avidyā*) of *nidāna* verse 3. Tsoṅ-kha-pa's rejection of this application of Yogācāra terms is consistent with how we may interpret those *Vajramālā* verses in its chapter 32. That is because, in terms of Buddhist Dependent Origination, the *Vajramālā* verses can be interpreted as setting *ālayavijñāna* equivalent to 3. *vijñāna* as a stream of consciousness which had undergone death's trauma and now (having 1. *avidyā* and 2. *saṃskāra*, as 'conditions') with reviving habit-energy is attracted to a new birthplace offering a field for evolving perceptions

That phase of attraction to the womb is stated in terms of *gandharva*-consciousness in Tsoṅ-kha-pa's *Sṅags rim chen mo* (f. 438a-4,5):

*| de las stoṅ chen ñer thob ste dri zaḥi sems so |*
*| de las thabs snaṅ ba mched pa ḥdod pa ñe bar len paḥi sems so |*
*| de las śes rab snaṅ ba ste skye ba gzuṅ baḥi sems so |.*

From that (Clear Light of Death) comes the great void, Culmination-of-Light, which is the *gandharva*-consciousness. From that, comes the means, Spread-of-Light, which is the indulgence-in-desire consciousness (**tṛṣṇopādāna-citta*). From that, comes the insight, Light, which is the seizing-of-birth consciousness (**janma-grāhaṇa-citta*).

The above passage has terminology associated with members 8-10 of Buddhist Dependent Origination: 8. craving (*tṛṣṇā*), 9. indulgence (*upādāna*), and 10. gestation (*bhava*). After considering the foregoing two selections from the *Vajramālā* and the *Sṅags rim*, it becomes credible that the three lights are the *Guhyasamāja* tradition of recasting the first three members of the 12-membered Buddhist Dependent Origination (*pratītya-samutpāda*); while the same three lights interpreted to start with *gandharva*-consciousness are explanatory of members 8, 9, and 10 of that same Dependent Origination.

To be explicit:—

| | *Dependent Origination* | *Bodhicitta stages* |
|---|---|---|
| 1. | nescience (*avidyā*) | Culmination-of-Light |
| 2. | motivations (*saṃskāra*) | Spread-of-Light |
| 3. | perception (*vijñāna*) | Light |
| 4. | name-and-form (*nāma-rūpa*) | |
| 5. | six sense bases (*ṣaḍāyatana*), | |
| 6. | contact (*sparśa*), | |
| 7. | feeling (*vedanā*); then, | |
| | *Dependent Origination* | *Rebirth consciousness* |
| 8. | craving (*tṛṣṇā*) | *gandharva*-consciousness |
| 9. | indulgence (*upādāna*) | indulgence-in-desire consciousness |
| 10. | gestation (*bhava*) | seizing-of-birth consciousness |

11. birth (*jāti*), and
12. old age and death (*jarā-maraṇa*).

// KA // *kaḥ khaṭidhātur āpaś ca tejo vāyus tathaiva ca /*
*upādāya tu vijñānaṃ jāyate tribhavālaye //8//*

What be the solid realm and of water; likewise that of fire and wind—using these, *vijñāna* takes birth in the womb of triple gestation.

*Mchan*: "At the time of transmigration, the *manovijñāna* uses as base the four elements within the 'semen-blood' entity and thus takes birth in the abode of triple gestation—superior, middling, and inferior destiny."

The grammatical formation of the first sanskrit line, with *ca.... tathaiva ca*, pairs the four elements in a manner consistent with astrology, wherein earth and water (the hard and soft 'heavy' elements) are mutually concordant, as are fire and wind (the hot and cold 'light' elements). Furthermore, the order of elements in the verse is that in which the equivalent goddesses Locanā, Māmākī, Pāṇḍarā, and Tārā ask their questions in the explanatory tantra *Caturdeviparipṛcchā*.

The four elements and their evolutes constitute the aggregate of form (*rūpa-skandha*) among the five aggregates. *Vijñāna* uses this aggregate of form to become embodied in the *ālaya* ('abode') which means the womb according to *Mchan ḥgrel* on the present verse. Hence, the verse practically defines the celebrated term *ālayavijñāna*, which thus means '*vijñāna* in (or toward) the womb' as the 3rd member of Dependent Origination or a phase of that member. The location of *vijñāna* in the womb is understood to be the place which becomes the heart of the new being. Thus, in his *Dkaḥ gnad* commentary on the *Guhyasamāja* (Lhasa ed., Vol. Ca, 10a-1), Tsoṅ-kha-pa starts by quoting passages about the supreme A, the indestructible syllable in the middle of the heart; and says, "In short, the very place where the *vijñāna* along with its 'together-born' (*sahaja*) wind enters amidst the 'semen-blood', is the heart. Also at the time of death it passes away from the heart when gathered in the expiring sequence" (/ mdor bsdu na daṅ por rnam par śes pa lhan cig skyes paḥi rluṅ daṅ lhan cig tu khu khrag gi dbus su gaṅ źugs pa de ñid sñiṅ ga yin la / ḥchi baḥi tshe ḥaṅ ḥbyuṅ ba rim gyis bsdus nas sñiṅ ga nas ḥchi ḥpho ba yin no /).

At that 'heart' site, according to the citations and discussion of *Sṅags rim*, f. 435a-2, ff., first the three primary channels of right, left and middle, are established. Then the five veins of the heart are originated. These veins are deified by goddesses, especially named in Mother Tantra tradition: Traivṛttā is form (rūpa), Kāminī is sound (śabda), Gehā is odor (gandha), Caṇḍikā is taste (rasa), and Māradārikā is *dharma*.

Māradārikā is in the middle and hence associated with the middle channel of Avadhūti; however, the five are separately counted to add up with the primary three to the total of eight, referred to as the eight petals of the heart. The other four goddesses are placed in the four directions and are said to be the self-existence of the four elements (*dhātu-svabhāva*). As the other cakras are established these goddesses transfer their essence accordingly; so it is theoretically possible to identify the four goddesses of the directions with the four of the *Guhyasamāja*, Locanā and so on. The numbers of petals in the other cakras are multiples of the original four directional veins of the heart. In the full list, according to the *Sṅags rim*, f. 436b-4, quotation from Abhayākaragupta's *Āmnāya-mañjarī*, there are 4 petals at the Uṣṇīṣa-cakra (crown of head at place of Brahmarandhra), 32 at the forehead cakra (sometimes misunderstood to be at the crown of the head because of the Tibetan word *spyi bo*), 16 at the throat, 8 as mentioned at the heart, 64 at the navel, 32 at the cakra of the sacral place, and 8 at the 'tip of the gem' (root of the penis). However, the intrauterine order of establishing the element bases, according to the *Sṅags rim* discussion, shows reversal within the pairs of the *nidāna* verse: 1st month 'water' vortex in heart; 2nd, 'earth' vortex in sacral region; 3rd, 'wind' vortex in navel; 4th, 'fire' vortex in throat (or neck). In the 5th month, '*ākāśa*' is invested throughout the body.

The *Sṅags rim* (f. 438a-6) cites the *Mahāmudrātilaka*, apparently as Āryadeva's quotation in his *Caryāmelāpaka*, with a different order of the elements:

*| rnam śes ṅo bo la brten nas |*
*| daṅ por ḥbyuṅ ba bźi po la |*
*| raṅ bźin ṅes par bskrun pa yis |*
*| de tshe raṅ gi gnas nas thim ||*
*| rnam śes las ni rluṅ skye ste |*
*| de las me ni yaṅ dag ḥbyuṅ |*
*| ḥdi las chu rnams yaṅ dag ḥbyuṅ |*
*| de las sa ni yaṅ dag ḥbyuṅ ||*
*| ḥdi rnams las kyaṅ phuṅ po ḥbyuṅ |*
*| de las skye mched rnams kyaṅ ṅo ||*
*| de las śes paḥi raṅ bźin can |*
*| drug cu lhag paḥi brgya rim pas |*

*| ji ltar skyes pa de ltar ḥdir |*
*| thim par ḥgyur ro raṅ bźin las || źes....*

When initially the form of *vijñāna* takes recourse to the four elements through the propagation of prakṛti(s), at that time it passes away from its own abode.
From *vijñāna* the wind arises; from that the fire; from the latter the waters arise, and from these the earth.
From these (four), in turn the personality aggregates (*skandha*) arise; from these the sense bases as well. From the latter, the holder of the prakṛtis of consciousness, in a sequence of 160, dissolves here in the same way as it was born, from the prakṛtis.

*|| SMIN || asmiṃś ca pañca saṃbhūtāḥ skandhās saṃskṛtilakṣaṇāḥ |*
*rūpavin nāma saṃskārā vijñānaṃ caiva pañcamaṃ ||9||*

And when this is present, the five skandhas arise with the characteristic of construction:—possessing 'form' is 'name'—the (three) saṃskāras, as is also perception (*vijñāna*), the fifth.

*Mchan* : "As previously stated, when this—the four elements—is present, the five *skandhas* arise. Arising with the characteristic of construction, the five are form (*rūpa*), feelings (*vedanā*), ideas (*saṃjñā*), motivations (*saṃskāra*), and perceptions (*vijñāna*)."

In the verse the word *saṃskāra* stands for the three middle *skandhas*—*vedanā*, *saṃjñā*, and *saṃskāra*—and labelled 'name' (*nāma*). The fact that in Buddhist Dependent Origination, the '*nāma*' of '*nāma-rūpa*' stands for the three middle *skandhas* of *vedanā*, *saṃjñā*, and *saṃskāra*, is an ancient teaching preserved in Buddhaghosa's *Visuddhimagga* in the chapter on Dependent Origination, section devoted to *nāma-rūpa*. On the other hand, when the term '*nāma-rūpa*' is employed for the five skandhas in discussions apart from Dependent Origination, it is standard for '*nāma*' to include *vijñāna* as well. *Guhyasamājatantra*, Chap. XVIII, verses 45-47, with emendation of verses 45, 46 :

*vijñānaṃ dveṣam ākhyātaṃ hetukāryadvayair dviṣāt |*
*rūpaṃ moham iti khyātaṃ jaḍabandhasvabhāvataḥ ||*
*vedanā ghaṭṭamānākhyā ahaṃkārasvabhāvataḥ |*
*saṃjñā saṃrāgam ātmanaṃ vastutaḥ Śaktilakṣaṇaṃ ||*

*saṃskāras tu sadā īrṣyā pratītya preraṇātmanām |*
*svabhāvaṃ bodhicittaṃ tu sarvatra bhavasambhavam ||*

Vijñāna is called 'hatred' because it is hostile to both cause and effect. Rūpa is called 'delusion' because its nature is insentient bondage. Vedanā is called 'stirring pride' because its nature is egoism. Saṃjñā is 'lust', having the character of attachment to things. Saṃskāra is always 'envy', being the instigation in dependence. (Their) intrinsic nature is *bodhicitta*, the source of gestation everywhere.

Celu-pā's *Ratnavṛkṣa-nāma-rahasya-samāja-vṛtti* (PTT, Vol. 63, p. 174-4) explains the attribution to *vijñāna* :

/ źe sdaṅ źes pa ni rgyu ḥbras gñis dbyer med par thugs su chud paḥi ye śes te / gñis kyi rnam pa la sdaṅ baḥi phyir ro // ji skad du / rgyu ḥbras gñis la sdaṅ bas na / rnam śes źe sdaṅ źes su bstan źes so // de ñid rigs te thog ma med pa nas rgyun chad pa med paḥi phyir ro /.

Called 'hatred' means it is the knowledge fully comprehending in an inseparable manner both cause and effect, because it hates the (separate) aspects of both. It is said, "Because it is hostile to both cause and effect, *vijñāna* is called 'hatred'." That is valid, because it (i.e. *vijñāna*) has been uninterrupted for immemorial time.

The idea seems to be that the notions of cause and effect require discontinuity—the cause must end so the effect may begin. But the 'stream of consciousness' (*citta-saṃtāna*), here the '*vijñāna*', is continuous, not discontinuous. So it is said (metaphorically) to hate cause and effect. Without this plausible explanation by Celu-pā, I would have supposed that the reason *vijñāna* is called hostile toward cause and effect is that the latter are inferred, not perceived, otherwise stated, *vijñāna* is the eternal *present*.

There is considerable commentarial material on the five skandhas, and since this topic is so important to the Tantras, more information is now given. There is (1) the order of treating the *skandhas*, (2) the locations attributed to the *skandhas*, (3) further explanation of the individual *skandhas*, and (4) the *skandhas* in the Intermediate State.

(1) For the order of the *skandhas*, we may refer to Alaṃkakalaśa's commentary on the *Vajramālā*, the *Gambhirārtha-dipikā*-

*nāma* (Vol. 61, p. 204-4) : "The basic nature (*ṅo bo ñid*) of the five skandhas is as follows :—

Prāṇa is vijñāna-skandha;
Apāna is vedanā-skandha;
Samāna is saṃjñā-skandha;
Udāna is saṃskāra-skandha;
Vyāna is rūpa-skandha." (This passage will be continued under the next *nidāna* verse).

While the *nidāna* verse calls *vijñāna* the 'fifth', it is usual in 'pregnant embryology' of the Tantras to assign vijñāna-skandha to the first lunar month, since in Buddhist dogmatics vijñāna is said to fall into the womb. The above passage from Alaṃkakalaśa's commentary states the traditional order of *skandha*-arising in the womb, namely during first through fifth lunar months. The old Buddhist order of stating the *skandhas*, to wit : *rūpa*, *vedanā*, *saṃjñā*, *saṃskāra*, *vijñāna*—is said by Buddhaghoṣa in *Visuddhimagga* (of course in terms of the Pāli equivalents) not to be the order of arising, rather to be the order of explanation difficulty, starting from the easiest to explain, namely *rūpa*. Hence, when it is a matter of giving definitions of the *skandhas*, that explanation order is followed.

(2) The locations of the *skandhas* is hinted at in a passage of the *Guhyasamājatantra*, Chap. XVI, verses 66-67A, which I discussed at length in my article, "The fivefold Ritual Symbolism of Passion," Part I. This is the passage :

*khavajramadhyagataṃ cintet mañjuvajraṃ mahābalam /*
*pañcabāṇaprayogeṇa mukuṭāgraṃ tu saṃsmaret /*
*pañcasthāneṣu mantrajñaḥ krūravajreṇa pātayet /*

The knower of *mantras* should contemplate in the middle of the diamond sky Mañjuvajra/ (=Mañjuśrī) of great power; he should recollect the crest pinnacle by the praxis of five arrows (which) he makes fall, by the diamond of ferocity, into five spots.

As that article explains, the *yogin* deposits five *mantras* in locations of the *skandhas* as targets for five arrows shot by a red Mañjuśrī in the sky (the Clear Light) to instill the essence of the five Tathāgatas, thus identifying the five *skandhas* with the five Tathāgatas. Those five *mantras* as germ syllables, with the respective *skandhas* and Tathāgatas, are set forth in Nāgārjuna's *Piṇḍikṛtasādhana*, verses 56-60. :

*Vairocaṇīyabījaṃ tv oṃkāraṃ śuklavarṇakam* /
*Rūpaskandhasvabhāvena nyasen mūrdhani mantravit* //
*Āḥkāram amitābhasya saṃjñāskandhasvabhāvakam* /
*Raktavarṇaṃ mukhe dhyātvā vāgaiśvaryam avāpnuyāt* //
*Akṣobhyasya tu hūṃkāraṃ rājāvartakasuprabham* /
*Vinyased dhṛdaye mantrī vijñānaskandharūpataḥ* //
*Svākāraṃ ratnanāthasya vedanāskandharūpataḥ* /
*Pītavarṇaṃ nyasen nābhau vedanā-śuddhihetukam* //
*Pādadvaye tu hākāraṃ saṃskāraskandhabhāvataḥ* /
*Haritābhaṃ nyasen mantrī karmanāthasya tattvataḥ* //

The knower of *mantras* will place at his head Vairocana's germ syllable Oṃ of white color, because it is the intrinsic nature of the personality aggregate of form.
Having contemplated in the throat Amitābha's red Āḥ, pertaining to the intrinsic nature of the aggregate of ideas, he attains lordliness of speech.
The *mantrin* should deposit in his heart Akṣobhya's Hūṃ, shining like the deep blue gem, as the form of the aggregate of perceptions. He should place at the navel a yellow Svā belonging to the Jewel Lord (=Ratnasambhava) and the cause of purifying feelings, because it is the form of the aggregate of feelings.
The *mantrin* then deposits in both feet a Hā of green light, as the reality of the Karma Lord (=Amoghasiddhi), because it is the nature of the personality aggregate of motivations.

(3) For further explanations of the skandhas, in fact there are many such in non-tantric Buddhist commentaries. Here it suffices to present the explanations in the Explanatory Tantra *Vajramālā*, Chapter 23 (PTT, Vol. 3, p. 214-1,2) :

/ phra rags la sogs dbye ba yis / / thogs bcas thogs med mtsham ñid daṅ / /ḥbyuṅ ba chen po bźiḥi dṅos / / ḥdi ni gzugs kyi phuṅ por gsuṅs / / der ni rnam snaṅ ṅo bo daṅ / /thams cad spros par byed . paḥi rgyu / / bde daṅ sdug bsṅal mchog tu źi / /graṅ daṅ dro ba mchog gi mchog / /gaṅ gis śin tu rig pa ni / / de ni tshor baḥi phuṅ por bśad / / rin chen ḥbyuṅ ldan ñid kyi mtshan / / de bźin gśegs paḥī spros bdag ñid / / glaṅ po boṅ bu lce sbyaṅ daṅ / /rta daṅ ri dags daṅ ni phag / / pha daṅ ma daṅ pha yi spun // mdzaḥ bo snag gi gñen tshan sogs // gaṅ gis yaṅ dag śes pa ni / / ḥdu śes phuṅ poḥi mtshan ñid ni / de bźin gśegs pa ḥod dpag med / / de ni spros pa kun nas gsal / ḥgro ba khyab par yoṅs su śes / / dge daṅ mi dgeḥi las ḥbras bu / / gźan yaṅ luṅ du ma bstan miṅ // de yi ḥdu byed du ni bśad // don yod spro baḥi raṅ bźin can / /ḥkhor ba dṅos daṅ dṅos med sogs / / kun rtog ḥbyuṅ baḥi bdag ñid can // rnam śes źes ni rnam par śes // mi bskyod spro baḥi bdag ñid can /

1. The characteristic of being obstructing and non-obstructing by division into subtle and coarse, etc.. and the substance of the four great elements—this is said to be the aggregate of form (*rūpa-skandha*). Therein is the nature of Vairocana and the basis of all manifestation.

2. Whereby one feels joy and suffering and the highest calm; cold, heat, and the furtherest supreme—that is explained as the aggregate of feelings (*vedanā-skandha*). It has the character of Ratnasambhava and the egoity of Tathāgata manifestation.

3. Whereby one recognizes a cow, an ass, a jackal, a horse, a deer, a hog; father, mother, brethren on the father's side; friends, relations on the mother's side, etc.—that characteristic of idea aggregate (*saṃjñā-skandha*) is the Tathāgata Amitābha and that clarifies the manifestation.

4. The thorough knowledge pervading the world, the fruit of good and evil deeds, besides being named the indeterminate (*avyākṛta*), what is explained as their motivations (*saṃskāra-skandha*) is Amoghasiddhi, the own-being (*svabhāva*) of the manifestation.

5. The perception of presences and absences of *saṃsāra*, etc.; what has the nature of *vikalpa*-arising, the (aggregate of) perceptions (*vijñāna-skandha*) is Akṣobhya, the soul of the manifestation.

The above is self-explanatory except in a few particulars which are explained in Alaṃkakalaśa's commentary (PTT, Vol. 61, p. 235-3). In the case of the *saṃskāra-skandha* he says, "Besides being named the indeterminate means that its intrinsic nature is indeterminate, because it generates the realms of form, formless, and so on" (gźan yaṅ luṅ ma bstan miṅ źes bya ba ni / luṅ ma bstan paḥi raṅ bźin te / gzugs daṅ gzugs med la sogs pa bskyed paḥi phyir ro). In the case of the *vijñāna-skandha*, he explains the 'presences' (*bhāva*) and 'absences' (*abhāva*) this way : "A 'presence' has the nature of efficiency (*arthakriyākāritva*) ; an 'absence' is the reverse of that" (dṅos po ni don byed nus paḥi bdag ñid can no / /dṅos med ni de las bzlog paḥo). This explanation is consistent with Tsoṅ-kha-pa's explanation of Mādhyamika philosophy in the *vipaśyanā* (discerning the real) portion of his *Lam rim chen mo*, where he defends the position at length that entities arise dependently, void of intrinsic nature but possessed of efficiency.

An intriguing feature of the above *Vajramālā* passage is that while it explains more about the *skandhas* it is not directly explanatory of the *Guhyasamājatantra*; for example, it does not explain the passage about the *skandhas* in chapter 18 (the Uttara-Tantra), e.g. that *vijñāna* is called 'hatred'. It does set forth the standard correspondence of *skandhas* to Tathāgatas, which is a matter of conceptual praxis in the next group of verses ('Bhagavān-Sarva'). This and other passages of the *Vajramālā* suggest that its 'explanatory' nature consists in giving more information consistent with the *Guhyasamāja*. In the present case, once the *skandhas* are so identified, one can proceed to correlate that chapter 18 passage with the current information to associate the Tathāgatas respectively with the defilements (*kleśa*), as follows : 'hatred'—Akṣobhya, 'delusion'—Vairocana; 'stirring pride'—Ratnasambhava; 'lust'—Amitābha; and 'envy'—Amoghasiddhi.

(4) The *skandhas* in the Intermediate State are already a teaching of non-tantric Buddhism in a scripture entitled *Ārya-nanda-garbhāvakrānti-nirdeśa* (in the collection called *Ratnakūṭa*) :

> /de la bar ma doḥi phuṅ poḥi dbyibs de yaṅ rnam pa gñis su gyur te/ kha dog sdug ciṅ mdzes pa daṅ / kha dog mi sdug ciṅ mi mdzes paḥo / / sems can dmyal ba rnams kyi bar ma doḥi srid paḥi kha dog mi sdug pa yin te / ḥdi lta ste dper na sdoṅ dum tshig pa daṅ ḥdraḥo//dud ḥgroḥi rnams kyi bar ma doḥi srid paḥi kha dog ni ḥdi lta ste / dper na dud pa daṅ ḥdraḥo / / yi dag kyi bar ma doḥi srid paḥi kha dog kyaṅ ḥdi lta ste / dper na chu daṅ ḥdraḥo / / lha daṅ mi rnams kyi bar ma doḥi srid paḥi kha dog ni ḥdi lta ste / dper na gser gyi kha dog daṅ ḥdraḥo / / gzugs kyi bar ma doḥi srid paḥi kha dog

ni dkar por ḥdug go / / gzugs med paḥi khams kyi lha rnams ni bar ma doḥi srid paḥi kha dog med de / ḥdi ltar de ni gzugs med paḥi phyir ro /

Now, that form of the Intermediate-State *skandha* is of two kinds—of pleasant, lovely color; and of unpleasant, ugly color. The color of the Intermediate State of sentient beings who are hell beings, is unpleasant, in this way; for example, like the burnt stump of a tree. The color of the Intermediate State of animals is this way : for example, like smoke. The color of the Intermediate State of hungry ghosts (*preta*) is this way : for example, like water. The color of the Intermediate State of gods and men is this way: for example, like the color of gold. The color of the Intermediate State of the 'realm of form' (*rūpa-dhātu*) is abiding white. The Intermediate State of the 'formless realm' (*arūpa-dhātu*) gods, has no color, for the reason that it is formless (*arūpa*) (i.e. since 'form' means shape, *saṃsthāna*, and color, *varṇa*).

The above description goes with the five-destiny list, omitting any reference to the *asura* destiny which in some lists brings the total to six.

// SA// *samatā pratyavekṣaṇā kṛtyānuṣṭhānam eva ca* /
*ādarśo dharmadhātuś ca asmin vijñānapañcakaḥ* //10//

Just (the knowledges) Equality, Discriminative, Procedure-of-duty; as well as (the knowledges) Mirror-like and Dharmadhātu. In this (knowledge-pentad) is the *vijñāna*-pentad.

*Mchan* does not help here, but mentions the theory that the Dharmadhātu kind is the basis of the other four knowledges. The solution that is faithful to the expression '*vijñāna*-pentad' should be the five proper functions of the sense organ of mind that correspond to the five knowledges as explained by Tsoṅ-kha-pa, *Pañcakrama* commentary (Vol. 158, p. 204-5) : (1) the bright appearance of objects like the bright reflection on a mirror; (2) equality consisting in the unified experience of the three kinds of feeling (i.e. pain, pleasure, and neutrality); (3) remembering the various names of beings, such as one's father and mother ; (4) remembering the deeds and needs of the world; (5) the transmutation (*parāvṛtti*) through elimination of impurity. Now, these are obvious references to the five *skandhas*, and consistent with the fact that this *nidāna* verse 10 groups apart the three middle knowledges on the first line (hemistich), comparable to the three middle skandhas being set apart in *nidāna* verse 9. This suggests that the term '*vijñāna*-pentad' means the five having *vijñāna* as salient member. This would permit the Mādhyamika type correspondence between the five skandhas and five knowledges. Thus, Alaṃkakalaśa's commentary on the *Vajramālā* (continued from citation under *nidāna* verse 9) states that when the personality aggregates (*skandha*) are pure, their equivalent winds correspond to the five knowledges as follows:

| *Wind* | *Skandha* | *Knowledge* |
|---|---|---|
| Prāṇa | vijñāna | dharmadhātu |
| apāna | vedanā | equality |
| samāna | saṃjñā | discriminative |
| udāna | saṃskāra | procedure-of-duty |
| vyāna | rūpa | mirror-like |

Of course the term '*vijñāna*-pentad' can also mean the five *vijñānas* based on the five 'door' senses, that ride on the five ancillary winds, as is shown elsewhere. In this case, the five *vijñānas* also correspond to the five knowledges by way of the five-Tathāgata correspondence to sense objects, presented under *nidāna* verse 21.

For individual explanations of the five knowledges, among many such there is a fine statement by Śrī Lakṣmī (*Pañcakrama* commentary, p. 29-1) :

> / ḥgyur ba med pa ni me loṅ lta buḥi ye śes te / dri ma med paḥi me loṅ bźin du tha dad med paḥi phyir ro / snaṅ ba med pa ni mñam pa ñid kyi ye śes ste / raṅ daṅ gźan gyi dbye ba so sor mi snaṅ phyir ro / / gñid med źes pa ni so sor rtog paḥi ye śes te / sgrib pa gñis rnam par dag paḥi phyir ro / / mchog ni bya ba nan tan grub paḥi ye śes te / dmigs pa med paḥi sbyor bas gźan gyi don mdzad paḥi phyir ro / / źi ba ni chos kyi dbyiṅs kyi ye śes te / bdag med pa gñis mṅon sum du mdzad paḥi phyir ro /.

> The mirror-like knowledge is unchanging, because there is no difference (i.e. it is a faithful reflection) in a clear mirror. The equality knowledge does not appear, because it has no appearance separately of a division

into oneself and another. The discriminative knowledge does not sleep, because it is the purity of the two hindrances (of defilement and the knowable). The procedure-of-duty knowledge is best, because it performs the goals of others by a praxis without aim. The Dharmadhātu knowledge is calm, because it produces in immediacy the two kinds of non-self (of *pudgala* and of *dharma*).

// MA // *manaāyatanaṃ caiva locane śravane tathā* /
*ghrāṇajihvā tataḥ kāyaś cety āyatanasaṃbhavaḥ* //11//

The sense base of mind, that of eye, so of ears, nose, tongue, then of torso—thus is the origination of the sense bases.

*Mchan* : By the condition (*pratyaya*) of accomplishing 'name-and-form' (*nāma-rūpa*) in the womb, the six sense bases arise—thus the origination of the sense bases in the womb.

*Mchan* alludes to the correspondence of ten lunar months to sequential development of five *skandhas* and then *āyatanas* in the womb. The sense base of mind arises in the fifth lunar month, then the five 'door' sense bases in the stated order of the verse during the lunar months sixth through tenth. In the traditional treatment, to the fifth lunar month are assigned both the *rūpa-skandha* and the *manaāyatana*.

Chapter 32 of the *Vajramālā* identifies the first five lunar months of the embryo with the first five Viṣṇu Avatars along with the sequential emergence of the five basic winds, and the second five with the emergence of the five secondary winds (Alaṃkakalaśa's commentary adds the second five Avatars). Table No. IV has some further data added from Rgyal-Tsḥab-Rje's *Dpyid thig zin bris* (Lhasa collected works, Vol. Ka, f. 7b-8a) /.

In the explanatory tantra *Caturdevatāparipṛcchā*, and accordingly in its commentary by Smṛtijñānakīrti, the *Upadeśa-pauṣṭika* (PTT, Vol. 66, p. 160-1) the discussion about the embryonic states of *mer-mer-po* (S. *arbuda*), etc., is followed immediately by mention of the nine orifices of the body :

/ don de gsuṅs pa sgo dgu la ni kun tu ḥgro źes pa ste , spyi bo tshaṅs paḥi bu ga daṅ / mig daṅ / rna ba daṅ sna daṅ / kha daṅ / sñiṅ ga daṅ / lte ba daṅ / gsaṅ ba daṅ / chu miṅ (*sic.* for chu mig) gi bu ga rnams dguḥo // de rnams la byaṅ chub kyi sems khyab par gyur to źes paḥi tha tshig go /

## IV. INTRA-UTERINE CORRESPONDENCES

| *Avasthā in womb* | *Skandha and āyatana perfected* | *Viṣṇu Avatar* | *Winds* | *Base of Wind or Orifice* |
|---|---|---|---|---|
| 1. | vijñāna | Fish | prāṇa | heart |
| 2. | vedanā | Tortoise | apāna | sacral region |
| 3. | saṃskāra | Boar | samāna | navel |
| 4. | saṃjñā | Man-Lion | udāna | neck |
| 5. | rūpa and mana-āyatana | Dwarf | vyāna | 12 great *dhātu* |
| 6. | locana | Paraśu-Rāma | nāga | eye |
| 7. | śravaṇa | The 2nd Rāma | kūrma | ear |
| 8. | ghrāṇa | Kṛṣṇa | kṛkila | nose |
| 9. | jihvā | Buddha | devadatta | tongue |
| 10. | kāya | Kalkī | dhanañjaya | torso |

The meaning stated as 'going every where in the nine orifices' is a reference to the *bodhicitta's* pervasion in those nine orifices, to wit : 1. brahmarandhra at the top of head, 2. eyes, 3. ears, 4. nose, 5. mouth, 6. heart, 7. navel, 8. the anus, 9. the urinary passageway.

*//YE// ye vai traidhātuke sattvāḥ prāṇāyāma-samāśritāḥ /*
*mantrarājaṃ japanty ajñā dhyānādhyāpana-varjitāḥ //12//*

The beings in the three worlds taking recourse to *prāṇāyāma* (breathing in and out) who recite the 'king of mantras' with ignorance, miss the 'mental reading'.

*Mchan* : 'Three worlds' means earth and below (*sa ḥog*), above the earth (*sa steṅ*), and the superior world (*sa bla*). *Prāṇāyāma* means breathing in (*prāṇa*) and breathing out (*āyāma*). 'Mental reading' is the *nītārtha* kind of mantra reading (*ṅes don gyi sṅags klog pa*). 'King of mantras' means Oṃ, etc. (i.e. Oṃ, Āḥ, Hūṃ). (Tsoṅ-kha-pa in his annotation also rejects a viewpoint of Skal-ldan-grags-pa that the 'pregnant doctrine of lust' (*ḥdod chags chos sbas*) occurs in the phase of 'diamond recitation' in the form of enjoying the consort).

The epithet '*mantrarāja*' for the three heart syllables is found earlier in the *Vajramālā* (PTT, Vol. 3, p. 211). According to the indications of *Mchan ḥgrel*, p. 51, the Oṃ is recited for entrance of the breath, Āḥ for the time the breath is held within, and Hūṃ for the outbreathing. The 'mental reading' of course is the recitation within the mind.

Smṛtijñānakīrti's *Caturdevatā-paripṛcchā-vyākhyāna-upadeśa-pauṣṭika* (PTT, Vol. 66, p. 160-2): " 'Earth and below' means Jambudvīpa (earth) downwards and hell upwards; 'superior world' means where the sun pervades; 'above the earth' means the peak of Mt. Meru" ( / de la sa ḥog ni ḥdzam bu gliṅ man chad dmyal ba yan chad do / / sa bla ni ñi mas gar khyab paḥo / / sa steṅ ni ri rab kyi rtse moḥo /).

The *nidāna* verse sets forth the praxis of *prāṇāyāma* proper to the stage of Generation. In this case, there are two important verses of the *Guhyasamājatantra* :

*pañcavarṇaṃ mahāratnaṃ sarṣapasthalamātrakam /*
*nāsikāgre prayatnena bhāvayed yogataḥ sadā* // III, 12 //

He should imagine a great five-colored jewel, no bigger in area than a mustard grain, on the tip of the nose, through continual *yoga* zealously.

*nāsāgre sarṣapaṃ cintet sarṣape sacarācaram* /
*bhāvayet jñānapadaṃ ramyaṃ rahasyaṃ jñānakalpitam* //VI,9 //
He should imagine a mustard grain at the tip of the nose, and the moving (sentient beings) and non-moving (receptacle worlds) in the mustard grain. He should contemplate the joyful realm of *jñāna* as the (highest) secret that is imagined by *jñāna*.

The foregoing two verses are cited consecutively by Nāgārjuna in his *Piṇḍīkṛtasādhana*, verses 199-200, and in his *Pañcakrama*, I, 10-11. The *Pradīpoddyotana* and *Mchan ḥgrel* (PTT. Vol. 158, pp. 36 and 37; *ibid*. p. 50) interpret them differently for the Stage of Generation and the Stage of Completion. In both cases, the enterprise is called 'subtle *yoga*' (*sūkṣmayoga*) and involves the reality of the wind and the reality of the *mantra*; and the five winds have the nature of the five knowledges and the five Tathāgatas. In the Stage of Generation the winds are the breathing in and out, as in *nidāna* verse 12 and the 'tip of the nose' is on the face. In the Stage of Completion, the winds are made to enter the central 'vein', along which there are three kinds of 'tip of nose', detailed in my introduction.

Concerning the recitation, *Guhyasamāja*, Chap. XVIII, p. 159, employs metaphorical language :

*puṣpam ity abhidhīyante navayoṣitkhadhātavaḥ* /
*kāyavākcittabhedena nyāsaṃ kuryāt kulakramaiḥ* //
The nine 'ladies' (*yoṣit*) and 'realm of space' (*ākāśadhātu*) are called 'flower'. One should 'arrange it' by division into body, speech, and mind in the order of the families (*kula*).

Tsoṅ-kha-pa (*Mchan ḥgrel*, p. 20-2) explains that the nine yoṣits are the nine winds while the ākāśadhātu is the tenth wind, *vyāna*; and that the verse refers to 'diamond muttering' of the three syllables (Oṃ, Āḥ, Hūṃ) of the three families (respectively Vairocana's Body, Amitābha's Speech, and Akṣobhya's Mind) to cause the (five) basic and (five) secondary winds to enter, stay, and rise (for leaving) (*ḥjug gnas ldaṅ*).

In its discussion of the 'Stage of Generation' kind of 'subtle yoga', the *Pradīpoddyotana* on Chapter Six cites the *Saṃdhivyākaraṇa* on Chapter Three (*Mchan ḥgrel*, p. 51) :

*pāṇḍarādijāpaḥ proktaḥ pañcaviṃśac chatadvaya* /
*caturbhir guṇitaṃ samyak caturyogaṃ śataṃ nava* //

> *navaśataṃ tu yad dṛṣṭaṃ caturviṃśatparikramaiḥ* /
> *pratyutpādāt bhavet atra dvyayutaṃ śataṣoḍaśam* //
> It is said that the recitation of Pāṇḍarā and the other goddesses involves 225 (wind recitations). When well multiplied by four (goddesses), the union with four is 900. Now that observed 900 by a series of 24 would increase here (for day and night) to 21,600.

When this same passage from the *Saṃdhivyākaraṇa* is quoted in *Sṅags rim*, f. 442a-1, Tsoṅ-kha-pa gives the explanation of the *Āmnāya-mañjari*, that when one is reciting the Pāṇḍarā wind, which is the (fire) wind of the Lotus-lord (Amitābha), then there are 225 of fiery Pāṇḍarā of fire, 225 of windy Tārā of fire, 225 of earth Locanā of fire, and 225 of watery Māmakī of fire. And one can understand the recitation of the other three the same way. The '24' comes from division of watches. ( / gos dkar la sogs źes pa ni pad ma mgon poḥi rluṅ la meḥi me gos dkar mo daṅ meḥi rluṅ sgrol ma daṅ meḥi sa spyan ma daṅ meḥi chu Mā-ma-kīḥi rluṅ ñis brgya ñer lṅa re yod paḥi dbaṅ du byas la des gźan gsum yaṅ śes par byaḥo / ḥdi la thun phyed pa ñer bźi źes man sñe las gsuṅs so / ). Since there are eight watches by day and night, the number '24' must result from multiplication with the three mantras. That this comes out commensurate with '24 hours' seems to be an accident. Dividing on this basis, we find that each shortest recitation takes 4 seconds. When one is reciting the wind of the Lotus-lord, he would recite first the fiery Pāṇḍarā of fire for four seconds of Oṃ, four seconds of Āḥ, and four seconds of Hūṃ. He continues this fiery Pāṇḍarā of fire recitation for 225 times (45 minutes) before going to the windy Tārā of fire, and so on to the other goddesses for a total of three hours. Then the instruction states to go through the process similarly in the case of the other three elements. This remark is clarified by observing that the *Saṃdhivyākaraṇa* verses in question are quoted in the *Pañcakrama* (krama No. 1; but the edited text by La Vallée Poussin numbering them 45-46 does not notice these as continuation of quotation). The commentary by Śrī Lakṣmī (PTT Vol. 63, p. 13) explains :

> / de la ñin mo thun daṅ po la mgrin par gnas paḥi padmaḥi meḥi dkyil ḥkhor las snaḥi bu ga gYas pa las kha dog dmar poḥi ḥod zer ḥbyuṅ ba ste / deḥi tshe dbaṅ gi las ḥgrub pa

yin no/ thun gñis pa la lte bar gnas paḥi rluṅ gi dkyil ḥkhor las / snaḥi bu ga gYon pa la kha dog sṅon poḥi ḥod zer ḥbyuṅ ba ste / deḥi tshe mṅon spyod kyi las ḥgrub pa yin no / ñi ma phyed las brtsams te / thun gsum pa la gsaṅ baḥi padmar gnas paḥi saḥi dkyil ḥkhor las gñis ka la kha dog ser poḥi ḥod zer ḥbyuṅ ba ste / deḥi tshe rgyas paḥi las ḥgrub pa yin no / thun bźi pa la sñiṅ gar gnas paḥi chuḥi dkyil ḥkhor las / kha dog dkar poḥi ḥod zer dal źiṅ dman par rgyu ba gñis ka las ḥbyuṅ ba ste / deḥi tshe źi baḥi las ḥgrub pa yin no / mtshan mo yaṅ de bźin du śes par byaḥo /

Here, during the first watch of day, a light of red color issues through the right nostril from the fire circle of the lotus based in the throat; at that time one can succeed in the rite of domineering magic. During the second watch, a ray colored green issues through the left nostril from the wind-circle based by the navel; at that time one can succeed in the rite of destructive magic. Starting at noon, in the third watch, a ray colored yellow issues through both nostrils from the earth-circle based in the lotus of the sacral place; at that time one is successful in the rite of prosperity. During the fourth watch, through both nostrils issues a slow and slight ray, colored white, from the water-circle based in the heart; at that time, one is successful in the rite of appeasing (the deities). The same order takes place during the night (watches).

Śrī Lakṣmī continues with explanation that those descriptions show the dominant ray, but that the other three are represented fractionally. This agrees with the foregoing manner of recitation, which obviously involves a permutation of the goddesses in the order of the four watches of the day, repeated in the four watches of the night. The total of recitations for the eight watches thus amounts to 21,600.

One may observe that these subdivisions are governed by the eight-watch system of classical times. There is evidence that in the B.C. period there was a system of six watches (three by day and three by night). This divided neatly with the *muhūrta* (48 minutes) unit; and recitation based thereon would be multiplied by five tattvas (or elements) in a *pañcikaraṇa* type of five-fold fractions similar to the above four-fold fractions.

Finally, Tsoṅ-kha-pa quotes *nidāna* verse 12 in the course of a comment that clarifies the relation of the generation cycle to the system of praxis, namely, in his *Pañcakrama* commentary (PTT. Vol. 158, p. 192-5 to 193-2):

> / ḥdi ni ḥchi baḥi dus kyi rluṅ ḥjig tshul dris paḥi lan yin la / de yaṅ ji ltar mes bsregs pa na śiṅ gi dṅos po med par ḥgro ba bźin du / ḥchi baḥi tshe yaṅ rluṅ rnams srog ḥdzin gyi bar du rim gyis thim nas ḥchi źiṅ / yaṅ śi baḥi ḥod gsal las las kyi rluṅ śar te / de daṅ rnam śes gñis lhan cig tu ḥjig rten gsum du gnas paḥi skye ba len no / / las kyi rluṅ de las kyaṅ chags pa la sogs paḥi kun rtog rnams skye la / des las bzaṅ ṅan gñis bsags nas yaṅ ḥchi źiṅ yaṅ skye ba ḥkhor lo bskor ba bźin du ḥgyur ro / / sṅon du bśad paḥi rdo rje bzlas pa sogs rim pa lṅa ni gźi dus kyi skye ḥchiḥi rim pa deḥi dbye bar ḥgyur ro źes gsuṅs so / / ḥgyur tshul ni / rluṅ ḥbyuṅ ḥjug rgyun ldan du byed pa ni gźiḥi rdo rje bzlas pa yin te / de ñid las / gaṅ yaṅ khams gsum sems can rnams / / srog daṅ rtsol ba la brten pa / / gsaṅ sṅags rgyal pa zlas bźin du / / mi śes bsam gtan klog pa spaṅs / / źes so / / de ltar ñin mtshan kun tu rluṅ gi bzlas pa byas paḥi mthar ḥchi ba ni / rluṅ phyi naṅ du rgyu ba log nas ḥbyuṅ ba rnams rim gyis thim ste / snaṅ mched thob gsum gyi ñams ḥohar ba ni sems dben gyi rim paḥo / / ñer thob kyi mthar ḥchi baḥi ḥod gsal ḥchar ba ni ḥod gsal gyi rim pa ste gźiḥo ohos sku źes kyaṅ byaḥo / / ḥchi baḥi ḥod gsal gyi mthar phuṅ po rñiṅ paḥi khrod na gnas paḥi rlun sems tsam las lus rñiṅ pa las logs su bye nas bar doḥi lus grub pa ni rgyu lus kyi rim pa ste gźiḥi loṅs sku źes kyaṅ byaḥo / / gźi la dag ma dag gi sgyu lus kyi rim pa so so ba gñis med kyaṅ / ḥdis lam dus kyi sgyu maḥi sku gñis ka mtshon nus pa ni ḥchad par ḥgyur ro / / gźiḥi bar do loṅs sku mig tha mal pa śaḥi mig gi yul du mi mthoṅ pa de / skye srid du skye ba blaṅs pa na mig deḥi yul du ḥgyur ba ni gźiḥi sprul skuḥo /

This (passage of the *Vajramālā*) answers the question about the dissolution of the wind at the time of death. Thus, just as when burnt by fire, the substance of the tree is annihilated, so also at the time of death the winds sequentially dissolve up to *prāṇa* (i.e. in the order, vyāna, udāna, samāna, apāna, prāṇa) and one dies. Then, from the Clear Light of Death the 'wind of action' arises, and the pair consisting of the latter together with *vijñāna*, takes birth somewhere in the three worlds. From that 'wind of action' the (80) *vikalpa*-s of 'desire', etc. arise, and therefrom one amasses good and evil, and the wheel of death and rebirth is so-to-say turned. The five stages (*pañcakrama*) of the aforementioned 'diamond muttering', etc. are said to differentiate the stages of birth and death pertaining to 'basic time'. The method of differentiating is as follows : The continuous activity of the wind's inhalation and exhalation is the 'basic' (1) 'diamond muttering', as said in the same work (the *Vajramālā*), "The beings in the three worlds taking recourse to *prāṇāyāma* (breathing in and out) who recite the 'king of mantras' with ignorance, miss the 'mental reading'." In that way, at the conclusion of the wind-recital during the whole day and night, 'death' occurs by the passage outward and inward of the wind being averted, followed by the serial dissolution of the elements, and then (2) stage of the secret state of mind (*cittaviveka*), wherein the three (gnoses)—Light, Spread-of-Light, and Culmination-of-Light, arise. The arising of the Clear Light of Death at conclusion of the Culmination-of-Light, is the (3) stage of Clear Light, also called 'basic Dharmakāya'. At the conclusion of the Clear Light of Death, a body formed of wind and mind-only emerges from the aged mass of personality aggregates (*skandha*), and from the aging of that body and consequent alteration the Intermediate-State body is produced, which is (4) stage of Illusory Body, also called 'basic Sambhogakāya'. As far as the 'basic (time)' is concerned, there is no differentiation of the stage of illusory body into pure and impure. However, as will be explained, for the time of the path, it is necessary to posit two sorts of illusory body. The basic Intermediate-State Sambhogakāya is not seen in the sense field of the fleshly eye, which is the ordinary eye. Upon taking birth through the birth process, what occurs in the sense field of that eye is (5) the basic (time) Nirmāṇa-kāya.

In that passage, Tson-kha-pa shows how to relate the five kramas of the Stage of Completion, that is, in the 'time of the path', with the sequence of ordinary generation in the cycle of death and rebirth, that is, in 'basic time'. The correspondence thus established can be listed as follows :

| | *Basic Time* | *Time of the Path* |
|---|---|---|
| 1. | Inhalation and Exhalation | Diamond Muttering |
| 2. | Dissolution of the elements | Purification of Mind |
| 3. | Clear Light of Death | Personal Blessing |
| 4. | Intermediate State body | Revelation-Enlightenment |
| 5. | Birth | Pair-united |

C. Bhagavān sarva (The Lord—All)

Candrakīrti's *Pradīpoddyotana* on Chapter XVII (*Mchan ḥgrel*, p. 152-5) cites this verse without identification :

> / *sarvayogo hi bhagavān vajrasattvas tathāgataḥ* /
> / *tasyopabhogaṃ sarvaṃ vai traidhātukam aśeṣataḥ* //
>
> For all yoga is the Bhagavat. The Diamond Being (*vajrasattva*) is the Tathāgata. His whole enjoyment is the three worlds without remainder.

Now the yogin advances to a more refined yoga, with minute partition of the world into partite realities (the 'hundred lineages') identified with the five Buddhas or Tathāgatas. This is the Atiyoga, or stage of the body-maṇḍala containing the bodies of all (*sarva*) the thirty-two deities emanated from the Lord (Bhagavat) as the *bodhicittavajra*. It corresponds in external ritual to the main part of the maṇḍala rite during which one employs the five colored threads representing the five Tathāgatas.

The usual commentarial explanations of the word 'Bhagavat', in both non-tantric and tantric Buddhist texts, refer to the six allotments (or good fortune, *bhaga*) and the defeat of the four Māras (temptors or metaphorical death). For the six allotments, there is the verse cited in *Sekoddeśaṭikā of Naḍapāda* (Nāropā), p. 3 :

> *aiśvaryasya samagrasya rūpasya yaśasaḥ śriyaḥ* /
> *jñānasyārthaprayatnasya ṣaṇṇāṃ bhaga iti smṛtiḥ* //
>
> It is taught that his 'good fortune' is of the six : lordliness, excellent form, fame, prosperity, knowledge, and zeal of the goal.

For the defeat of the four Māras, this tradition has special features such as explaining the defeat of the skandha-māra in terms of the body-maṇḍala, as in Alaṃkakalaśa's *Vajramālā* commentary, p. 164-4 :

/ de la bdud bzi bcom pa ḥam dbaṅ phyug la sogs paḥ'i yon tan drug daṅ ldan pas na / bcom ldan ḥdas so / / de la stoṅ pa ñid bsgoms pas ḥchi bdag gi bdud bcom mo // lha sum cu rtsa gñis kyi bdag ñid can gyi dkyil ḥkhor gyi ḥkhor loḥi rnam pa raṅ gi lus la yoṅs su śes pas phuṅ po bdud bcom mo / /de bźin gśegs pa lṅaḥi rnam pas ñon moṅs pa lṅa yoṅs su śes pas ñon moṅs paḥi bdud boom mo / bgegs skrad paḥi dus na dbaṅ po la sogs paḥi phyogs bcuḥi ḥjig rten skyoṅ ba la phur bus btab pas rnam par bcom paḥi phyir lhaḥi buḥi bdud bcom mo /. By reason of defeating the four Māras or of having the six qualities of lordliness, and so on, he is the Bhagavat. By contemplation of voidness he defeated the Mṛtyu-māra ('Death' māra). By fully recognizing his own body as the circular form of the *maṇḍala* having the embodiment of the thirty-two gods, he defeated the Skandha-māra ('Personality-aggregate' māra). By fully understanding the five defilements as the aspects of the five Tathāgatas, he defeated the Kleśa-māra ('Defilement' māra). At the time of frightening away the hindering demons, because he defeated Indra and the other ten Lokapālas by applying the magic nail, he defeated the Devaputra-māra ('Son-of-the-gods' māra).

Concerning the 'All' (sarva), *Pradipoddyotana* on Chapter XIII, first sentence, comments on the epithet *muni* : "He is called *muni* because he lives in the mind of all the Tathāgatas" (*sarvatathāgatamanovarttitvād munim*). Besides, all the deities are an expression of the Buddha's 'mind of enlightenment' (*bodhicitta*), a term which also means the male-female *bindu* in the central channel and the mysterious substance tasted in the 'Secret Initiation' of the Stage of Completion. This 'all'-inclusive character of the *bodhicitta* is portrayed in some verses of Tsoṅ-kha-pa, in his "Rnal-ḥbyor dag-paḥi rim pa" (PTT, Vol. 160, p. 85) :

*/ gaṅ źig gzugs daṅ tshor ba ḥdu śes ḥdu byed daṅ /*
*/ rnam par śes daṅ skye mched drug daṅ dbaṅ po drug /*
*/ sa chu me daṅ rluṅ daṅ nam mkhaḥ thams cad ni /*

*| byaṅ chub sems ḥdra rgya chen de la phyag ḥtshal lo ||*
*| gti mug ñes pa ḥdod chags rdo rje chos bcas gaṅ |*
*| rig paḥi sbyor ba lasbyuṅ rtag tu rab ḥbrel bar |*
*| rnam pa sna tshogs dgaḥ bas myos paḥi dṅos gyur pa |*
*| byaṅ chub sems ḥdra rgya chen de la phyag ḥtshal lo ||*
*| sdud daṅ dgaḥ daṅ rnam pa de bźin mi ḥgyur daṅ |*
*| rgyu daṅ ḥbras buḥi raṅ bźin sems su rjes thogs chos |*
*| rmoṅs daṅ źe sdaṅ ḥdod chags sgrib pa rdo rje ste |*
*| byaṅ chub sems ḥdra rgya chen de la phyag ḥtshal lo ||*
*| źes pas lha sum cu so gñis la phyag byaḥo |.*

I bow to that expanse like *bodhicitta*—all that is rūpa, vedanā, saṃjñā, saṃskāra, and vijñāna; the six (external) sensory bases, and the six sense organs; earth, water, fire, and wind and space.

I bow to that expanse like *bodhicitta*—any fault of delusion along with the nature of diamond lust; which by continual union arisen from association with the consort (*vidyā*) becomes an element intoxicated by variegated ecstasy.

I bow to that expanse like *bodhicitta*—the reunification, the ecstasy, the aspect, the unchanging Thusness; the intrinsic nature of cause and effect as a nature afterwards obtained in the mind; the diamond obscuration of delusion, hatred, and lust.

With those verses one bows to the thirty-two gods.

In the first of those three verses, the five personality aggregates (*rūpa*, etc.) are the five skandha-Tathāgatas; the six (external) sensory bases are the five goddesses called *vajrā* and also *sems ma* (for the sixth sense object, some goddess would do double duty); the six sense organs are six of the Bodhisattvas; the five elements (earth, etc.) are the four goddesses Locanā, etc. (the *dhātu-mudrā*) and the Ākāśadhātu. That list includes all the deities which are subject to division into five aspects, namely : (a) five *skandha-Tathāgata* (*nidāna* verse 14). (b) four *dhātu-mudrā* (verse 15), six *indriya-bodhisattva* (verse 16), and (d) five *viṣaya-vajrā* (*nidāna* verse 20). Tsoṅ-kha-pa explains (PTT, Vol. 158, p. 205-3) that the ten *krodha* or wrathful gods, in the ten limbs, and the bodhisattvas Maitreya and Samantabhadra, in the joints and veins, are counted among the thirty-two gods for the purpose of 'arcane body' (*kāya-viveka*), but are not each divided into five aspects because they were not so indicated in the basic Tantra.

The hundred subdivisions are listed by Āryadeva in his *Caryāmelāpakapradīpa* (PTT, Vol. 61, p. 295-5, line 7, to 297-5, line 8). In my annotation I follow the subdivisions as presented in Tsoṅ-kha-pa's *Pañcakrama* commentary *Gsal baḥi sgron me* (PTT, Vol. 158 pp. 204 and 205) and a few differences with the lists in that Peking edition of Āryadeva's work may be due to the fact that Tsoṅ-kha-pa employed all translations of this work in Tibetan, as I pointed out in "Notes on the Sanskrit Term *Jñāna*" p. 267, note 59. Āryadeva, *op. cit.*, p. 295-5, merely cites the *Candraguhyatilaka* (*zla gsaṅ thig le*) as mentioning the term 'hundred lineages'. Tsoṅ-kha-pa's exposition always uses the order Vairocana, Ratnasambhava, Amitābha, Amoghasiddhi, and Akṣobhya; and means this order in many other places by saying 'Vairocana etc.' This shows the *Guhyasamāja* traditional correspondences to the *skandhas* to agree with the old Buddhist statement of the *skandhas* (cf. *nidāna* verse 9, above), and this gives rise to the table in Tucci (*Tibetan Painted Scrolls*, I, p. 240), where the standard jurisdictional activity of the Buddha families is given in the same order : moha (delusion), abhimāna (pride), rāga (lust), īrṣyā (envy), krodha (wrath). While this work was being printed, the author temporarily in Japan heard that a scholar wondered about the consistency of the *Guhyasamājatantra* to have Akṣobhya as the chief deity and yet apparently in another place assigning this role to Vairocana. But by reference to the Akṣobhya-maṇḍala translated above it will be noticed that the placement of Akṣobhya in the center gives Vairocana the assignment to the East. In this Tantra Akṣobhya has the role of emanating, as though from above downwards, the whole maṇḍala. The human candidate has to work from downwards upward and he does this by the correspondences which start from the East, so there is no inconsistency.

The subdivisions amounting to a hundred lineages as well as other lists in the annotation of these verses, are somewhat tedious, unless the reader can sense the interesting sidelights on Indian civilization suggested by the way of sectioning the 'worlds' into these partite realities grouped under the five Tathāgatas as 'building-blocks' of the world, which is made up of them in various permutations and combinations. To help the reader to this point of view, four summarizing tables have been included under the respective *nidāna* verses (Nos. 14, 15, 16 under 'Bhagavān sarva' and No. 20 under 'Tathāgata'). By way of easing the reading of this annotation set, I have omitted the Tibetan passages for the 'partite realities' and 'hundred lineages', since this subsection is already swollen with technical details.

> *//BHA// bhaviny asmin prakṛtayo rāgārāgādikāḥ punaḥ /*
> *tābhya(ḥ) śubhāśubhaṃ karma tato janma-samudbhavaḥ //13//*
> In this gestation are the *prakṛtis* desire, aversion, and so on; as a result of those, auspicious and inauspicious *karma*; therefrom the origination of (re)birth.

*Mchan* : 'In this gestation' means the three lights. Auspicious *karma* leads to birth in a good destiny (*sugati*), inauspicious *karma* to birth in a bad destiny (*durgati*). Again, after amassing the two kinds of *karma* one experiences the Clear Light of Death, then undergoes the Intermediate State (*antarābhava*), and is reborn through a womb or by some other means of birth. In further explanation, after the amassing of *karma*, when facing death, earth dissolves in water, water in fire, fire in wind, the wind which stirs up the (80) *vikalpa*-s in Light, that in Spread-of-Light, that in Culmination-of-Light, and that in the Clear Light of Death. This sequence of dissolution is the direct order (*anuloma-krama*) and describes the 'secret state of mind' (*citta-viveka, sems dben*).

*Pañcakrama*, 2nd krama, 44-47 ; Śrī Lakṣmī (*op. cit.*), p. 27-3, ff.:

> *kṛtvā śubhāśubhaṃ karma bhramanti gatipañcake //*
> *ānantaryādikaṃ kṛtvā narakeṣu vipacyate //*
> *śubhaṃ dānādikaṃ kṛtvā svargādiṣu mahīyate /*
> *anantajanmasāhasraṃ prāpya caivaṃ punaḥ punaḥ //*
> *pūrvakarmavipāko 'yam iti śocati mohataḥ /*
> *prakṛtyābhāsayogena yena kliśyanti jantavaḥ //*
> *jñātvā tam eva mucyante jñānino bhavapañjarāt /*
> *prajñāsvabhāva evāyaṃ candramaṇḍalakalpanā //*
> Having done good and evil deeds they wander in the five destinies; having committed the sins of immediate retribution, they roast in the hells; having done the good deeds of giving and the like, they thrive in heaven and other (good destinies):—Again and again this happens during their uncountable lives. This maturation of former

deeds distresses because of delusion; the beings are tormented by way of the (eighty) *prakṛti* lights. The knowing ones who know that, are liberated from the net of generation. This intrinsic nature of *prajñā* is (represented in the 'Stage of Generation' as) the imagination of the lunar disk.

While the *Mchan* annotation and the above citation from the *Pañcakrama* treat the entire cycle of *karma* and fruit in generalities, the *nidāna* verse 13 in fact emphasizes birth or rebirth. This is consistent with the observation in the Introduction III, E. 'Grouping the nidāna kārikas', that the stage of Atiyoga, the body-maṇḍala, corresponds to birth. This *nidāna* verse therefore corroborates the remark in Tsoṅ-kha-pa's *Don gsal ba* on the *Guhyasamāja* (PTT, Vol. 160, p. 124-1, 2) that the Stage of Generation corresponds to the development of the men of the first aeon : first, a condition of 'death' corresponding to the generation of the palace in Yoga; second, a condition of 'intermediate state' corresponding to the generation of the primeval lord in Anuyoga; third, a condition of 'birth' corresponding to the body-maṇḍala as though in the generation cycle of the womb during Atiyoga. According to Tsoṅ-kha-pa in that place, this 'birth' is illustrated by the descent from the Tuṣita heaven of the Bodhisattva for his last life. Referring to the correspondence of five stages at the close of the preceding group of verses ('Ekasmin samaye'), 'birth' corresponds to the fifth krama, 'pair-united (*yuganaddha*), and so to the 'pair-united with training' (*śaikṣa-yuganaddha*). This *yuganaddha* phase of course occurs in the Stage of Completion, not in the present Stage of Generation.

|| GA || *gatiḥ saṃbhavati skandhaḥ pañcabuddhātmakaḥ punaḥ* | *pañcākārābhisaṃbodhir iti nāma pracoditaḥ* || 14 ||

A *skandha* occurs as a destiny (*gati*), also as (one of) the five *buddhas*, and exhorted as (one of) the *abhisaṃbodhi* of five kinds.

*Mchan* : 'As a destiny (gati)' means belonging to the six families (*rigs drug gi*). The contemplation of the skandhas as equivalent to the Buddhas is the 'arcane body' (*kāyaviveka*).

Tsoṅ-kha-pa's remark about 'destiny' means the standard Buddhist doctrine that the five *skandhas* can appear in any one of six destinies, those of gods and men; of asuras; and of animals, hungry ghosts, hell beings. The correspondence of *skandhas* to Buddhas is standard (cf. Guiseppe Tucci. *Tibetan Painted Scrolls*. I, p. 238) : *rūpa* (Vairocana), *vedanā* (Ratnasambhava), *saṃjñā* (Amitābha), *saṃskāra* (Amoghasiddhi), *vijñāna* (Akṣobhya). The contemplation of the correspondences takes place in the Stage of Generation; the identification in fact is the achievement of the Stage of Completion.

The five kinds of *abhisaṃbodhi* mean here the five of the Stage of Generation rather than the five of the Stage of Completion (*nidāna* verse 36). In the present case, fortunately we can use the correspondences from *Mkhas grub rje's Fundamentals of the Buddhist Tantras*, Chapter One. There the moon corresponds to Akṣobhya, the second (the red moon) to Ratnasambhava, the germ syllable to Amitābha, the hand symbol to Amoghasiddhi, and the image to Vairocana. Since the five Tathāgatas have already been indicated in terms of the *skandhas*, the five *abhisaṃbodhis* of 'moon,' and so forth, are in turn made to correspond.

In their undivided correspondence to the Tathāgatas, the five *skandhas* are said to have 'partite reality', in terms of their correspondence to the five defilements given above under 'Smin,' with *rūpa-skandha* called 'delusion' (*moha*). Tsoṅ-kha-pa, "Rnal ḥbyor dag paḥi rim pa" (Vol. 160, p. 91) : "Having purified 'delusion,'... (etc.), one is transferred to the rank of Vairocana, etc.; thus the partite reality of the (respective) Tathāgata (*gśegs pa dbyuṅ ba ḥi de ñid*)." Thus the defilement (*kleśa*) brings the yogin to a particular Buddhahood, by his purifying that very defilement going with that Buddha.

The authority for the 'hundred lineages' subdivisions of *skandhas* is *Guhyasamājatantra*, XVII, p. 137 :

> / *pañcaskandhāḥ samāsena pañcabuddhāḥ prakīrtitāḥ* /
> The five *skandhas* are proclaimed in short to be the five Buddhas.

Tsoṅ-kha-pa's *Pañcakrama* commentary (Vol. 158, p. 204) :

"Among them, when dividing up the *rūpa-skandha* = Vairocana,—(1) *Shape*, long and short, etc., whether inner, outer, or both; (2) *aspect* of oneself, other or both; (3) *color*, blue, etc., whether inner or outer; (4) *lustre* of sun, moon, etc., whether inner or outer; (5) *form* which lacks representation—have in the given order, the Vairocana, the Ratnasambhava, the

Amitābha, the Amoghasiddhi, the Akṣobhya—of Vairocana.

"When dividing up the *vedanā-skandha*—Ratnasambhava (1) impartiality and indifference; (2) (feeling) arisen from bodily phlegm and wind; (3) joy and suffering; (4) (feeling) arisen from meeting (of perception, sense organ, and sense object); (5) feeling arisen from bile,—have in the given order, the Vairocana, etc., of Ratnasambhava.

"When dividing up the *saṃjñā-skandha* = Amitābha—(1) (ideas of) the non-moving and the unchanging; (2) (ideas of) the four-footed stage; (3) (ideas of) the footless stage; (4) (ideas of) the multiple-footed stage; (5) (ideas of) the two-footed stage—have in the given order, the Vairocana, etc., of Amitābha.

"When dividing up the *saṃskāra-skandha* = Amoghasiddhi,—(1) (motivations of) the body; (2) (motivations of) the three realms; (3) (motivations of) speech; (4) (motivations of) liberation; (5) (motivations of) the mind—have in the given order, the Vairocana, etc., of Amoghasiddhi.

"When dividing up the *vijñāna-skandha* = Akṣobhya,—(1-5) the perceptions based on eye, etc. down to body—have in the given order, the Vairocana, etc., of Akṣobhya."

This multiplication of each Tathāgata by each Tathāgata yields the number $5 \times 5 = 25$, the number of twisted threads outlining the palace in the maṇḍala-rite. Also, Tsoṅ-kha-pa, "Rnal ḥbyor dag paḥi rim pa" (PTT, Vol. 160, p. 89-2) states: "The five colors of the *maṇḍala* are the purity of the five *skandhas*" (*phuṅ po lṅa rnam par dag pa ni dkyil ḥkhor kha dog lṅa*).

## V. PARTITE REALITIES OF THE FIVE TATHĀGATAS IN THE FIVE SKANDHAS

| Skandha (Tathāgatas) | Vairocana | Ratnasambhava | Amitābha | Amoghasiddhi | Akṣobhya |
|---|---|---|---|---|---|
| rūpa | shape | aspect | color | lustre | (unrepresented) form |
| vedanā | impartiality | from phlegm and wind | joy and suffering | from sense contact | from bile |
| saṃjñā | of the inanimate | of the four-footed | of the footless | of the multiple footed | of the two-footed |
| saṃskāra | of body | of three realms | of speech | of liberation | of the mind |
| vijñāna | eye | ear | nose | tongue | body |

*|| VĀṄ || vāyus tejo jalaṃ (bhūmir) locanādicatuṣṭayam |*
*jñānatrayātmakajñeyaṃ buddhabodhipradāyakam* || 15 ||

Wind, fire, water, earth, are the quaternion Locanā and so on, which is to be known by one with the nature of the three gnoses as conferring the enlightenment of the Buddhas.

*Mchan* : 'One with the nature of the three gnoses' means one who has experienced the three—Light, Spread-of-Light, Culmination-of-Light in meditative attainment after being engaged in subtle contemplation of the 'lower orifice' (*ḥog sgoḥi phra mo bsgoms pa*). 'Which is to be known' means after having realized the inseparable 'bliss-void' (*sukha-śūnya*) one returns to experience of external objects along with the 'subsequent attainment' of knowing them in the manner of the three gnoses = the three lights. This involves contemplating the five progenitor-Buddhas in each of the four elements. This is the 'arcane body' (*kāya-viveka*) in terms of elements (*dhātu*).

The four goddesses are assigned intermediate directions in the *maṇḍala*. South-east (*āgneya*), etc. are Locanā, etc. Thus, Locanā, south-east; Māmakī, south-west; Pāṇḍarā, north-west; and Tārā, north-east. Since Locanā, etc. means, in correspondential terms, earth, etc., *nidāna* verse 15 states the goddesses in reverse order. The verse indicates that one must be cautious in interpreting the phrase 'Locanā, etc.' since a series may be meant that does not really begin with the correspondence to Locanā. This is also a problem in the respective jurisdiction of the goddesses, as follows :

Tsoṅ-kha-pa, "Rnal ḥbyor dag paḥi rim pa," (Vol. 160, p. 91) : "The jurisdictional activity (*sgos mdzad pa*)... of the four goddesses Locanā, etc. is in order :

1. Appeasing (*śāntika*) the sentient beings tormented by illness and demons.
2. Protecting and making prosper (*pauṣṭika*) those troubled by hindering elements.
3. Pacifying and guarding against the demons which oppress sentient beings.
4. Dominating (*vaśīkaraṇa*) all sentient beings.

"Thus the partite reality of the (respective) Tathāgata consort." According to the information presented under *nidāna* verse 12, it is clear that the correspondence does not take No. 1 as going with Locanā, despite the 'Locanā, etc.' Indeed, the jurisdiction order is Māmakī for No. 1, 'Appeasing' (*śāntika*); Locanā for No. 2, 'Prosperous' (*pauṣṭika*); Tārā for No. 3, 'Overpowering' (*abhicāraka*); and Pāṇḍarā for No. 4, 'Dominating' (*vaśikaraṇa*).

At the beginning of Candrakīrti's *Pradipoddyotana* on Chapter XIV, he mentions that one performs the appeasing rite (white), facing North; prosperity rite (yellow), facing East; overpowering rite (black), facing South; and dominating rite (red), facing West. (Therefore, the jurisdictional order of the goddesses is clockwise in terms of the direction being faced.) Candrakīrti goes on to cite an unnamed explanatory tantra:

> / yathoktaṃ bhagavatā vyākhyātantre / vajrapāṇir āha / adhyātmikā velā iti bhagavan kim ucyate / bhagavān āha / adhyātmikā velā nāma vajrapāṇe mahāguhyātiguhyam atisūkṣmaṃ bodhicittādhiṣṭhitaṃ jñānaṃ mokṣāya sattvānāṃ mantrāṇāṃ siddhisādhane śānti-pauṣṭika-karma ca / tathā vaśyābhicārake / agrāhyo bhagavān / śāntaḥ cittadhātus tathāgataḥ / yathā puṣpe bhaved gandhaḥ tathā sattvahṛdisthitā vihared ardhayāmikā velā paripāṭyā yathākramaṃ / agnivāyavyamāhendra-vāruṇe pratimaṇḍale / raktā kṛṣṇā tathā pītā sitā caiva samāsata iti /
>
> The following was said by the Lord in the Explanatory Tantra: Vajrapāṇi said, "Lord, what is said to be the 'inner interval'?" The Lord spoke, "Vajrapāṇi, the 'inner interval' is among great secrets still more secret, highly subtle—the gnosis empowered by the *bodhicitta* for the liberation of sentient beings, and the rites of appeasing and prosperity, so also, of overpowering and dominating, in the accomplishment of *siddhis* going with *mantras*. The Lord is imperceptible, calm; the Tathāgata is the realm of consciousness. As in the flower is perfume, so in the heart of sentient beings dwells the half-watch interval, in short, red, black, so also yellow, white, in sequence according to their order, in the several *maṇḍalas* (*cakras* of the body), to wit, fire, wind, earth, and water.

The meaning of 'half-watch interval' is clear by the data under *nidāna* verse 12, that one recites each goddess in periods of 45 minutes. Therefore, the 'red, black' is two such periods or the

$1\frac{1}{2}$ hours constituting a half-watch; so also 'yellow, white'.

It is of interest to observe that the sequence of jurisdiction by the goddesses over the four rites is the same order in which their respective elements are said to arise in lunar months in the information under *nidāna* verse 8; and of course, the very reverse of this order is the recitation sequence of the four goddesses.

The 'hundred lineages' authority for the four goddesses is *Guhyasamājatantra,* Chap. XVII, p. 137 :

> *pṛthivī locanā khyātā abdhātur māmakī smṛtā |*
> *pāṇḍarākhyā bhavet tejo vāyus tārā prakīrtitā ||*
>
> Locanā is earth; Māmakī, water; Pāṇḍarā, fire; Tārā, wind.

Tsoṅ-kha-pa's *Pañcakrama* commentary (Vol. 158, p. 204) :

"Among them, when dividing up the earth element = Locanā, by external and personal, (a) the personal are : (1) the essence of head hair, bone, excrement, liver; (2) the essence of body hair, nails, pus; (3) the essence of teeth, skin, flesh(?); (4) the essence of tendons, flesh, ribs; (5) the essence of filth, intestines, bile; . . and, (b) the external are: (1) Mount Meru; and (2-5) the South, West, North, and East Continents. The five personal and external groups have in the given order the Vairocana, etc. of Locanā. (Vairocana, etc. means Vairocana, Ratnasambhava, Amitābha, Amoghasiddhi, and Akṣobhya).

"When dividing up the water element = Māmakī, (a) the personal are: (1) phlegm, along with tears; (2) menses and blood; (3)(semen); (4) lymph; (5) urine; and (b) the external are: (1) waterfalls; (2) rivers; (3) springs; (4) ponds; (5) oceans. Both groups have, in the given order, the Vairocana, etc. of Māmakī.

"When dividing up the fire element = Pāṇḍarā, (a) the personal are : (1-5) the heat of (1) the head, (2) the (secret) navel, (3) all the limbs, (4) the belly, (5) the heart (the chest ?); and (b) the external are: (1-4) fire from (1) stones, (2) burning crystal, (3) wood, and (4) forests; (5) fire placed in continual series (as in Dīvāli ?). Both groups have, in the given order, the Vairocana, etc. of Pāṇḍarā.

## VI. THE TWENTY PERSONAL-EXTERNAL PAIRS REPRESENTING PARTITE REALITIES OF THE FIVE TATHĀGATAS WITHIN THE FOUR ELEMENTS

| Element-Goddesses: | Earth (Locanā) | Water (Māmakī) | Fire (Pāṇḍarā) | Wind (Tārā) |
|---|---|---|---|---|
| Vairocana | head hair, bone, excrement, liver | phlegm and tears | head heat | vyāna |
| | Mount Meru | waterfalls | fire from stones | upper winds |
| Ratnasambhava | body hair, nails, pus | menses and blood | heat of (secret) navel | apāna |
| | South Continent | rivers | fire from burning crystal | south winds |
| Amitābha | teeth, skin, flesh | (semen) | heat of all the limbs | udāna |
| | West Continent | springs | fire from wood | west winds |
| Amoghasiddhi | tendons, flesh, ribs | lymph | heat of the belly | samāna |
| | North Continent | ponds | forest fire | north winds |
| Akṣobhya | filth, intestines, bile | urine | heat of the heart (the chest)? | prāṇa |
| | East Continent | oceans | fire placed in continual series | east winds |

"When dividing up the wind element = Tārā, (a) the personal are : (1) vyāna, (2) apāna, (3) udāna, (4) samāna, (5) prāṇa; and (b) the external are : (1) upper, (2) south, (3) west (4) north, (5) east—winds. Both groups have, in the given order, the Vairocana, etc. of Tārā.

"Granted that if one counts separately the personal and external subdivision among the four elements it adds up to twice twenty. Nevertheless while thus dividing the earth element, etc. into personal and external elements, (for purposes of 'one hundred lineages') the total is taken as twenty."

Besides the above materials, which draw out the implications of *nidāna* verse 15 in terms of the praxis in the Stage of Generation, that *nidāna* verse requires further annotation to explain how those goddesses confer the enlightenment of the Buddhas as a conceptualization in the Stage of Generation and as an actual accomplishment in the Stage of Completion. *Mchan's* annotation suggests that the particular phase of the Stage of Generation in which such a conceptualization takes place is taught by *nidāna* verse 19 which deals with the 'subsequent attainment'. There are two matters to be discussed : (1) the conferring of enlightenment, (2) *Mchan's* remark about 'subtle contemplation of the lower orifice'.

(1) One explanation for the statement that those goddesses confer the enlightenment of the Buddhas is that the explanatory tantra *Caturdevīparipṛcchā*, in the commentary of Smṛti (PTT, Vol. 66, p. 155-2), shows that the four steps of *sādhana* are identified with the four goddesses: 1. sevā = Locanā; 2. upasādhana = Māmakī; 3. sādhana = Pāṇḍarā, 4. mahāsādhana = Tārā. However, the chief explanation would be in the *Guhyasamājatantra*, Chap. XV, the chapter devoted to dreams and other auspices. Verses 32-34 can be understood as the auspice of the later role of the four goddesses to be treated in verse group 'Diamond Ladies of the Heart'; those three verses are here translated in *Pradīpoddyotana* context (Mchan ḥgrel, p. 123) :

*jñānasattvaprayogeṇa madhye bimbaṃ prabhāvayet |*
*catuḥsthāneṣu mantrajño yoṣitaṃ sthāpayet sadā ||*
*sarvālaṅkārasampūrṇāṃ sarvalakṣaṇalakṣitām |*
*padmaṃ prasāritaṃ kṛtvā idaṃ mantraṃ vibhāvayet ||*

// *Hūṃ* //

*pañcaraśmiprabhaṃ dīptaṃ bhāvayet yogaṃ vajriṇaḥ* /
*kāyavākcittavajreṣu pātayan bodhim āpnuyāt* //

By the praxis of the Knowledge Being, he should contemplate the image (of Mahāvajradhara's Body appearing instantly) in the center (of the lotus). The mantra-knower should always place the 'lady' (i.e. Locanā, etc.) in the four spots (corners, i.e. intermediate directions) who has the full range of ornaments and who bears all the (ladylike) characteristics. Having made the lotus (of his own heart, svahṛtpadma, and of the doors, mukhakamala) wide-open, he should contemplate this mantra :

// Hūṃ //

He should contemplate the blazing light of five rays as the *yoga* of the *vajrin*. Falling into the diamonds of his body, speech, and mind, it attains enlightenment.

The actual experience so indicated belongs to the phase Stage of Completion with the praxis called 'without prapañca' (*niṣprapañca*, T. *spros bral*), which involves the experience of the three light stages whether in the forward or reverse direction.

(2) The 'subtle contemplation of the lower orifice' is discussed at length in Tsoṅ-kha-pa's commentary on the *Pañcakrama* called "Gdan rdzogs kyi dmar khrid" (PTT, Vol. 159, pp. 120 and 121). It is the 'arcane body' as a practice in the Stage of Completion; therefore it does not involve experience of the three Lights, which is called 'arcane mind' (*cittaviveka*); rather, it is a preparation for that experience of the Lights. The 'lower orifice' refers to the lower orifice of the central vein (the *avadhūti*), which Tucci (*Tibetan Painted Scrolls*, I, p. 241) identifies as the perineum. In Tsoṅ-kha-pa's work (*op. cit.*, p. 120-2) the 'lower orifice' seems to be equivalent to the 'middle of the gem' (*nor buḥi dbus*) or 'tip of the gem (*nor buḥi rtse*). In the male this is the root of the penis. The 'subtle contemplation' (*ibid.*, p. 120-4) involves contemplating at that spot a small solar disk and on it a 'drop' (*thig le*, S. bindu) of substance having three features : its color is blue; its shape is round; its size is no bigger than a tiny grain such as barley and seen as the form of one's presiding deity (*adhideva*) brilliantly shining with five rays. In the basic Tantra this contemplation is alluded to in Chapter Six, verse 15 ('Documents'). In Tsoṅ-kha-pa's

*Mthaḥ gcod* on Chapter Seventeen (PTT, Vol. 156, p. 58-3), the same spot seems to be called 'site of the vajra' (*rdo rjeḥi sa gźi*), which he explains as 'the lotus of the woman which is the basis of the *vajra* (i.e. penis) in the sacral place' (*gsaṅ gnas kyi rdo rjeḥi rten yum gyi padma*). In the light of this terminology, when the yogin imagines there a *bindu* as above described, it can be described mystically as depositing the seed in the 'woman'. Accordingly, one could expect some different terminology in the case of an actual woman. Such seems to be the implication of Tsoṅ-kha-pa's citation from the *Vajramālā* (its chapter 16) in his commentary on the *Vajrajñānasamuccaya* (PTT, Vol. 160, p. 153-4, and p. 154-1). The verse citation as follows is not transparent :

> / *bśaṅ sgo gsaṅ baḥi dbus na gnas* /
> / *miṅ ni ma skyes rtsa chen no* /
> / *de yaṅ rnam śes uaṅ bral ba* /
> / *ye śes lus ni bdag med pa* /
> / *der ni skye ba srog gi mchog* /
> / *srog chags rnams kyi mchog tu brjod* /

> It is situated in the middle of the sacral place by the excrement orifice. Its name is 'Great Unborn Root'. It is free from *vijñāna*. The Knowledge-Body, selfless, is the best of life born there, and is said to have the best of animated beings.

Tsoṅ-kha-pa's commentary (based on Alaṃkakalaśa's) explains the 'Great Unborn Root' as the womb of the mother, the place where one takes birth. It is unconscious, insentient matter, hence free from *vijñāna*. The Knowledge-Body of the Intermediate State, which is selfless because devoid of any ego substance that craves rebirth, so also devoid of the coarse body (the *vipāka-kāya*) that undergoes states, is the best of life born there, and rides on the *prāṇa*-wind which is the best of animated beings. (That discussion may point to the yoga-praxis of a woman as distinct from that of a man).

> // *SA* // *sarvatathāgataḥ kāyaś caturmudrayā mudritaḥ* /
> *cakṣurādyātmanā tatra kṣitigarbhādijinaurasāḥ* // 16 //

> Every Tathāgata body is sealed by four seals. By means of the eye, etc. identifications, in that (body) are the Bodhisattvas Kṣitigarbha, etc.

*Mchan* : The four seals are the samayamudrā of Mind, the

dharmamudrā of Speech, the mahāmudrā of Body, and the karmamudrā of Action. The Bodhisattva Kṣitigarbha is imagined in the eye; Vajrapāṇi in the ear; Khagarbha in the nose; Lokeśvara (or : Avalokiteśvara) in the tongue; Sarvanivaraṇaviṣkambhin in the body surface; Mañjuśrī in the mind (*manas-indriya*). This is *kāyaviveka* in terms of the (six) sense organs (*indriya*).

*Prakāśikā* on SA, p. 293-4 : "The four seals (*mudrā*) have the characteristic of attracting from that (realm of light), drawing in, tying, and subduing. Some (Tathāgata body) does the attracting, etc. of the knowledge being (*jñānasattva*). Also, the four goddesses, Locanā, etc. are the four seals" ( / de las dgug pa daṅ/gźug pa daṅ / bciṅ ba daṅ / dbaṅ du bsdu baḥi mtshan ñid can phyag rgya bźi poḥo / / gaṅ gis ye śes sems dpaḥ dgug pa la sogs bya baḥo / / yaṅ na spyan la sogs pa bźi po ni phyag rgya bźi ste /...). *Pañcakrama*, II, 50 :

> *prajñopāyasamāyogāt jāyate devatākṛtiḥ /*
> *caturmudrābhir āmudrya devatāgarvam udvahan //*
>
> Through the union of *prajñā* and *upāya* the configuration of deities is generated—sealing with by four seals, conveying the pride of divinity.

The following directions are assigned to the eight Bodhisattvas in the *Akṣobhya-maṇḍala*, translated previously :

| | | |
|---|---|---|
| Maitreya and Kṣitigarbha | — | Eastern paṭṭikā |
| Vajrapāṇi and Khagarbha | — | Southern paṭṭikā |
| Lokeśvara and Mañjughoṣa | — | Western paṭṭikā |
| Sarvanivaraṇaviṣkambhin and Samantabhadra | — | Northern paṭṭikā |

The rite of imagining the Bodhisattvas in the respective places is depicted in the *Guhyasamājatantra*, first half of chapter 11, where the emphasis is on the Mahāmudrā, or body of deity.

In regard to the 'four seals' of the *nidāna* verse, the dharmamudrā, samayamudrā, mahāmudrā, and karmamudrā, are explained in these passages of Tsoṅ-kha-pa's *Don gsal ba* (PTT, Vol. 160, p. 141-4): "The syllables Hūṃ, etc. are the dharmamudrā (seal of the law). The thunderbolt (*vajra*), etc. are the samayamudrā (symbolic seal). Akṣobhya, etc. constituting the circle of deities, are the mahāmudrā (great seal)." (Hūṃ la sogs pa ni chos kyi phyag rgyaḥo / / rdo rje la sogs pa ni mtshan maḥi phyag rgyaḥo / mi bskyod pa sogs paḥi lhaḥi ḥkhor lo ni phyag rgya chen poḥo / .... (According to one view :) "The wondrous action accomplishing the aim of all sentient beings by diverse appearances of the gods—is the karma-mudrā (seal of action)." (lha rnams kyi gzugs sna tshogs kyis sems can thams cad kyi don byed ciṅ sgrub paḥi phrin las ni las kyi phyag rgyaḥo/).

Tsoṅ-kha-pa, "Rnal ḥbyor dag paḥi rim pa," Vol. 160, p. 91-2: "The jurisdictional activity.... of the eight, Maitreya, etc., is, in the usual order, purifying the (1) veins; purifying (2-7) the sense bases of (2) eyes, (3) ears, (4) nose, (5) tongue, (6) mind, (7) body; and purifying (8) the joints—of all sentient beings. Thus the partite reality of the Bodhisattvas." (The order is seen by the assigned directions, above, or else by the *mchan* note).

The 'hundred lineages' subdivisions in terms of the Bodhisattvas is based on *Guhyasamājatantra*, XVII, p. 137 :

> / *vajra-āyatanāny eva bodhisattvāgryamaṇḍalam iti* /
> Precisely the adamantine sense bases are called 'best maṇḍala of bodhisattvas'.

Tsoṅ-kha-pa, *Pañcakrama* commentary (Vol. 158, p. 204-4) :

"Among them, when dividing up the eye = Kṣitigarbha,—(1) grasping the three kinds of form (cf. verse 19) by means of the eye; (2) the white part around the pupils of the eye; (3) form seen through a corner of the eye ; (4) movement of the eye; (5) an eye organ no bigger than a grape or corn—have in the given order the Vairocana, etc. of Kṣitigarbha.

"When dividing up the ear = Vajrapāṇi,—(1) the intrinsic nature of the ear; (2) grasping the three kinds of sound; (3) the ear orifice; (4) the ear root; (5) an ear organ like a twisted, cut-off ravine—have, in the given order, the Vairocana, etc. of Vajrapāṇi.

"When dividing up the nose = Khagarbha,—(1) the own-being of nose; (2) inside of nose; (3) grasping the three kinds of odor; (4) orifice of the nose; (5) nose organ like a thin spoon for antimony—have, in the given order, the Vairocana, etc. of Khagarbha.

"When dividing up the Lokeśvara of the tongue,—(1) the own-being of the tongue; (2) its root; (3) its tip; (4) grasping the three kinds of taste; (5) tongue sense organ shaped like a half moon—have in the given order the Vairocana, etc. of Lokeśvara.

"When dividing up the body = Sarvanivaraṇaviṣkambhin,—(1) the sense organ of body; (2) the skeleton of the body; (3) the own-being of flesh; (4) the own-being of skin; (5) grasping the (three kinds of) tangible—have, in the given order, the Vairocana, etc. of Sarvanivaraṇaviṣkambhin.

"When dividing up the sense organ of mind = Mañjuśrī, where is gathered the three, Light, Spread-of-Light, and Culmination-of-Light—the five knowledges: (1) mirror-like, (2) equality, (3) discriminative, (4) procedure-of-duty, (5) dharmadhātu—have the Vairocana, etc. of Mañjuśrī."

## VII. THE PARTITE REALITY OF THE FIVE TATHĀGATAS WITHIN THE SIX SENSE ORGANS

| The Six Senses (Bodhisattvas) | Vairocana | Ratnasambhava | Amitābha | Amoghasiddhi | Akṣobhya |
|---|---|---|---|---|---|
| eye | grasping the three kinds of form | white part around the pupil of the eye | form seen through a corner of the eye | movement of the eye | eye organ no bigger than a grape |
| ear | own-being of ear | grasping the three kinds of sound | ear orifice | ear root | ear organ like a twisted cut-off ravine |
| nose | own-being of nose | inside of nose | grasping the three kinds of odor | orifice of the nose | nose organ like thin spoon for antimony |
| tongue | own-being of tongue | root of tongue | tip of tongue | grasping the three kinds of taste | tongue organ shaped like a half moon |
| body | sense organ of body | skeleton of body | own-being of flesh | own-being of skin | grasping the three kinds of tangible |
| mind | mirror-like knowledge | equality knowledge | discriminative knowledge | procedure-of--duty knowledge | dharmadhātu knowledge |

*|| RVA || arvanti ye tu tuṣṭā vai krodharājamahābalāḥ |*
*tān digvidik-svabhāveṣu bhujādyaṅgeṣu lakṣayet* || 17 ||

As for the mighty Fury Kings who run delighted, one should depict them in their natural abodes of the quarters and intermediate directions and in the limbs such as the arms.

*Mchan* : 'Who run delighted' means that they subdue the hostile spirits. This contemplation is *kāyaviveka* in terms of the *rakṣā-cakra*, the protective circle.

The Fury Kings are ten in number, as named in the *Vajramālā*, chapter 23. Their directions are stated in the *Akṣobhya-maṇḍala*, body positions given in Nāgārjuna's *Piṇḍikṛta-sādhana* 66-67, taking Prajñāntaka = Aparājita, Padmāntaka = Hayagrīva, Vighnāntaka = Amṛtakuṇḍali.

| | *Fury Kings* | *Directions* | *Position in Body* |
|---|---|---|---|
| 1. | Yamāntaka | East | Right arm (savya-bhuja) |
| 2. | Prajñāntaka | South | Left arm (apasavya-bhuja) |
| 3. | Padmāntaka | West | Mouth (mukha) |
| 4. | Vighnāntaka | North | Face (vaktra) |
| 5. | Acala | Agni (S.E.) | Right side (dakṣiṇa-bhāga) |
| 6. | Ṭakkirāja | Nairṛta (S.W.) | Left side (vāma-bhāga) |
| 7. | Nīladaṇḍa | Vāyu (N.W.) | Right knee (dakṣiṇa-jānu) |
| 8. | Mahābala | Īśāna (N.E.) | Left knee (vāmajānu) |
| 9. | Uṣṇīṣacakravartin | Above | Crown of head (mūrdhan) |
| 10. | Sumbha (rāja) | Below | Both feet (pādānta-dvaya) |

Tsoṅ-kha-pa, "Rnal ḥbyor dag paḥi rim pa," Vol. 160, p. 91 : "The jurisdictional activity... of the ten, Yamāntaka, etc., is, in the usual order, destroying (1) the demons of senses, etc. (2) the demons of *yama*, *ma-mo*, etc., (3) the demons of song and *genius loci*, (4) the demons of *yakṣa*, *gaṇapati*, etc., (5) the demons of *agni*, (6) the demons of *nairṛta*, (7) the demons of *vāyu*, (8) the demons of *iśāna*, (9) the demons of *brahmā* and *deva*,

(10) the demons of stationary and mobile poison (e.g. of herbs and of snakes, resp.), *nāga*, and *genius loci*. Thus the partite reality of the krodhas."

## D. *Tathāgata* (*Thus-Gone*)

The last stage of *sādhana*, the Mahāyoga, includes the two *samādhis* called 'Triumphant maṇḍala' and 'Victory of the Rite'. In the *Guhyasamājatantra* (Chapter One), the 'Triumphant maṇḍala' is the thirteen-deity maṇḍala (Tsoṅ-kha-pa, *Don gsal ba*, p. 144-1), because it is the revelation of the Buddha to the retinue of Tathāgatas. Similarly in this phase the master reveals the maṇḍala to the disciple, who is then initiated in it. In fact, the Tathāgata verses fall into two of Tathā for the 'Triumphant maṇḍala' and two of Gata for the 'Victory of the Rite'. There are two interpretations of Tathā (the same way): (a) displaying (the same way) for the sake of sentient beings (*nidāna* verse 18); (b) 'afterwards ... should dwell' (the same way) (verse 19). There are also two interpretations of Gata (gone) : (a) gone (as a divinity) to sense objects (for supernormal faculties) (verse 20); (b) gone, rendered up to, the Tathāgatas (verse 21).

There are five Tathāgata families (*Guhyasamāja*, Chapter I, p. 6) :

> *dveṣamohau tathā rāgaś cintāmaṇisamayas tathā* /
> *kulā hy ete tu vai pañcakāmamokṣaprasādakāḥ* //
> Hatred and delusion; likewise lust, wish-granting gem, and symbol-pledge are the families. And they arrange the liberation in terms of the five 'desires' (sense objects).

*Mchan ḥgrel* (p. 26-5) : "Hatred (*dveṣa*) is Akṣobhya's Family; delusion (*moha*), Vairocana's; lust (*rāga*), Amitābha's; wish-granting gem (*cintāmaṇi*), Ratnasambhava's; and symbol-pledge (*samaya*), Amoghasiddhi's. 'Liberation in terms of five desires (sense objects)' means the ultimate *akṣara-mahāsukha* (incessant great ecstasy)." According to our earlier indications ('The two stages'), the verse can be understood to mean that the Tathāgatas arrange in the Stage of Generation for the later liberation in the Stage of Completion.

Also this literature attributes to each Tathāgata a superintendence or empowering (*adhiṣṭhāna*), Vairocana of Body, Amitābha of Speech, Akṣobhya of Mind, Ratnasambhava of Merits (*guṇa*), and Amoghasiddhi (called the *karmanātha*) of Acts (*karma*).

Following is a summary of the 'hundred lineages' in terms of the partite realities allotted to each Tathāgata on three tables in the previous group of verse comments and here under verse 19:

Vairocana: Shape, impartial feeling, idea of the inanimate, motivation of body, eye perception—among *skandha-Tathāgatas*. Head hair, etc. and Meru; tears and waterfalls; head heat and fire from stones, vyāna and upper winds—among *dhātu-mudrās*. Grasping three kinds of form; own-being of ear, of nose, of tongue, of body sense; and mirror-like knowledge—among six *indriya-Bodhisattvas*. Barely visible form, sound inside ear, diffuse odor, sweet taste, and tangible of sitting on mat—among five *viṣayavajrās*.

Ratnasambhava: Aspect, feeling from phlegm and wind, idea of the four-footed, motivation of three realms, ear-perception—among *skandha-Tathāgatas*. Body hair, etc. and South Continent; menses and rivers; secret navel heat and burning-crystal fire; apāna and south winds—among *dhātu-mudrās*. White part around eye-pupil, grasping three kinds of sound, inside of nose, root of tongue, skeleton of body, equality knowledge—among *indriya-Bodhisattvas*. Form clung to, song, specific odor, astringent taste, tangible of embracing—among *viṣaya-vajrās*.

Amitābha: Color, joy and suffering, idea of the footless, motivation of speech, nose-perception—among *skandha-Tathāgatas*. Teeth, etc. and West Continent; semen and springs; heat of all limbs and fire from wood udāna and west winds—among *dhātu-mudrās*. Form seen through eye-corner, ear orifice, grasping three kinds of odor, tip of tongue, own-being of flesh, discriminative knowledge—among *indriya-Bodhisattvas*. Form of three kinds, pleasurable, etc.; palatal, labial, and voiced sound; odor of three kinds; salty taste; tangible of kissing—among *viṣaya-vajrās*.

Amoghasiddhi: Lustre, feeling from sense contact, idea of the multiple-footed, motivation of liberation, tongue-perception—among *skandha-Tathāgatas*. Tendons, etc. and North Continent; lymph and ponds; belly heat and forest fire; samāna and north winds—among *dhātu-mudrās*. Movement of eye, ear root, orifice of the nose, grasping three kinds of taste, own-being of skin, and procedure-of-duty knowledge—among *indriya-Bodhisattvas*. Form accomplishing duties, nature's music, savory odor, sour taste, tangible of inhalation—among *viṣaya-vajrās*.

Akṣobhya : Unrepresented form, feeling from bile, idea of the two-footed, motivation of the mind, and body-perception —among *skandha-Tathāgatas*. Intestines etc. and East Continent; urine and oceans; heat of heart and fire in series; prāṇa and east winds—among *dhātu-mudrās*. Eye organ size of grape, ear organ like ravine, nose organ like spoon for antimony, tongue organ like half-moon, grasping three kinds of tangible, and dharmadhātu knowledge—among *indriya-Bodhisattvas*. Sensual form, incantations, foul odor, pungent and bitter taste, tangible of copulation—among *viṣaya-vajrās*.

*|| TA || tattatkulasamudbhūtā devā devyaḥ pṛthagvidhāḥ |*
*na te santi na tāḥ santi sattvārthaṃ pratidarśitāḥ || 18 ||*

Of the different gods and goddesses generated by him and his family, neither the gods nor the goddesses exist, but are displayed for the sake of sentient beings.

*Mchan* : They do not exist separately : all those gods and goddesses are unified in the family of Vajradhara. This is *kāyaviveka* in terms of Mahāguhya Vajradhara.

The families are detailed at the end of the *Akṣobhya-maṇḍala*, previously translated, but I follow here Nāgārjuna's commentary on the basic Tantra (Derge, Sa, 30a-1, ff.). The Tathāgata families include the following deities :

| *Tathāgata* | *Family Mother* | *Sense Object* | *Bodhisattva* | *Krodha* |
|---|---|---|---|---|
| Vairocana | Locanā | Rūpavajrā | Kṣitigarbha and Maitreya | Yamāntaka and Acala |
| Ratnasaṃbhava | Māmakī | Śabdavajrā | Vajrapāṇi | Prajñāntaka and Ṭakkirāja |
| Amitābha | Pāṇḍarā | Gandhavajrā | Khagarbha | Padmāntaka and Nīladaṇḍa |
| Amoghasiddhi | Tārā | Rasavajrā | Lokeśvara | Vighnāntaka and Mahābala |
| Akṣobhya | (Māmakī) | Sparśavajrā | Sarvanivaraṇa-viṣkambhin, Mañjuśrī, and Samantabhadra | Uṣṇīṣacakra-vartin and Sumbharāja |

Those deities are all involved in what Bhavyakīrti calls in his commentary on the *Pradīpoddyotana* (PTT, Vol 60, p. 275-2) the 'Tantric options' (*ḥdam kha*), citing in this connection *Guhyasamāja*, XIII, verse 56 (second hemistich here considerably èmended) :

> *kāyavākcittavajrais tu svamantrārthaguṇena vā /*
> *athavauṣṇiṣasamayair ājñācakraprayojanam //*
>
> There is application of the 'command-circle' (*ājñācakra*) either by means of the diamonds of body, speech, and mind; by the purpose and the merit of one's own *mantras*; or by the pledges of the *uṣṇiṣa*.

According to the *Pradīpoddyotana* on Chapter XIII (*Mchan ḥgrel*), p. 100-2, 3), the 'command' is used against the demonic elements. When by the diamonds of body, speech, and mind—the five Tathāgatas are meant; and the 'command circle' belongs to the goddesses, Locanā, etc., of the five families. When by the purpose and the merit of one's own *mantras*, i.e. the yogin families of Vairocana, etc.—the associated eight Bodhisattvas, Maitreya, etc., are meant; the "command circle' belongs to their purpose (*artha*) the *mahāmudrā* form generated from the five *abhisambodhis* in the phase of *prathama-prayoga* and belongs to their merit (*guṇa*), the fierce aspect of Vajrasattva arising from the transformation of the Bodhisattvas in the phase of Victorious *maṇḍala*'. When by the pledges of the *uṣṇiṣa*—the ten *krodhas* starting from Uṣṇīṣacakravartin are meant; and one applies their 'command circle'.

Besides, the generation phase of *nidāna* verse 18 can be illustrated both by the method of Chapter One and by the method of the master revealing to the disciple. In the first case, there is *Guhyasamājatantra*, Chap. I, p. 3 :

> */ atha bhagavān bodhicittavajras tathāgataḥ*
> *sarvatathāgatakāyavākcittavajrasamayodbhava-vajraṃ nāma*
> *samādhiṃ samāpadyemāṃ mahāvidyāpuruṣamūrtiṃ*
> *sarvatathāgata-sattvādhiṣṭhānam adhiṣṭhānam adhiṣṭhāpayām āsa/*
> *samanantarādhiṣṭhitamātre sa eva bhagavān bodhicittavajras*
> *tathāgatas trimukhākāreṇa sarvatathāgataiḥ saṃdṛśyate sma /*
>
> Then the Bhagavat, the *vajra* of *bodhicitta*, the Tathāgata ('come' or 'gone' 'the same way'), immersing himself in the samādhi named Diamond of the Body, Speech, and Mind of all the Tathāgatas and Diamond of symbolic

generation, blessed the body of the great incantation person to have the blessing of the *sattvas* belonging to all Tathāgatas. No sooner was that blessed, than the Bhagavat, the *vajra* of *bodhicitta*, the Tathāgata, was seen by all the Tathāgatas to have three heads.

*Mchan ḥgrel* (p. 22-5)— 'Diamond of Body, Speech, and Mind,' means respectively the syllables Oṃ, Āḥ, Hūṃ. 'Diamond of symbolic generation' means deific generation through the five *abhisaṃbodhis*, namely, generating from those three syllables the pair 'hand symbol' [Anuyoga] and 'finished body' [Atiyoga]. 'Great incantation' means the three syllables; and the body of a person of those syllables means a *mantra*-body. The method of generating is through the four *yogas* called (a) yoga, (b) anuyoga, (c) atiyoga, (d) mahāyoga, which goes up through the generation of the three *sattvas*. 'Seen to have three heads' means seen by all the candidates in the world.

In the second case, there is *Guhyasamājatantra*, X, p. 40; *Mchan ḥgrel*, Vol. 158, p. 73-4, 5 :

*svamantrapuruṣaṃ dhyātvā catuḥsthāneṣu rūpataḥ* /
*trimukhākārayogena trivarṇena vibhāvayet* //

Having meditated upon oneself as the incantation-person, one should contemplate in the manner of form (bodily color, hand symbol, etc. of Vairocana, Ratnasambhava, Amitābha, Amoghasiddhi) in four places (the cardinal directions) by way of three-faced aspect (the three, lust, etc.; the three lights; and so on) and by means of the three syllables (Oṃ, Āh, Hūṃ).

The second passage makes it clear that the three heads can be understood as the white light, red light, and dark light respectively of Light, Spread-of-Light, and Culmination-of-Light.

Concerning the 'sattvas' of the first passage, which *Mchan ḥgrel* expands as the 'three sattvas', there is this passage in Nāgārjuna's *Piṇḍīkṛtasādhana* (Ratnākaraśānti's commentary, PTT Vol. 62, pp. 80 and 81):

Oṃ sarvatathāgatakāyavākcittavajrasvabhāvātmako 'ham
91. adhiṣṭhāyaivam ātmānaṃ śaśimaṇḍalamadhyagam
ṣaḍbhiś cihnaiḥ samāyuktaṃ cintet samayasattvakam
92. hṛnmadhyasaṃsthitaṃ sūkṣmaṃ jñānasattvaṃ vibhāvayet
samādhisattvasaṃjñaṃ ca hūṃkāraṃ taddhṛdi nyaset

93. niṣpādyaivaṃ mahāyogaṃ trisattvātmakam ātmavān
anena vidhiyogena mahāsādhanam ārabhet
"Oṃ, I am the nature of the Body, Speech, and Mind diamonds of all the Tathāgatas."

Having in that way empowered himself, he should contemplate a Symbolic Being (*samayasattva*) endowed with six signs (*vajra*, etc., as listed in the *Akṣobhya-maṇḍala*) and located in the middle of a moon-disk. He should contemplate as stationed in the middle of its heart a tiny Knowledge Being, and should place in the latter's heart (here, meaning first at the crown of head) a Hūṃ referred to as a Concentration Being (samādhisattva). The self-possessed one in that way completes the Mahāyoga identical to three *sattvas*. With such a praxis of rite he should enterprise the Mahāsādhana.

The contemplation of the three sattvas is stated briefly in *Guhyasamāja*, Chapter XII, verses 46-47 ('Documents'). Nāgārjuna refers to this portion of Chapter XII in his *Guhyasamāja-mahāyoga-tantrotpattikrama-sādhana-sūtramelāpaka-nāma* (PTT, Vol. 61, p. 274-2) and continues with a citation from *Guhyasamāja* Chapter XI, which apparently justifies the verse 92 of his *Piṇḍikṛta-sādhana*. The *Guhyasamāja* verse is No. 16 in that chapter :

*khavajramadhyagaṃ cintet vajramaṇḍalam uttamam* |
*niṣpādya svamantrapuruṣaṃ Hūṃkāraṃ cittasaṃsthitam* ||

He should imagine in the middle of the diamond sky the supreme diamond maṇḍala, and complete his Mantrapuruṣa as a Hūṃ formed of *citta*.

In *Mkhas grub rje's Fundamentals of the Buddhist Tantras*, pp, 296-7 (footnote), there is the citation from Padmavajra's *Vāhikaṭīkā* on the *Śrī-Ḍākārṇava* : "The Dharmakāya of the *yogins* is the Samādhi Being; the Saṃbhogakāya, the Knowledge Being; the Nirmāṇakāya, the Symbolic Being, because one creates (those Beings) in direct vision in this world by means of those Bodies that way."

In his *Dkaḥ gnad*, Tsoṅ-kha-pa (Lhasa ed., Vol. Ca, f. 10a-6) shows the dissolution sequence of those same three sattvas, and uses the term 'article of purification' (*sbyaṅ gži*) which means the affiliation to the three bodies of the Buddha as in the foregoing identification by Padmavajra : "In the time of contemplating the Stage of Generation, the arising of the 'articles of purification' being consistent with the sequence of dissolution—the Samayasattva dissolves in the Jñānasattva; the latter dissolves in the Samādhisattva, whereupon (the yogin) enters the *nāda* Clear Light, his gaze fixed thereon" ( / bskyed rim sgom paḥi dus su sbyaṅ gźiḥi ḥbyuṅ ba thim paḥi rim pa daṅ mthun par dam tshig sems dpaḥ ye śes sems dpaḥ la thim / de tiṅ ṅe ḥdzin sems dpaḥ la thim pa nas nā-da ḥod gsal la źugs paḥi bar yaṅ gnas der dmigs pa gtod ciṅ... ). Alaṃkakalaśa's commentary on the *Vajramālā* (Derge Kanjur, Gi, f. 166b-3) says, "The expression '*nāda*' means the aspect of the A-letter" (nā-da ni źes bya ba ni A yig gi rnam paḥo).

Thus, finally the yogin reaches the extreme non-*prapañca* (*atyanta-niṣprapañca*) in the letter A, wherein neither the gods nor the goddesses exist.

> // *THĀ* // *sthātavyaṃ viṣayeṣv asmād yogināḍvayadarśinā* /
> *hīnamadhyapraṇīteṣu jñānatrayanidarśanāt* // 19 //
>
> Afterwards the yogin who sees the non-duality should be dwelling upon sense objects 'inferior', 'intermediate', and 'superior' by seeing the triple gnosis.

*Mchan* : 'Sees the non-duality' means:—sees directly the non-dual knowledge of bliss-void (*sukha-śūnya*) while experiencing the three light stages.

Each of the sense objects is of three kinds according to the *Guhyasamājatantra*, Chapter VII; see B. Bhattacharyya's edition, pp. 27-8: rūpaṃ vijñāya trividhaṃ pūjayet pūjanātmakaḥ, etc. The three kinds are now to be stated as 'inferior', 'intermediate' and 'superior'.

The *Mchan ḥgrel* on *Pradīpoddyotana*, Chapter VII (Vol. 158, p. 56-1) mentions that *rūpa* is of three kinds—pleasurable, repulsive or displeasing, and neutral. Thus, they correspond to the prakṛtis of the three lights (=three jñānas), i.e. 'desire'—'lust' for pleasurable form; 'aversion'—'hatred' for repulsive form, while 'indifference' is said to be 'intermediate'. Furthermore, *ibid.*, p. 55-3, the 'superior' kind of the sense object is the one seen as its own Buddha Family, and one should have 'desire' for that kind. For example, the superior 'form' (*rūpa*) is Vairocana and the deities generated by him.

The idea here is alluded to in the *Guhyasamāja*, Chapter XVIII, p. 158 (Sanskrit cited in history introduction):

The 'desires' (i.e. the five strands of desire, *pañcakāma-*

*guṇa*) 'form', 'sound', etc.—pleasurable, painful, and neutral—continually generate in the heart the source (respectively) of 'lust', 'hatred', and 'delusion'.

Since the yogin experiences the three light stages, this is the second kind of *caryā*, the 'non-*prapañca*' kind.

The 'hundred lineages' subdivisions in terms of deified sense objects are based on *Guhyasamāja*, Chapter VII, verse 14 (edited text corrected by authority of both Tibetan and Chinese):

*|rūpaśabdādibhir mantri devatā bhāvayet sadā|*

The *mantrin* should always contemplate as a divinity by means of form, sound, etc.

Tsoṅ-kha-pa, Vol. 158, p. 205-1, ff.: "According to that (*Guhyasamāja*) passage, the arcane basis (*dben gźi*) of the *kāya-viveka* in terms of sense domains, is the five sense domains (themselves); and the contemplation of those five as the five diamantine goddesses (*vajrā*) is the *kāyaviveka* (itself).

"Among them, the *rgyu ba* wind, based on the eye, assists in seeing the five kinds of form; and when dividing up the visible form = Rūpavajrā—when it (the wind) is based on the set of three conditions (*pratyaya, rkyen*), (1) the barely visible form; (2) that clung to; (3) that of the three kinds, pleasurable, repulsive, neutral; (4) that one accomplishing duties; (5) sensual form, namely, vulgarly carefree, playful, and coquettish—have in the given order the five families, Vairocana, etc. of the goddess Rūpavajrā.

"The *rnam par rgyu ba* wind, based on the ear, assists in hearing sound; and when dividing the heard sound = Śabdavajrā—(1) the sounds inside the ear, and those of the head and its hair, (2) the sounds of song and (tinkling) ornaments; (3) palatal, labial, and voiced sounds; (4) musical sounds of glades, rivers, claps of the palms, drums of earthen ware, etc., (5) mild and fierce sounds of syllables such as Hūṃ—have, in the given order, the five, Vairocana, etc., of the goddess Śabdavajrā.

"The *yaṅ dag par rgyu ba* wind, based on the nose, assists in the selection of odors; and when dividing up the smelt odor = Gandhavajrā—(1) a general odor, (2) specific odors, (3) the three kinds of odor, (4) savory odor, (5) foul odor—have, in the given order, the five, Vairocana, etc., of the goddess Gandhavajrā.

"The *rab tu rgyu ba* wind, based on the tongue, assists in enjoying tastes; and when dividing up the enjoyed taste = Rasavajrā—(1) sweet, (2) astringent, (3) salty, (4) sour, (5) pungent and bitter, tastes—have, in the given order, the five, Vairocana, etc. of the goddess Rasavajrā.

"The *ṅes par rgyu ba* wind, based on the torso, assists in enjoying tangibles; and when dividing up the enjoyed tangible = Sparśavajrā—(1) that of sitting on a single mat, (2) that of embracing, (3) that of kissing, (4) that of inhalation, (5) that of copulation—have, in the given order, the five, Vairocana, etc. of the goddess Sparśavajrā."

The five ancillary winds, mentioned above successively by their alternate names in Tibetan, are further treated under *nidāna* verse 20.

## VIII. PARTITE REALITIES OF THE FIVE TATHĀGATAS IN THE FIVE SENSE OBJECTS

| *Sense Objects (Goddesses)* | *Vairocana* | *Ratnasambhava* | *Amitābha* | *Amoghasiddhi* | *Akṣobhya* |
|---|---|---|---|---|---|
| Form | barely visible | clung to | of three kinds, pleasurable, etc. | that accomplishing duties | sensual form |
| Sound | inside ear | of song | palatal, labial and voiced | musical sounds | mild and fierce incantations' |
| Odor | diffuse | specific | three kinds | savory | foul |
| Taste | sweet | astringent | salty | sour | pungent and bitter |
| Tangible | of sitting on a mat | of embracing | of kissing | of inhalation | of copulation |

*//GA// gacchann asty indriyas tat tat svayaṃ svaviṣayaṃ prati/ ābhāsamātrakaṃ tat tad yad yad indriyagocaram //20//*

While each and every sense organ is going by itself toward its own sense object, whatever be the sense organ and its range, each of them is 'light only' (*ābhāsamātra*).

*Mchan* : 'Each of them is light only' means that both the sense organ and its range (*gocara*) is merely the combination bliss-void along with the knowledge of the three lights.

Cf. *Guhyasamājatantra*, Chapter XI (2nd half), beginning with text, p. 46, line 12; now text, p. 47, *Mchan ḥgrel*, p. 80-1-5:

*/trivajrasamayadhyānena trivajraketusamo bhaved ity āha bhagavān ratnaketuvajraḥ/*

By the meditation consolidating the three *vajras* (here: odors—pleasurable, repulsive, and neutral) one would be equal to Three-Diamond Glory (Trivajraketu)'—so says the Lord Ratnaketuvajra. (Three-Diamond-Glory is hence the Bodhisattva Khagarbha generated in the nose by a Ratna-Oṃ; compare *nidāna* verse 16 above). (This meditation leads to supernormal faculty regarding odor).

Likewise, Sanskrit text, p. 47: "By the meditation consolidating the three *vajras* (here : the three tastes) one would be equal to Three-Diamond-Immeasurable" (hence the Bodhisattva Lokeśvara generated in the tongue by a Dharma Oṃ, and leading to supernormal faculty regarding taste).

Following is a summary of the five meditations that lead to supernormal faculty (*abhijñā*) by consolidating the three *vajras* (*Guhyasamāja*, XI, p. 46. 12, ff., with corrections in names of the Oṃ's) :

| *Three Vajras of sense objects (i.e. pleasurable, repulsive, and neutral)* | *Bodhisattva or Buddha* | *Oṃ by which is generated the abhijñā* | *Organ in which it is generated* |
|---|---|---|---|
| Sound | Vajrapāṇi | Jñāna-Oṃ | ear |
| odor | Khagarbha | Ratna-Oṃ | nose |
| taste | Lokeśvara | Dharma-Oṃ | tongue |
| tangible | Sarvanivaraṇa-viṣkambhin | Samaya-Oṃ | body (surface) |
| form | Vairocanavajra | Trikāya-Oṃ | eye |

*Pradīpoddyotana* and *Mchan ḥgrel* (p. 81.4) : "Previously, by the stage of generation (utpatti-krama) one places the seed-syllables and (merely) points to the accomplishment of the five *abhijñā*-s, because the Stage of Completion (*saṃpanna-krama*) demonstrates the actual accomplishment."

*Guhyasamāja*, Chapter XI, p. 48, and *Mchan ḥgrel* (p. 81-4) :

> *pañcaśūlaṃ mahāvajraṃ pañcajvālavibhūṣitam/*
> *pañcasthānaprayogeṇa pañcābhijñasamo bhavet//*
>
> By the praxis of the five abodes (the objects, form, etc.), the great thunderbolt (*mahāvajra*) (which cannot be warded off) with five prongs (the five sense organs piercing their objects like spears) adorned with five flames (the five ancillary winds proceeding through sense orifices to objects and returning as vehicles of *vijñāna*), would be tantamount to the five *abhijñā*-s

| *Ancillary wind* | *Alternate name and color* | *Passing through which orifice* | *Piercing which sense object* |
|---|---|---|---|
| Nāga | rgyu ba, red | eye | form |
| Kūrma | rnam par rgyu ba, blue | ear | sound |
| Kṛkila | yaṅ dag par rgyu ba, yellow | nose | odor |
| Devadatta | rab tu rgyu ba, white | tongue. | taste |
| Dhanañjaya | ṅes par rgyu ba, green | torso (surface) | tangible |

Note : In the foregoing table the order of the ancillary winds is the traditional order and the same in which they are supposed to arise in the intrauterine states, lunar months 6th through 10th. The five colors are given by Tsoṅ-kha-pa, Vol. 159, commentary on *Pañcakrama*, p. 7-5-5, and ascribed to a precept of Rje-ḥgos.

According to *Mchan ḥgrel* on *Pradīpoddyotana*, Chapter XV, verse 125, there is a dream auspice of the mundane *siddhi* :

> */sarvālaṅkārasampūrṇaṃ surakanyāṃ manoramām/*
> */dārakaṃ dārikāṃ paśyan sa siddhim adhigacchati//*

When he sees the delightful daughter of the gods replete with all ornaments, the lad, (or) the maiden, He gains the occult power (*siddhi*).

As to where one practises those meditations:—

*Guhyasamājatantra*, Chapter XI, p. 48 :

*|parvateṣu vivikteṣu nadīprasravaṇeṣu ca|*
*|śmaśānādiṣv api kāryam idaṃ dhyānasamuccayam||*

The set of meditations is done on lonely mountains, at flowing streams, and in cemeteries, etc.

*Pradīpoddyotana* on the above :

In hinted meaning (*neyārtha*), 'lonely mountains' are mountain peaks graced with flowers and fruit; 'flowing streams' are glades with flowing streams; 'cemeteries, etc.' means (for the 'etc.') isolated tree, empty house, temple, and so on.

(Note that the three main categories go with three kinds of magical practice—a. appeasing deities, b. promoting prosperity, c. destructive magic).

In evident meaning (*nītārtha*), the 'lonely' of 'lonely mountains' means free from reliance by other men, and 'mountains' can refer to *maternal women*. 'Flowing streams' are frequented by all men, and so are the *dissolute women*. Worldly persons are like 'cemeteries', and so these are *outcaste women*, washerwoman, and so on.

(Note that they are the goddess in three forms : the mythological 'Mother', 'Whore'; 'Devouring Earth').

*||TA|| tattadindriyamārgeṇa viṣayaṃ prāpya sādhakaḥ |*
*tathāgatebhyas sakalaṃ prīṇanāya nivedayet ||21||*

While the *sādhaka* is reaching the sense object by way of this and that sense organ, he should make offering completely satisfying the Tathāgatas.

*Mchan* : The verse indicates the secret state of body (*kāya-viveka*) consisting in contemplating the five sensory objects as the adamantine goddesses (*vajrā*). Tsoṅ-kha-pa, "Rnal ḥbyor dag paḥi rim pa," Vol. 160, p. 91 :

"The jurisdictional activity... of Rūpavajrā, etc., is, in the usual order, purifying the longings for form, sound, odor, taste, (tangible); and then bring offerings to the Jinas as the pleasure of form, etc. Thus, the partite reality of the *sems-ma* (the *vajrā*)." *Mchan ḥgrel*, pp. 55 and 56-1, 2:—For example, when reaching the sense object 'forms' by way of the eye, he offers the lady Rūpavajrā, who is the *nāga*-wind, completely satisfying Vairocana. An analogous offering is made in the case of the other sense organs and sense objects, i.e.

| | | |
|---|---|---|
| Śabdavajrā | to | Ratnasambhava |
| Gandhavajrā | to | Amitābha |
| Rasavajrā | to | Amoghasiddhi |
| Sparśavajrā | to | Akṣobhya |

The goddesses are also referred to as offering flowers in *Guhyasamāja*, Chapter VIII, p. 33 :

*padmaṃ pañcavidhaṃ jñātvā utpalaṃ ca vicakṣaṇaḥ /*
*jātikāṃ trividhaṃ kṛtvā devatānāṃ nivedayet //*
*karṇikārasya kusumaṃ mallikāyūthikāṃ tathā /*
*karavīrasya kusumaṃ dhyātvā pūjāṃ prakalpayet //*

A wise person, knowing the *padma* and the *utpala*, of five kinds; and having prepared the three kinds of *jāti*, should offer them to the gods. Having imagined the Karṇikāra, Mallikā, Yūthikā, and Karavīra flowers, he should contemplate them as worship.

Celu-pā's *Samāja-vṛtti* (p. 185-4) explains that the five lotuses, *utpala*, etc. are the five goddesses of the senses, Rūpavajrā, etc.; that the three kinds of *jāti* are Dharmavajrā who pervades the three birthplaces; and that Karṇikāra is Locanā, Mallikā is Māmakī, Yūthikā is Pāṇḍarā, and Karavīra is Tārā. The *Pradīpoddyotana* on Chapter VIII (*op. cit.*), p. 64-1, explains that the five lotuses have the five colors going with the five Tathāgatas, and that *jāti* is made into three colors. Among those words for flowers, *jāti* is the Jasminum grandiflower ; Karṇikāra, flower of Pterospermum acerifolium (Hibiscus mutablis, with red flowers); Mallikā, the Jasminum Zambac; Yūthikā, a kind of Jasmine; and Karavīra, the Oleander.

## II. STAGE OF COMPLETION

### E. *Kāyavākcitta* (*Body, Speech, and Mind*)

In the introductory discussion of the four Tantras, it was pointed out that the Anuttarayoga-tantra is preeminently inner samādhi. This description is justified by the Stage of Completion, which begins with *nidāna* verse 22. According to *Guhyasamājatantra*, XVII, p. 142:

> *caityakarma na kurvīta na ca pustakavācanam /*
> *maṇḍalaṃ naiva kurvīta na trivajrāgravandanam //*
>
> He should not engage in the rite of *caitya*, or in the recitation of books; he should not make a *maṇḍala*, or praise the best of the three diamonds.

On the preceding, *Pradīpoddyotana* in *Mchan ḥgrel* edition says (PTT, Vol. 158, p. 160-3): "This refers to the great *yogin* (*Mchan*: 'belonging to the Stage of Completion'). Regarding his secret body, speech, and mind :... he should not engage in the rite of *caitya* (e.g. circumambulation), including (preparation of) the site and (removal of) gravel, etc., because it is not right (*Mchan*: 'for a person on the Stage of Completion who himself is all Tathāgatas') to have craving for *caitya*-worship; he should not recite books, because it is not right for one who has aroused the spontaneous diamond recitation to lend his voice to a different (recitation); he should not make an external *maṇḍala*, because when the *maṇḍala* is one's own body, it is not a case of the (stationary) earth-*maṇḍala*; he should not worship the best of diamonds, namely, the *śrāvakas*, *pratyekabuddhas* (concretely or their images), or the (image of) Samyaksambuddha, because it violates himself being all Tathāgatas (in the steady state of comprehending bliss-void);...."

In this phase there is also the practice called '*vidyā-vrata*' (defined in Appendix III).

The authoritative passage is in the *Guhyasamājatantra*, Chapter XVI: (*Mchan ḥgrel*, p. 147-2, 3):

> *kāyavākcittavajrāṇāṃ kāyavākcittabhāvanam /*
> *svarūpeṇaiva tatkāryam evam siddhir avāpyate // 89 //*
> *tatredaṃ svakāyavākcittavidyāvratam /*

*jaṭāmukuṭadharaṃ bimbaṃ sitavarṇanibhaṃ mahat* /
*kārayet vidhivat sarvaṃ mantrasaṃvarasaṃvṛtam* // 90 //
*kandamūlaphalaiḥ sarvaṃ bhojyaṃ bhakṣyaṃ samācaret* / 94A//

The task is the contemplation of a body, speech, and mind belonging to (i.e. issuing from) the Body-, Speech-, and Mind-diamonds and precisely like one's own appearance. Just so is the *siddhi* (of Mahā-mudrā) attained.

Herein is the '*vidyāvrata*' of one's own body, speech, and mind. The Great One, white in color, his (divine) form (of Vairocana) bearing a crown of matted locks, practises everything in ritual manner, restrained by the *mantra*-vow.

By means of bulbs and fruits, he subsists on all food and drink.

In Tsoṅ-kha-pa's commentary on the *Pañcakrama* (PTT, Vol. 159, p. 74-3, 4, 5), there is a lengthy discussion of what is meant by the phrase 'precisely like one's own appearance'. This is frequently alluded to in Buddhist Tantra *sādhanas* by the term '*svābha*' ('like oneself'). The solution appears to be that the consort is one of the goddesses Locanā, etc. having the same dress as oneself as the yogin of one or another Buddha. The consort is described in that Chapter XVI, verse 91, as the 'sixteen-yeared girl'. The meaning apparently is that the yogin is accompanied by a goddess-consort who has issued from his own body, speech, and mind which have been identified with the Body, Speech, and Mind of the Tathāgatas. Tsoṅ-kha-pa explains the phase as 'without prapañca (*niṣprapañca*).

Turning to the separate treatment of 'kāya', 'vāk', and 'citta', according to previous indications the 'arcane body' as *pratyāhāra* and *dhyāna* among the six members of yoga, is treated under the 'Kāya' verses (see Śrī Lakṣmī's comment under 'YA'). In that same *Pañcakrama* commentary (the "Gsal baḥi sgron me"), PTT, Vol. 158, p. 205-4, Tsoṅ-kha-pa continues his discussion of the 'hundred lineages' of 'arcane body' to show how to condense them into 'elements'. Among them, the 20 lineages belonging to the Vairocana-kula, that is, from the lineage of *rūpa-skandha* up to the lineage of the 'tangible diamond goddess', are condensed into the element of earth. Similarly the 20 parts of Ratnasambhava lineage are condensed into the element of water; the 20 of Amitābha lineage, into fire; the 20 of Amoghasiddhi, into wind; and the 20 of Akṣobhya lineage into the element of *vijñāna.* Tsoṅ-kha-pa mentions that the classification into five groups is further reduced into three 'secret' families by the method of including Ratnasambhava in the *kāya-vajra* family of Vairocana; Amoghasiddhi in the *vāg-vajra* family of Amitābha; and the 'sixth Tathāgata' Vajradhara in the *citta-vajra* family of Akṣobhya. The three families considered as three *vajras* when taken as indivisible, yield the sixth *adhideva* Vajradhara, which is the ultimate of *kāyaviveka* ('arcane body').

The 'arcane speech' as *prāṇāyāma*, third of the six members, is included in 'VĀK'. Nāgārjuna starts his five stages here, with 'diamond muttering' (*vajrajāpa*). The praxis which begins with VĀK is stated succinctly by Tsoṅ-kha-pa in his commentary on the *Vajrajñānasamuccaya*, Vol. 160, p. 159-3: "The generality in that regard is that the means of generating the three knowledges (*jñāna*) has the inner (subjective) condition of contemplating *prāṇāyāma* and the outer (objective) condition of resort to a *mudrā* ('seal', partner)." He explains the first as the three kinds of *prāṇāyāma* based on three differently located *bindus* (see under VĀK), and the second as the generation of the four 'joys' (see under VA, verse 30). Therefore, the goddess companion previously mentioned in connection with 'vidyāvrata' has the function of helping the *yogin* generate the four 'joys'.

The 'arcane mind' as *dhāraṇā*, the fourth member, is included in CIT-TA. Nāgārjuna's system is more explicit, because it allows a whole *krama*, the 'purification of consciousness' (*cittaviśuddhi*), for CIT—the three light stages; and another whole *krama*, the 'personal blessing' (*svādhiṣṭhāna*), for TA—entrance of the illusory body into the Clear Light.

> *|| KĀ || kāyatrayaṃ samuddiṣṭaṃ pṛthagbhāvena tāyinā |*
> *ekākāraṃ punar yāti niṣpannakramayogataḥ || 22 ||*
> The Protector (i.e. the Buddha) well taught the three Bodies as being different. Moreover, their unity occurs through the *yoga* of *niṣpanna-krama.*

*Mchan* : (When the three bodies are taught to be different, they are:) (1) Dharmakāya associated in the Clear Light (of Death) with a goddess; (2) Sambhogakāya generated from the five *abhisambodhi* as the 'primeval lord' (*ādinātha*);

(3) the latter converted into the Nirmāṇakāya. This is taught in the Stage of Generation.

*Mchan*: In the basic time, (the unity occurs through) accomplishing the primordial body (*ādideha*) from wind-and-mind-only belonging to the Clear Light of death. Accordingly, in the time of the path, there is the secret of *saṃvṛti-māyā*—accomplishing the illusory body from wind-and-mind-only belonging to the Symbolic Clear Light (*dpeḥi ḥod gsal*).

*Mchan* : In the case of the first *krama* (the Stage of Generation), there is only a mental orientation to conviction, but the path is lacking because there is no *yoga* of the three bodies. (In the case of the second *krama*,) by *yoga* unifying the three bodies it is not a matter of figments of imagination. (These remarks apply respectively to the two foregoing passages of *Mchan* annotation).

This *nidāna* verse ('KĀ') and the next one ('YA') continue and conclude the 'arcane body' (*kāyaviveka*) of the foregoing Stage of Generation. According to the *Pradipoddyotana* on XII, 60-64, and its *Mchan ḥgrel* ('Documents'), the kind of 'arcane body' is called 'purification afterwards obtained'. This, then, is the reflex in the Stage of Completion of the preceding praxis. Hence the commentators are allowed the latitude of using the verse 'KĀ' and 'YA' to compare the two stages in the matter of the innate body, which is the basis of the present praxis rather than the coarse body seen by the eye of flesh. 'KĀ' can be understood as *pratyāhāra* ('Withdrawal'), the first member. To show the continuity of the Stage of Generation into the Stage of Completion, *Pañcakrama*, 2nd krama, 48-50; Śrī Lakṣmī, Vol. 63, p. 27-5, ff., has the following:

> *cittam evaṃ svayaṃ paśyet svam eva śaśibimbavat |*
> *atha candraṃ samālambya vajracihnaṃ prakalpayet ||*
> *upāyasūcakaṃ hy etad vajrādyutpattiyoginām |*
> *candravajrādisaṃyogāc cittacaitasasaṃgamaḥ ||*
> *prajñopāyasamāyogāj jāyate devatākṛtiḥ |*
> *caturmudrābhir āmudrya devatāgarvam udvahan ||*
>
> He should so regard his own mind as itself like a moon-reflection; then, he should imagine the *vajra*-sign taking its support on the moon.
>
> The (five)-pronged *upāya* belongs to the *yogins* of (the Stage of) Generation of the *vajra*, etc. From the Generation union

of the *vajra*, etc. and the moon there (results) the Completion combination of *citta* (=*prajñā*) and *caitasa* (=*upāya*). From the union of *prajñā* and *upāya* there arises the configuration of deity,—sealing with four seals, conveying divine pride.

The meaning of '*vajra*, etc.' is shown under *nidāna* verse 18, referring back to the six signs listed in the *Akṣobhya-maṇḍala*. Hence the above verses show the continuation of the Mahāsādhana phase of the Stage of Generation into the outset of the Stage of Completion.

It is this union of *prajñā* and *upāya* that unifies the three Bodies, according to *Guhyasamājatantra*, IX, p. 36; *Pradīpoddyotana* and *Mchan ḥgrel*, PTT. Vol. 158, p. 68-1 :

*dvayendriyaprayogeṇa sarvāṃs tān upabhuñjayet* /
*idaṃ tat sarvavajrāṇāṃ trikāyābhedyabhāvanam* //

By the union of the two organs (that of *vajra* and of *padma*), he would enjoy all those (goddesses). This contemplation of the inseparable three Bodies (Dharma-, Sambhoga-, and Nirmāṇa-kāya) belongs to all '*vajras*' (*sādhakas* of Buddhahood).

Furthermore, the *Pradīpoddyotana* explanation of *pratyāhāra* ('Documents') brings in the three kinds of each sense object, and so in turn, according to earlier explanations, is consistent with *Pañcakrama*, 2nd krama, verse 37; Śrī Lakṣmī, Vol. 63, p. 26-5 :

*rāgaś caiva virāgaś ca dvayor antar iti trayam* /
*dvīndriyasya samāpattyā vajrapadmasamāgamāt* //

Desire (=the middle knowledge), aversion (=the first knowledge), and 'between the two' (the combination of the prior two)—are the three, (as symbolized) by union of the two organs and by combination of *vajra* and *padma*.

But what is the meaning of having a *mudrā* or partner in this case ? Tsoṅ-kha-pa writes in his commentary on the *Caturdevīpariprcchā* (Lhasa ed., Vol. Ca, *Bźis źus*, f. 25a-6) :

*| dgoṅs pa luṅ stoṅ las | | ḥdu śes can daṅ ḥdu śes med | | sems can du b(r)tags ḥdi gnas pa | de rnams rluṅ las byuṅ ba ste | | rluṅ las slar yaṅ ḥgag pa yin | źes gsuṅs so | gñis pa ni | | rluṅ daṅ sems kyis moḥi gzugs daṅ phoḥi gzugs sprul nas gnas paḥi thabs śes mñam par sbyor baḥi rnal ḥbyor pa rnams la ni phyag rgya de ñid bbe ba chen poḥi go ḥphaṅ mchog ḥthob paḥi gnas su ḥgyur te |*

> It is expressed in the *Saṃdhivyākaraṇa* (in fact, Chapter II, p. 236-1): "Those with this abode who are imagined as ideational and non-ideational sentient beings, arise from wind and again pass away in the wind." Second: the yogins who by wind and mind (-only) materialize the form of female and the form of male, and unite the means (*upāya*) and insight (*prajñā*) with abode, have as the abode that very *mudrā* which achieves the best station of great ecstasy (*mahāsukha*).

Also, the resort to a partner points to a celebrated verse of the *Pañcakrama*, 2nd krama, verse 36; Śrī Lakṣmī, Vol. 63, p. 26-3,4:

> *sarvāsām eva māyānāṃ strīmāyaiva viśiṣyate* /
> *jñānatrayaprabhedo 'yaṃ sphuṭaṃ atraiva lakṣyate* //
> Of all illusions (*māyā*), the illusion of woman is supreme; just here the variety of three gnoses is differentiated clearly.

According to Śrī Lakṣmī, the verse concerns differentiation of the three gnoses by sequence of 'partner' (*mudrā*) (*phyag rgyaḥi rim pas*) as contrasted with the differentiation by sequence of 'incantation' (*mantra*) (*sṅags kyi rim pas*). According to Śrī Lakṣmī, 'just here' (*atraiva*) means, according to the precepts (*man ṅag*)—in the time of the Secret Initiation (*guhya-abhiṣeka*), when the disciple is conferred the *prajñā* by the *guru* (*śes rab kyi dbaṅ gi* dus su bla mas śes rab sbyin paḥi slob ma....). First, the *bodhicitta* drips down from the *brahmarandhra* (aperture in crown of the head); and, with non-apperception of the thirty-three *prakṛtis*, there is an instant of the gnosis of Light, pure like moon-rays. Next, that *bodhicitta* pervades the elements (*dhātu*) of all the limbs; and with non-apperception of the forty *prakṛtis*, there arises the gnosis Spread-of-Light, like sun-rays. Then, that *bodhicitta*, spreads to the 'tip', the center of the *vajra* (*rdo rjeḥi dbus ma* / *rtse mor...*) (in the male, the root of the penis); and with non-apperception of the seven *prakṛtis*, there arises the gnosis Culmination-of-Light, like twilight. Hence the word 'clearly' (*sphuṭam*) in the verse line, "Just here the variety of three gnoses is differentiated clearly." This graphic description by Śrī Lakṣmī clarifies the Initiation in the conventional *bodhicitta-maṇḍala*. According to the discussion under *nidāna* verse 15 of the 'subtle contemplation of the lower orifice', when the *bodhicitta* arrives at the 'tip of the *vajra*' it is in the 'lotus of the woman', which is the 'woman' always in that spot of the yogin. However, according to Śrī Lakṣmī, it is precisely here that arises the androgyne Culmination-of-Light, which is the 'dark light'. When the *bodhicitta* is in that spot, presumably that place is what is called the 'place of androgynes'.

And if the preceding is not sufficiently mysterious, note the *Guhyasamājatantra*, XVII, p. 141:

> *dvayendriyaprayogeṇa svaśukrādiparigrahaiḥ |*
> *pūjayet vidhivat sarvān buddhabodhim avāpnuyāt ||*
>
> By the union of the two organs, and by conceiving their *śukra*, etc. ('etc.' = *rakta*, etc.), one should worship all (the Buddhas) according to the rules, and may attain the enlightenment of the Buddhas.

On the preceding, *Pradīpoddyotana*, *Mchan-ḥgrel* ed., Vol. 158, p. 159-4, explains: This is the secret worship of the Body, Speech, and Mind of all the Tathāgatas (*sarvatathāgata-kāyavākcittapūjārahasya*). The verse says, 'by the union of the two organs,' 'meaning, by the union of diamond (*vajra*) and lotus (*padma*) (*Mchan* : through the realm of deific brightness of 'Father-Mother,' *yab yum gyis lhar gsal baḥi ṅaṅ nas*). The verse says, 'by conceiving their *śukra*, etc.', means that one conceives his own semen and the partner's (*vidyā's*) menstrual blood (*rakta*) becoming transformed into the (intrauterine) states *mer-mer-po*, etc. (*Mchan*: the five states of the womb, which are the five progenitors = Tathāgatas, and then giving birth to a son, nephew, etc., which one protects, nourishes, and so on, according to the rules. Thereby one worships and obtains.)

Having been brought into existence, they (the Tathāgatas) are made to lose their individual life. They are said to have been engendered by sexual union and finally killed. This is the message of Chapter VII, context of verse 33, here translated from corrected Sanskrit with the help of *Pradīpoddyotana* and *Mchan ḥgrel*, p. 59.

> *tatra kathaṃ samayānusmṛtibhāvanā ?*
> *| samayāt kṣarenduvidhinā vidhivat phalakāṃkṣiṇaḥ |*
> *| mārayet tathāgataṃ vyūhaṃ sutarāṃ siddhim āpnuyāt ||*
>
> And what is the contemplation with recollection of the union? In the manner of the rite of overflowing drop from the

union, after desiring the fruit according to the rules, one should kill the Tathāgata array and obtain the highest siddhi.

According to the *Pradipoddyotana*, the diverse deities by the sequence of re-unification are drawn into the Paramārtha-maṇḍala.

But that union of *prajñā* and *upāya* is not the union of the two sex organs. Indrabhūti writes in his *Jñānasiddhi* (GOS ed., p. 57):

*sukhaṃ dvindriyajaṃ kecit tattvam āhur narādhamāḥ* /
*tac cāpi mahāsukhaṃ naivaṃ pravadanti jinottamāḥ* //
*pratityotpādasambhūtaṃ na tattvaṃ jāyate kvacit* /

Some vile men say that the pleasure born from the two (sex) organs is reality (*tattva*). But the Buddhas deny that it is Mahāsukha. Nothing engendered in Dependent Origination is reality.

Along the same lines, it is said in the *Hevajratantra* (I, x, 40c-d; 41a-c):

/*tasmāt saukhyaṃ na tattvākhyaṃ mahābhūtaṃ yataḥ sukham* /
/ *sahajātyāṃ yad utpannaṃ sahajaṃ tat prakīrtitaṃ* /
/ *svabhāvaṃ sahajaṃ proktaṃ...*

Whenever pleasure is of the Mahābhūta sort (i.e. derived from the four elements), then the pleasure is not called 'reality'. Whatever (pleasure) arises in 'together-birth', that is called 'together-born'. The self-existent kind is said to be 'together-born'.

The *Sṅags rim chen mo*, f. 288a-2., quotes the fifth *mañjari* of Abhayākaragupta's *Āmnāya-mañjari* : "Thus, the reality arising from the 'together-born' (pleasure)is the *bodhicitta* that is the inseparability of voidness (*śūnyatā*) and compassion (*karuṇā*)" (/de ltar lhan cig skyes pa las byuṅ baḥi de kho na ñid byaṅ chub kyi sems stoṅ pa ñid daṅ sñiṅ rje dbyer med paḥo /).

That terminology which seems to imply an external consort of a woman, and yet which is denied to so intend, is partially explained by Tsoṅ-kha-pa in his *Pañcakrama* commentary "Gsal baḥi sgron me" (PTT, Vol. 159, p. 77-4) :

/ phyag rgyaḥi khyad par ni spyod bsdus las / de bas na phyi rol gyi bud med spaṅs nas sñiṅ khar gnas paḥi ye śes kyi phyag rgya daṅ lha cig sñoms par ḥjug nas śin tu myur bar rdo rje ḥchaṅ thob par byaḥo sñam du dmigs te / gcig pu kho nar spyod pa bya bar gsuṅs paḥi ye śes kyi phyag rgyaḥo /

The superior *mudrā* is the *jñānamudrā* ('knowledge consort') referred to in the *Caryāmelāpaka* (*-pradīpa*), when it says: Therefore, he bears in mind, that spurning an external woman and entering into union with the Jñānamudrā located in the heart, he will speedily attain (the rank of) Vajradhara; so he is to practise in complete solitude.

*Mchan*: Concerning that (unifying) path, the phase in which it occurs is now stated:

*//YA// yat satyaṃ saṃvṛtiḥ proktaṃ buddhānāṃ kāyalakṣaṇaṃ /*
*sa eṣo niṣpannayoga(ḥ) syāt prabhāsvaraviśuddheḥ //23//*

Whatever body characteristic of the Buddhas has been stated to be 'conventional truth' (*saṃvṛti-satya*), the *niṣpannayoga* would be it through purification in the Clear Light.

*Mchan*: 'Whatever body characteristic' means:—body ornamented with the major characteristics and minor marks of Vajradhara. 'Stated to be conventional truth' means: — stated as the illusory body (*māyā-deha*). That '*niṣpannayoga*' means: — that yoga unifying the three bodies, of the Stage of Completion (*sampanna-krama* = *niṣpanna-krama*).

There are two kinds of *māyā* to be considered in this case. The following passage clarifies that *nidāna* verse 23 refers to the first kind of *māyā*.

*Pañcakrama*, 3rd verses 26-27 (with emendations); Śrī Lakṣmī, Vol. 63, p. 38-4, 5:

*iyaṃ eva hi saṃlakṣyā māyānirdeśalakṣaṇā /*
*māyaiva saṃvṛteḥ satyaṃ kāyaḥ saṃbhogasyāpi ca //*
*saiva gandharvasattvaḥ syād vajrakāyaḥ sa eva hi /*
*vajrasattvaḥ svayaṃ tasmāt svasya pūjāṃ pravartayet //*

For the characteristic describing *māya* is precisely a thing to be differentiated: that very *māyā* as the truth of convention, and as the Body of Sambhoga.

That very (māyā) could be a *gandharvasattva*, as well as the 'diamond body' (*vajra-kāya*).

Therefore, Vajrasattva prompts by himself his own worship.

Śrī Lakṣmī (pp. 38-5 to 39-1): Vajrasattva, being all the

Buddhas, worships himself when those Buddhas honor him. "The worship (*pūjā*) is to be conducted with *pratyāhāra* and *dhyāna*, and not with any other stages" (mchod pa ni yaṅ so sor sdud pa daṅ / bsam gtan dag gis bya ba yin te / rim pa gźan gyis bya ni ma yin no).

Tsoṅ-kha-pa discusses the differentiation of these two kinds of '*Māyā*' in his *Mthaḥ gcod* on Chapter One (PTT, Vol. 156, p. 26-4, 5); and to get the point one should refer back to the table in our section 'The Two Stages,...'. On the line 'Intermediate State' under 'Time of the Path' there is Illusory Body and Yuganaddha-deha. The Illusory Body as the 'truth of convention' (*saṃvṛti-satya*) is that 'gandharvasattva'; and the Yuganaddha-deha as the Sambhogakāya is that 'diamond body'. In the first case, the state of 'māyā' lacks the 'precepts' of skill in the means (*thabs la mkhas paḥi man ṅag*) and so in the condition of gandharvasattva is headed for rebirth, i.e. reoccupation of five personality aggregates in the ordinary way. In the second case, the 'māyā' is attended with the precepts of skill in the means involving the winds and mind-only, and so the diamond body can appear in the world as a Nirmāṇakāya. An important point about the terminology is that the illusory body can be called the diamond body when there is present the precepts of skill in managing the situation.

Concerning the major characteristics and minor marks, I abstract these, with the latter commenting on the former—drawn originally from Śākyamitra's *Kosalālaṃkāra*—as presented in my article "Thirty-two Characteristics of the Great Person," in most cases omitting the presumed original Sanskrit terms in the following:

Associated with the characteristics (*lakṣaṇa*) 'each hair of the head curled to the right' (*ekaikakeśa pradakṣiṇavarta*) and 'having a proof of authority on the head' (*uṣṇiṣa śiraskatā*) are the twelve secondary distinctions (*anuvyañjana*): head umbrella-shaped, curly tips on the head hair, hair of head thick, hair of head black, hair of head fragrant, hair of head not disordered, hair of head not shaggy, hair of head lovely, hair of head soft, hair of head glossy, hair of head regular, hair of head appearing like bees.

Associated with the characteristic 'treasure of hair' (*ūrṇā-kośa*) are the eight secondary distinctions: forehead large, forehead unwrinkled, eye-brows black, eye-brows like bows, eye-brows long, eye-brows of uniform hair, eye-brows of equal width (?), nose prominent.

Associated with the characteristics 'eyes dark blue' and 'eye-lashes bovine', are the five secondary distinctions : eyes as though smiling, eyes large, eyes clear, eyes long, eyes pure.

Associated with the characteristic 'jaws leonine' are the secondary distinctions : ears uniform, ear flaps thick and long.

Associated with the seven characteristics 'tongue long and slender', 'voice pure', 'teeth very white', 'teeth without gaps', 'teeth 40 in number'. 'teeth equal in size', and 'taste perfect' are the six secondary distinctions : face sweet-smelling, face leonine, lips red like the Bimba fruit, eye-teeth regular, eye-teeth sharp, disk of face circular and broad.

Associated with the characteristic 'shoulders gently curved' is the secondary distinction : throat like the neck of a flask.

Associated with the eight characteristics 'standing, not bending himself', 'hands which hang low', 'skin delicate', 'skin of golden hue', 'upper part of body leonine', 'broad-shouldered,' 'rounded like a Banyan tree', and 'seven mounds on his body', are the eighteen secondary distinctions : veins not showing, joints not showing, joints as strong as those of Nārāyaṇa, body clean, body not crooked, body regular, body well-rounded, body smooth, members and limbs well-proportioned, body well-controlled, body soft, whose signs are consummated, abdomen well-rounded, abdomen without folds, belly slender, abdomen as though polished, body devoid of freckles or dark spots, ever beautiful.

Associated with the characteristic 'secret of privities drawn into a recess' are the three secondary distinctions: navel deep, navel well-rounded, recess of navel filled-up.

Associated with the characteristic 'legs like those of an antelope' is the secondary distinction, knee-caps well-rounded and beautiful.

Associated with the characteristic 'each hair of body turning to the right side' is the secondary distinction, each hair pore emitting delightful perfume.

Associated with the characteristic 'fingers and toes long' are the six secondary distinctions: nails elevated, nails copper-coloured, nails smooth, fingers and toes well-rounded, fingers and toes full, fingers and toes regular.

Associated with the six characteristics 'hands and feet marked by a wheel rim', 'feet well-planted', 'hands and feet soft and tender', 'webs joining (the fingers and toes on) his hands and feet', 'heels broad', and 'ankle joints inconspicuous', are the seventeen secondary distinctions : lines in the hands non-intermittent, lines in the hands alike, lines in the hands deep, lines in the hands not crooked, lines in the hands glossy, palms and soles red like copper; on his hands, the lion's seat (*siṃhāsana*), fish (*mīna*), banner of victory (*dhvaja*), thunderbolt (*vajra*), the hook (*aṅkuśa*), the flask (*kalaśa*), the Nandyāvartta, the Śrīvatsa, the conch shell (*śaṅkha*), the lotus (*padma*), and the Svastika.

It is obvious that the characteristics and secondary distinctions (minor marks) as presented by Śākyamitra are ordered by starting from the top of the head and proceeding down to the legs, and showing last of all the pores, hands and feet. His minor marks go with a *static* figure and appear to suit the Buddha as a great *yogin*.

> *||VĀK|| vākpathasyaiva viṣayaḥ kāyo jñānamayaḥ prabhuḥ |*
> *sarvasattvahitāc cāpa dṛśyate śakracāpavat ||24||*
>
> 'The speech-path's topic, (namely) the Lord — the body made of knowledge — is seen like a rainbow, as well as apart from the benefit of all sentient beings.

*Mchan* : 'The speech-path's topic' means : — the topics of 'illusion' (*māyā*), etc. conveyed to the disciple. . . . Those remarks teach the 'illusory body' (*māyā-deha*) to be the body of Vajradhara, a rainbow body — the body of knowledge born from wind-and-mind-only of the Clear light.

In regard to the words 'as well as apart' (*ca-apa*), which were not translated into Tibetan, cf. *Guhyasamāja*, Chapter XVII, p. 134; *Mchan ḥgrel*, p. 153-5:

> *svabhāvaśuddhanairātmye dharmadhātunirālaye |*
> *kalpanā vajrasaṃbhūtā gīyate na ca gīyate ||*
>
> The imagination arisen from the *vajra* (of Body, Speech, and Mind) expresses in the case of the selflessness (= Clear Light) of the intrinsically pure (moving and stationary

life), and also does not express in the case of the full womb of *dharmadhātu* (with the *vajra* of *bodhicitta*).

*Pradipoddyotana* and *Mchan ḥgrel*:—'expresses' because it can appear like a rainbow, then teach the *dharma*; 'does not express' because discursive analysis does not reach reality.

The above appears to explain the two alternatives of verse 24, to wit: (1) 'seen like a rainbow,' and (2) 'apart from the benefit'. Furthermore, since the 'illusory body' when purified in the Clear Light is the Sambhoga-kāya located in, or made to correspond to, the 'speech center' of the throat, verse 24 alludes to this by saying "the speech-path's topic, (namely) the Lord."

The *Guhyasamājatantra*, Chapter III, has two celebrated mantras which point to the rainbow body of Vajradhara. The first (III, p. 14) begins the chapter :

> atha bhagavān kāyavākcittavajras tathāgataḥ sarvatathāgata-spharaṇameghavyūhaṃ nāma samādhiṃ samāpadyedaṃ vajravyūhaṃ nāma samādhipaṭalam udājahara /
>
> // *OM ŚŪNYATĀJÑĀNAVAJRASVABHĀVĀTMAKO 'HAṂ* //
>
> Then the Bhagavat, 'Diamond of Body, Speech, and Mind', the Tathāgata, immersing himself in the samādhi called 'array of clouds with the vibration of all the Tathāgatas,' proclaimed this samādhi-mass named 'diamond array':
>
> "Oṃ. I am the intrinsic nature of the knowledge diamond of voidness !"

The second (II, p. 15) runs as follows :

> atha bhagavān kāyavākcittavajras tathāgataḥ dharmadhātusvabhāvavajraṃ nāma samādhiṃ samāpadyedaṃ kāyavākcittādhiṣṭhānamantram udājahāra /
>
> // *OM DHARMADHĀTUSVABHĀVĀTMAKO 'HAM* //
>
> Then, the Bhagavat, 'Diamond of Body, Speech, and Mind', the Tathāgata, immersing himself in the samādhi named 'intrinsic-nature diamond of the *dharmadhātu* (=*Clear Light*)' proclaimed this mantra which blesses the body, speech, and mind :
>
> "Oṃ. I am the intrinsic nature of the Dharmadhātu !"

In the 'evident meaning' (*nītārtha*) interpretation of the *Pradīpo-*

*ddyotana*, both mantras incorporate the five Tathāgatas and a sixth Buddha; in the former case, identified with the five winds by name, and the sixth (Aham) identified with Vajrasattva, who is the incessant *bindu* of the heart (*Mchan ḥgrel* p. 35-4); in the latter case, identified with the five winds by the colors, constituting the rainbow of the verse 'VĀK', and the sixth, (Aham) identified with Vajradhara, as the gnosis of the Supreme Entity. In illustration let me translate the second mantra, according to *nītārtha* (*Pradīpoddyotana*, *Mchan ḥgrel* edition PTT, Vol. 158, p. 36-2):

> Then the Bhagavat, 'Diamond of Body, Speech and Mind' (=Vajradhara), the Tathāgata, immersing, himself in the samādhi (gazing at the Clear Light) named 'intrinsic nature diamond of the *dharmadhātu* (=Clear Light) proclaimed this *mantra* which blesses the body, speech, and mind :
>
> OṂ—(Vairocana as a blue-rayed wind serving as the mount of the gnosis of the Clear Light of the [Absolute] Object).
>
> DHARMA—(Ratnasambhava, as a yellow-rayed wind).
>
> DHĀTU—(Amitābha, as a red-rayed wind).
>
> SVABHĀVA— (Amoghasiddhi, as a green-rayed wind).
>
> ĀTMAKO—(Akṣobhya, as a white-rayed wind).
>
> AHAM—(Vajradhara, that gnosis itself of the Clear Light of the [Absolute] Object).

*Mchan ḥgrel* on the preceding : "This mantra expresses both the gnosis of the Clear Light of the Absolute Object and the five rays of wind which are its mount."

Since 'VĀK' refers in the praxis to the 'diamond muttering' a brief indication is given now about that. *Mchan ḥgrel*, p. 51-4-1, on Chapter Six ('Documents'), mentions that verses 15-18 concern the subtle yoga of the Stage of Completion, of which verse 15 is here repeated with Sanskrit :

> *nīlotpaladalākāraṃ pañcaśūlaṃ viśeṣataḥ |*
> *yavamātraṃ prayatnena nāsikāgre vicintayet ||*
>
> He should imagine with perseverance at the tip of his nose a five-pronged (thunderbolt) appearing like a blue lotus petal and in the advanced degree the size of a tiny barley grain.

The *Pradīpoddyotana* and *Mchan ḥgrel* clarify that the tip of the nose (among the three possible ones in the Stage of Completion) here meant is the one in the sacral place, now identified as the 'tip of the gem', i.e. the root of the penis (the svādhiṣṭhāna-cakra of the Hindu tantras). And in the advanced degree (*viśeṣataḥ*), he reduces the lotus to the size of a tiny barley grain. According to verse 16, the yogin then imagines the red eight-petalled lotus of that *cakra*, no bigger than a chick-pea, which is the lotus of the yogin's 'woman', his own *dharmodaya* ('source of dharmas'). Verse 17 mentions the still more subtle contemplation of a wheel therein. Finally (verse 18), the yogin can draw forth the 'Dharma word marked with body, speech, and mind,' consistent with the *nidāna* verse 'VĀK'.

The theory that the yogin's 'woman' is found at the base of the penis seems parallel with the womb in the woman found at the end of the vaginal tube. The Buddhist Anuttarayoga-tantra seems concerned with the symbolism of that base in the male and that womb in the woman rather than with what respectively leads up to them.

> //CIT// *cittaṃ caitasikāvidyā prajñopāyopalabdhikam.* /
> *śūnyātiśūnyamahāśūnyam iti cāpi pragiyate* //25//
>
> Thought (*citta*), thought derivative (*caitasika*), and nescience (*avidyā*) are also called respectively, Insight (*prajñā*), Means (*upāya*), Culmination (*upalabdhika*); as well as Void (*śūnya*), Further Void (*atiśūnya*), and Great Void (*mahāśūnya*).

*Pañcakrama*, 2nd krama, 7 :

> *ālokaś śūnyaṃ prajñā ca cittaṃ ca paratantrakam* /
>
> Light is Void, is Insight, is thought, is dependence (*paratantra*).

*Ibid.*, 2nd krama, 15 :

> *ālokābhāsaṃ ity uktam atiśūnyam upāyakaṃ* /
> *parikalpitaṃ tathā proktaṃ proktaṃ caitasikaṃ tathā* //
>
> Spread-of-Light is Further Void, is Means, also called 'imagination' (*parikalpita*) and called 'thought derivative'.

*Ibid.*, 2nd krama, 23 :

> *ālokasyopalabdhiś ca upalabdhaṃ tathaiva ca* /
> *pariniṣpannakaṃ caiva avidyā caiva nāmataḥ* //
>
> The Culmination-of-Light, likewise 'the culminated' also named 'perfection' (*pariniṣpannaka*) as well as 'nescience' (*avidyā*).

Tsoṅ-kha-pa's commentary on *Pañcakrama*, Vol. 159, p. 31-2

Synonymous terms for the Three Lights: ... those three (i.e. *prajñā*, *upāya*, and *avidyā*); the three *citta*, *manas*, *vijñāna*; the three, *parikalpita*, *paratantra*, *pariniṣpanna*; the three, hatred, lust, delusion; and the three *svabhāvas*. Among those, *upāya* is Spread-of-Light, *prajñā* is Light, the combination of those two as hermaphrodite (or androgyne) is Culmination-of-Light. Among the two, ecstasy and void, 'Light' is the preponderance of void mentality (*buddhi*); 'Spread-of-Light' the reverse thereof; 'Culmination-of-Light' those two (ecstasy and void) in equal parts.

Tsoṅ-kha-pa's commentary on the *Pañcakrama* called "Gsal baḥi sgron me" (PTT, Vol. 199, p. 31-4) faces the problem of why the three lights have as synonyms the terms *parikalpita*, *paratantra*, and *pariniṣpanna* (which are the well-known three *svabhāvas* or three *lakṣaṇas* of Yogācāra terminology). The following explanation may have been developed in Tibetau traditions :

/ rim lṅa las / snaṅ ba gźan dbaṅ daṅ / mched pa kun brtags daṅ / ñer thob la yoṅs grub tu gsuṅs la / de ltar bśad pa ni gzuṅ ḥdzin gñis rgyaṅs ched du snaṅ baḥi snaṅ gźi ni gźan dbaṅ daṅ / de ltar snaṅ ba la brten nas gsuṅ ḥdzin rjes tha dad par sgro btags pa kun brtags daṅ / ḥgyur ba med paḥi yoṅs grub mṅon du byas paḥi dor / kun brtags daṅ g ñis snaṅ gñis kas dben pa bźin du stoṅ pa rnams kyi thog maḥi gźi snaṅ ba daṅ / de la brten nas mched pa ḥbyuṅ ba daṅ / ñer thob kyi tsho sṅa ma gñis ka log nas thobs śes gnis ka log nas thabs śes gñis ka log nas thabs śes mñam par ḥjug paḥi chos mthun la brten nas yin nam sñam ste dpyad par byaḥo / The *Pañcakrama* says (respectively at II, 7; II, 15; and II, 23) that Light is *paratantra* ('dependent'), Spread-of-Light is *parikalpita* ('imaginary'), and Culmination-of-Light is *pariniṣpannaka* ('perfect'). One should ponder whether this is the explanation: The basic Light which shines when severing the distance between the thing perceived and the perceiver is 'dependent'. Having in that way taken recourse to Light, the subsequent difference between, and affirmation of thing perceived and perceiver,

> is 'imaginary'. The casting away of the two lights—'imaginary' and the other light—has incessant 'perfect' immediacy. Therefore, according to the particular secret state: — Light is the initial basis of the voids; on that basis Spread-of-Light arises; and at the time of Culmination-of-Light, having averted the former two—i.e. having averted both 'means' and 'insight', one takes recourse to the common *dharma* of uniting 'means' and 'insight'.

The three lights constitute the fourth of the five signs presented in the *Guhyasamāja*, Chapter XVIII and included in Candrakīrti's comments ('Documents', PART ONE). The first sign, a mirage, manifests through dissolution of earth into water. The second, smoke, through dissolution of water into fire. The third, fire-flies, through dissolution of fire into wind. The fourth, a changeable lamp, through dissolution of wind into the three lights. Through sequential dissolution of the three lights, there is the fifth sign, the Clear Light like a cloudless sky.

Vitapāda, in his commentary *Sukusuma-nāma-dvikrama-tattva-bhāvanā-mukhāgama-vṛtti* (PTT, Vol. 65, p. 58-4, 5) explains the signs in accordance with the preceding *prāṇāyāma* involving the *bindu*:

> Now, what happens at first when that yogin turns back his discursive thought (*vikalpa*) ? He should know that at first there is the sign which is a manifestation like a mirage. One should understand that phase this way: the rays from that *bindu* have a pattern both bright and not bright, appearing like a mirage. This is an illusory appearance allowed in one's stream of consciousness that should be warded off, because one is attached to it if he has the pride of thinking that he knows the sign. The same applies to the others. It is like smoke when brighter than the mirage, while lacking colors such as green, white, and so on. The 'fireflies' or lights in space, are brighter than the smoke and of different type. The sign 'shining like a lamp' is superior to the fireflies and of different type. Those are seen in the manner of rays, with each one brighter than the preceding one. Concerning the phrase, "like the meaning of non-duality of the profound and the bright," the body is considered to be like smoke,

> because it is not genuine. Moreover, what is the manifestation? "Bright like a cloudless sky" means a cloudless sky that manifests with special brilliance.

The above shows the difference between the 'Ārya' and the 'Buddhajñānapāda' schools of the *Guhyasamāja*. The 'Ārya' tradition understands the mystic signs to be related to sequential dissolution of the elements, and takes the fourth sign 'shining like a lamp, to stand for three light stages. The other tradition explains the signs as resulting from contemplation of the *bindu*, does not relate them to the elements, and does not subdivide the sign 'shining like a lamp'.

A remarkable ability to describe the praxis is found in Āryadeva's *Caryāmelāpaka-pradīpa* (quoted in Tsoṅ-kha-pa's *Sṅags rim chen mo*, f. 456b-4), where we read a most lucid statement of the sequence:

> / spyod bsdus las / /de nas skye ba gcig nas gcig tu goms pas bdag med paḥi chos la bslabs pas rnam par dag paḥi sbyor ba khoṅ du chud nas raṅ b źin gyi snaṅ ba daṅ gcig tu ḥdre bar bya ste rim pa ḥdis don dam paḥi bden pa la dmigs par byaḥo / deḥi rim pa ḥdi yin te phuṅ po la sogs pa ni khams phra ba la gźug go / khams phra ba ni yaṅ sems la gźug go / sems ni yaṅ sems pa la gźug go / sems pa ni yaṅ ma rig pa la gzug ste de ltar spyad nas gñid log par byed do / de la dus ḥdir ni sems daṅ sems pa ma rig pa la rab tu źugs paḥi skad cig la draṅ pa brjod paḥo / phyis ni brjod pa yaṅ med paḥi ye śes kyi ṅo bo ñid ni ḥod gsal baḥo / yaṅ grol ba na rluṅ gi raṅ bźin rñed de gaṅ gi tshe rmi lam gźan dag ḥbyuṅ ba na ji srid du rnam par śes pa mi gYo ba de srid du gñid log nas ḥod gsal ba la blta ste / de ni so sor raṅ g is rig pa lus daṅ ṅag daṅ bral baḥi don dam paḥi bden pa naṅ gi mṅon par byaṅ chub pa źes byaḥo / źes gsuṅs te...
>
> Then, by meditative repetition from one life to the next, and by training in the self-less natures, he comes to fully understand the right praxis: how to mix together with the Light of intrinsic nature; how to visualize the Supreme Truth (*paramārtha-satya*) by this sequence. The sequence of it, is as follows : The personality aggregates (*skandha*) and so on, should be merged into the subtle element (**sūkṣma-dhātu*) (i.e. wind); the subtle element, in turn,

merged into consciousness (*citta*); consciousness, in turn, merged into mentals (*caitta*); mentals, in turn, merged into nescience (*avidyā*); and so practising he creates deep sleep (*suṣupti*). Now, in this life, he expresses the truth at the instant when *citta* and *caitta* are absorbed in *avidyā*. At the next instant there is the Clear Light with the intrinsic nature of the inexpressible gnosis. Even when it is released, he has attained the intrinsic nature of wind; and at whatever time other dreams occur, then as long as his perception (*vijñāna*) is immobile (*acala*) i.e. one-pointed, in *samādhi*, the deep sleep (*suṣupti*) (is also present) and he sees the Clear Light. That introspection is called 'inner revelation of the Supreme Truth that is free from Body and Speech'.

The meaning of this remarkable passage is exposed in Tsoṅ-kha-pa's commentary on the 'Six Laws of Nāro-pā' (PTT, Vol. 161, pp. 7-8 and p. 12). Here we learn a distinction between the Clear Light of the waking state (*jāgrat-prabhāsvara*) and the Clear Light of deep sleep (*suṣupti-prabhāsvara*). The waking state Clear Light is also distinguished as subjective (*viṣayin*), the Jñāna-Dharmakāya, and the objective (*viṣaya*), the unconstructed (*asaṃskṛta*) Dharmakāya. The subjective type I understand by former terminology as 'Clear Light of True Mind' or Symbolic Clear Light (of three gnoses or Jñāna lights, namely, Light, Spread of Light, and Culmination of Light, referred to by Āryadeva as, respectively, *citta*, *caitta*, and *avidyā*). The objective type is the Clear Light of the Absolute Entity. The Clear Light of deep sleep is similarly distinguished into the subjective deep sleep which is heavy (*ḥthug po*) or light (*srab mo*), 'lost' (*ñams*) (to memory) or 'comprehended' (*rtogs pa*), and the objective 'ground' (*gži*) Clear Light of death. In the waking state category is the 'son Clear Light' contemplated with praxis of 'bliss-void' (*sukha-śūnya*) (*bde stoṅ sbyor yin bsgoms paḥi buḥi ḥod gsal*) which is the Clear Light of the path. In the deep sleep category is the 'mother Clear Light' which is the 'ground' Clear Light of death (*gžiḥi ḥchi baḥi ḥod gsal ni maḥi ḥod gsal*). As I understand this yoga praxis, the intention is to make the 'son' Clear Light break through to subjective waking state, and to make the 'mother' Clear Light break through to subjective deep sleep (*suṣupti*) as a *samādhi*. Then the yogin should be capable of mixing the 'mother' and 'son' Clear Lights (*ḥod gsal ma bu gñis bsre thub pa*). All the preceding appears to be intended in Āryadeva's passage.

Further details of the process are sketched in C. C. Chang's *Teachings of Tibetan Yoga*, pp. 94-104. A fuller treatment is found in Tsoṅ-kha-pa's *Mthaḥ gcod* on chapter seven (PTT, Vol. 156, p. 45) and in his *Don gsal ba* on the *Guhyasamāja* (PTT Vol. 160, pp. 146 and 147). This exposition by Tsoṅ-kha-pa, of the *dhāraṇā-aṅga* is based on the *Saṃdhivyākaraṇa* and *Pradipoddyotana* on Chapter VII, the *Vajramālā* and its commentary by Alaṃkakalaśa, and Āryadeva's *Caryāmelāpaka-pradipa*. Previously, under *nidāna* verse 4, a passage was quoted from Nāgārjuna's *Piṇḍikṛta-sādhana* (43-44A), which in fact stems from the *Vajramālā*. The theory is to draw the $5 \times 5 = 25$ entities into the Clear Light as the *paramārtha-maṇḍala*. There are five each of *skandhas*, *dhātus*, *indriyas*, *viṣayas*, and *jñānas*. The first group to dissolve is of course the one with earth element (*dhātu*) since this gives rise to the first sign, a mirage. With dissolution of the earth element, the entire body is desiccated (i.e. thirsts for water). Individual explanations are given for dissolution of the form-skandha (*rūpa-skandha*), mirror-like knowledge, eye-organ (*indriya*), form-object (*viṣaya*)

The second group includes the element of water, the dissolution of which, yielding the sign of smoke, involves the drying up in one's body of spittle, perspiration, urine, menstrual blood, semen, and so on. Besides, the *skandha* of feeling, equality knowledge, ear organ, and sense object of sound, are dissolved.

The third group includes the element of fire, the dissolution of which, yielding the sign of fire-flies, involves loss of ability to eat, drink, and digest. Besides, the *skandha* of ideas, discriminative knowledge, sense of smell, and odors, are dissolved.

The fourth group includes the element of wind, the dissolution of which, yielding the sign of a changeable lamp, involves the transfer from their individual places of the ten winds, the *prāṇa*, etc. Besides, the *skandha* of motivations, the procedure-of-duty knowledge, organ of taste, and tastes, are dissolved.

Also, as Tsoṅ-kha-pa points out, at the time of dissolution of each group, the deities of the corresponding Tathāgata family are drawn into the Clear Light together with the other members of the group. Thus, the 'Fury Kings' (*nidāna* verse 17) and other members of the family (*nidāna* verse 18) are sequentially so drawn into the Clear Light of Death. In the case of the first group, Vairocana's family; second group, Ratnasambhava's family; third group, Amitābha's family; fourth group, Amogha-siddhi's family.

Finally, there is the dissolution indicated by that passage of the *Piṇḍikṛta-sādhana*, i.e. of the upper and lower Fury Kings, of the twice-eighty prakṛtis, and of Akṣobhya's family; whereupon 'perception' (*vijñāna*) passes "to the Clear Light, also called 'universal void with *nirvāṇa*' and 'Dharmakāya'."

> //TA// *tataścaryāṃ prakurvita prakṛtyābhāsabhedavit* /
> *karmakāyaṃ parityajya vajradehatvam āpnuyāt* //26//
>
> Then, knowing the differences of the *prakṛtis* and the Lights, one should engage in the *caryā*, (namely), abandoning the body of works (*karmakāya*), he would obtain the diamond body (*vajradeha*).

*Mchan*: Knowing the differences of the eighty *prakṛtis* and the three Lights (=three gnoses), the time has come for one to engage in the *caryā* ('praxis') part of the Stages of Completion. He takes recourse to contemplation of the profound means of piercing the centers in the body. Then he takes recourse to experiencing the generation of the voids by the dissolution seauence of the winds. Thus he has certainty in the methods of arousing the three Lights and the (eighty) *vikalpa*-s. However, the verse takes for granted that one has achieved the Lights of 'arcane mind' (*cittaviveka*), then alludes to the subsequent (1) *caryā* for the aim of accomplishing the Illusory Body (*māyā-deha*), as well as to the (2) *caryā* for the aim of *śaikṣa-yuganaddha* after attaining the characteristics of the Illusory Body; but the verse does not allude to the (3) third *caryā* for the purpose of *aśaikṣa-yuganaddha* after attaining the *śaikṣa-yuganaddha*. (1) Thus the *sādhaka* engaged in the *caryā*, abandoning the 'maturation' (*vipāka*) body propelled by former deeds (*karma*), obtains the illusorv body called 'diamond body'. (2) Having obtained that, he attains the *śaikṣa-yuganaddha*, wherein the 'diamond body' is uninterruptedly affiliated (*rigs ḥdra rgyun mi ḥchad par rdo rje sku*). This illusory body is a topic of the third krama of the *Pañcakrama* called *Svādhiṣṭhāna-krama*.

The *Pradīpoddyotana* on Chapter VI (*Mchan ḥgrel*, p. 53) quotes the *Vajrahṛdayālaṃkāra-tantra* :

*evaṃ samādhiyuktena nirvikalpena mantriṇaḥ |*
*kālāvadhiṃ parityajya prāpyate 'nuttaraṃ padam ||*

When one thus abandons the limitation of time by non-discursiveness joined to the samādhi of a mantrin, he attains the incomparable rank.

Here the expression 'limitation of time' (*kālāvadhi*) seems to refer to the 'maturation body'.

About that 'non-discursiveness', there is the important verse 3 in Chapter II of the *Guhyasamājatantra*:

*abhāve bhāvanābhāvo bhāvanā naiva bhāvanā |*
*iti bhāvo na bhāvaḥ syād bhāvanā nopalabhyate ||*

When there is an absence, there is no contemplation (because there is nothing to contemplate). (But also,) a contemplation is not a contemplation (of reality). That being so, whether it be a presence (for contemplation) or an absence (for no contemplation), the contemplation is not perceptively reached.

From the various interpretations in the *Pradīpoddyotana* (*Mchan ḥgrel*, pp. 31 and 32), we present here the 'pregnant sense':

When there is an absence (because of dissolution in the central channel), there is no contemplation. The contemplation (of the impure illusory body=*saṃvṛti-satya*) is not a contemplation (of the Clear Light). That being so, whether it be a presence (the illusory body) or an absence (disappearance in the central channel), the contemplation (of the two truths, *saṃvṛti* and *paramārtha*) is not perceptively reached (in either case).

Tsoṅ-kha-pa quotes the above *nidāna* verse 26 in his *Pañcakrama* commentary. Vol. 159, p. 51-5, to emphasize that this *caryā* is indispensable for becoming a Buddha in this present life. If there is this aim, one must apply himself to the *caryā* of the two *dhyānas* called 'contraction' (*piṇḍagrāha*) and 'expansion (*anubheda*), set forth in *Pañcakrama*, Abhisambodhi-k., IV,25-27:

*prāptopadeśakaḥ śiṣyo dvidhā yoga athābhyaset |*
*piṇḍagrāhakrameṇaiva tathā caivānubhedataḥ ||25||*
*śirasaḥ pādato vāpi yāvad dhṛdayam āgataḥ |*
*bhūtakoṭiṃ viśed yogi piṇḍagrāha iti smṛtaḥ || 26 |*
*sthāvaraṃ jaṅgamaṃ caiva pūrvaṃ kṛtvā prabhāsvaram |*
*paścāt kuryāt tathātmānam anubhedakramo hy ayam || 27 ||*

The disciple who has secured the precepts then applies

> himself unremittingly to *yoga* of two sorts : by the sequence of 'contraction' as well as by 'expansion'.
> Drawing (the winds) from head down, and from feet up, into the heart, the yogi enters *bhūtakoṭi* (the true limit): this is called 'contraction'.
> Having first rendered the stationary and the moving life into the Clear Light, he then renders that into himself : this is the stage of 'expansion'.

Again, Tsoṅ-kha-pa's *Pañcakrama* commentary, Vol. 159, p. 52-1 and p. 53-5, explains that those are comparable to the (Mother Tantra terminology) '*yogas* of transfer (*ḥpho ba*=S. *saṃkrānti*) and entrance to the city (*groṅ ḥjug*, S. *purāvatāra*)'. Hence the praxis proceeds along two lines : the first involves the manipulation of winds to separate the five basic winds from the five secondary winds; the second involves a separation of 'mind-based perception' (*manovijñāna*) from the five outer-sense based perceptions. Thus, the separation of the 'intrinsic body' from the 'body of maturation' has the aspects of wind and mind, aimed at separating the subtle from the coarse, to yield the body formed of 'wind and mind only'.

*Pañcakrama*, Svādhiṣṭhāna-krama, III, 19 :

> *tad eva vāyusaṃyuktaṃ vijñānatritayaṃ punaḥ* |
> *jāyate yoginā mūrtir māyādehas tad ucyate* ||
> Precisely that vijñāna-triad joined to the winds then arises as a body by a *yogin*. That is called 'illusory body'.

*Pañcakrama*, 3rd krama, 23 :

> *darpaṇapratibimbena māyādehaṃ ca lakṣayet* |
> *varṇāṃ indrāyudhenaiva vyāpitvam udakendunā* ||
> One characterizes the Illusory Body by the image in a mirror, the colors by a rainbow, the spread by the moon in the waters (Cf. Śrī Lakṣmī's commentary, p. 35- 3: the rainbow body means having the five colors).

The *Vajrajñānasamuccaya* contains twelve similes of illusion concerning that body:—(1) phantom (*sgyu ma*), (2) moon in the waters (*chu zla*), (3) shade (*mig yor*), (4) mirage (*smig rgyu*), (5) dream (*rmi lam*), (6) echo (*brag cha*), (7) cloud (*dri zaḥi groṅ khyer*), (8) hallucination (*mig ḥphrul*), (9) rainbow (*ḥjaḥ tshon*), (10) lightning (*glog*), (11) water bubble (*chuḥi chu bur*), (12) image in a mirror (*me loṅ gi gzugs brñan*). Tsoṅ-kha-pa's commentary on that Tantra, Vol. 160, p. 160-4, 5, is in this case apparently based on the *Caryāmelāpaka-pradīpa* : 1. It is like a phantom (illusory man) because, although it has a full complement of main and secondary limbs when generated as the body of Vajradhara from wind and mind-only, it is nothing but wind and mind-only. 2. It is like the moon in the waters wherever it is spread. 3. It is like a shade, i.e. the shadow body of a man, because it lacks flesh, bone, and so on. 4. It is like a mirage, because it shifts by the instant. 5. It is like a dream body because, as a body accomplished from wind and mind-only, it is (similar to) a body in a dream which is imputed distinctions that differ from what it properly is. 6. It is like an echo, because, although it belongs to the same stream of consciousness as the 'maturation body' (*vipāka-kāya*), it appears elsewhere. 7. It is like a cloud, because that body possesses the maṇḍala of residence (*ādhāra*) and of residents (*ādheya*). 8. It is like a hallucination, because being single it appears multiple. 9. It is like a rainbow, or 'Indra's bow', since that body appears with five colors that are unimpeded and unmixed. 10. It is like the lightning bursting from the cloud, from its location within the personality aggregates of the maturation body. 11. It is like a water bubble in very clear water when it suddenly emerges from the realm of the void. 12. It is like the image of Vajradhara in a mirror, because of simultaneous completion of all the major and minor limbs.

One of the problems of the commentarial tradition is to relate the theory of the two *dhyānas* known from the *Pañcakrama* back to the basic *Guhyasamājatantra*. Tsoṅ-kha-pa, *Pañcakrama* commentary, Vol. 159, p. 57-1, ff., points out that regarding the contemplation (or cultivation) of the two *dhyānas* by way of the illusory body (*sgyu lus pas bsam gtan gñis sgom pa la*), the Mar-pa school does not explain it in terms of piling up the three *sattvas* of the three *vajras*. Tsoṅ-kha-pa goes on to highly approve the precept handed down from Ḥgos (*ḥgos lugs*), that the *caryā* of both *dhyānas* is indicated in *Guhyasamājatantra*, chapter eleven, verses 40-44 (with emendations):

*buddhamaṇḍalamadhyasthaṃ kāye vairocanaṃ nyaset* |
*Oṃkāraṃ hṛdaye dhyātvā mantravijñānaṃ bhāvayet* ||
*nirodhavajragataṃ citte yadā tasya prajāyate* |
*sa bhavec cintāmaṇiḥ śrīmān sarvabuddhāgrasādhakaḥ* ||
*buddhamaṇḍalamadhyasthaṃ vajrākṣobhyaṃ prabhāvayet* |

*Hūṃkāraṃ hṛdaye dhyātvā cittaṃ bindugataṃ nyaset* /
*buddhamaṇḍalamadhyasthaṃ amitābhaṃ prabhāvayet* //
*Āḥkāraṃ hṛdaye dhyātvā vajraṃ bindugataṃ nyaset* //
*idaṃ tat samayāgrāgryaṃ trivajrābhedyabhāvanam* /
*nirodhasamayajñānaṃ buddhasiddhiṃ samāvahet* //

He should place in (his own) body the Vairocana abiding in the middle of the Buddha-maṇḍala. Having meditated on the Oṃ in his heart, he should contemplate the *vijñāna* in the *mantra*.

At the time he engenders the state of cessation-*vajra* in his *citta*, he becomes the 'wishing gem', 'glorious one', best *sādhaka* of all the Buddhas.

He should contemplate a diamond Akṣobhya in the middle of the Buddha-maṇḍala. Having meditated on the Hūṃ in his heart, he should place the *citta* in the form of a *bindu*.

He should contemplate Amitābha stationed in the middle of the Buddha-maṇḍala. Having meditated on the Āḥ in his heart, he should place the *vajra* in the form of a *bindu*.

This, the chief of best pledges, the contemplation of the inseparable three *vajras* (of one's own body, speech, and mind), the knowledge of the cessation-pledge, brings the success of the Buddhas.

Tsoṅ-kha-pa also mentions that some persons claimed that the above verses portray the *dhyāna* of 'contraction' while the subsequent *Guhyasamāja* verses (XI, 45-47) portray the 'expansion'. Tsoṅ-kha-pa denies this theory and states that both *dhyānas* are portrayed in the above verses, and that the following verses 45-47 simply expand on the same topic.

In preparation for this *caryā*, according to the indication of *Mkhas grub rje's Fundamentals of the Buddhist Tantras*, the candidate is conferred the 'Prajñā-jñāna Initiation'. This is the initiation concerned with the *cakras* or *bhagas*. These *bhagas* become the centers of associating four voids (the four lights) with four ecstasies. Abhayākaraguptapāda's *Upadeśamañjari-nāma* (PTT, Vol. 87, p. 82) associates the lights with ecstasies as follows : Light (*āloka*) with ecstasy (*ānanda*); Spread-of-Light (*ālokābhāsa*) with high ecstasy (*paramānanda*); Culmination-of-Light (*ālokopalabdhi*) with extraordinary ecstasy (*viramānanda*); Clear Light (*prabhāsvara*) with consubstantial ecstasy (*sahajānanda*). The same identification is made in the *Mahāmudrātilaka-tantra*, Chapter Five, according to quotation in *Snags rim*, f. 408a-5. Tsoṅ-kha-pa's *Pañcakrama* commentary "Gsal baḥi sgron me" (PTT, Vol. 159, p. 2, 3, discusses this association of voids (= lights) with ecstasies (*ānanda*), and *ibid*, p. 2-4, cites the *Vajramālā* for the direct order (*rjes lugs ḥbyuṅ*) and reverse order (*lugs ldog rim pa*) of the four ecstasies. In the direct order *ānanda* starts at the Mahāsukha-cakra of the head, down to the Sambhoga-cakra of the throat, where starts *paramānanda*; that down to the Dharma-cakra of the heart, where starts *viramānanda*; that down to the *Nirmāṇa-cakra* of the navel, where starts *sahajānanda* (continuing down to the 'tip of the thunderbolt gem', already identified as the root of the penis, according to the Prajñā-jñāna initiation as portrayed in Mkhas grub rje's-work). In the reverse order, there is *ānanda* up to the Nirmāṇa cakra; *paramānanda* up to the Dharma-cakra; *viramānanda* up to the Sambhoga-cakra; and *sahajānanda* up to the Mahāsukha-cakra. Again, according to Mkhas grub rje's initiation section, this reverse order is prepared for by the Fourth Initiation.

### F. *Hṛdayavajrayoṣid* (*The Diamond Ladies of the Heart*)

In terms of six-membered yoga this is 5. *anusmṛti* ('recollection') and in the *Pañcakrama* system, it is Abhisaṃbodhi-krama, the fourth. Besides, according to the *Pradīpoddyotana* it is included in *yuganaddha*, and therefore is the initial 'śaikṣa-yuganaddha' ('the pair-united where there is learning'). It is the ability to come forth from the Clear Light (equivalent to going through the portals of death) as a yogin in command of the situation.

When the Illusory Body has been purified in the Clear Light and emerges to pass in reverse order through the three lights, it is treated by the simile of a fish, in *Pañcakrama*, 4th krama (Abhisaṃbodhi), verse 31:

> *yathā nadījalāt svacchān mīna utpatito drutam* /
> *sarvaśūnyāt tathā svacchān māyājālam udīryate* //
>
> Like a fish quickly springing up from a clear stream,
> so the net of illusion emerges from the clear universal void.

For this phase there is the Fourth Initiation (there is no further one), which the *Guhyasamājatantra*, Chapter XVIII, describes as just like the Prajñā-jñāna initiation. This is because here the yogin experiences the reverse order of the very same combination of voids with ecstasies.

The activities and symbolism are centered about the heart. Three nidāna verses are devoted to this : HṚ, the place of aim and creativity; DA, the yield or accomplishment; YA, the after-realization. Both the diamond (*vajra*) and the lady (*yoṣit*) symbolism are associated with the heart in Indrabhūti's *Jñāna-siddhi*: hṛdayaṃ jñānaṃ tad eva vajrayoṣit ('the Diamond Lady is just that heart gnosis'). The diamond (or thundebolt) has two aspects according to *Guhyasamāja*, Chap. XVIII, 39 (with considerable emendation suggested by Nāgārjuna's commentary, PTT, Vol. 60, p. 7-5, which mentions the two syllables 'Va' and 'Jra'), that is, a destructive aspect of VA and a holding or positive aspect of JRA,

> *pañcahetiś ca vetīti vajram ity abhidhīyate |*
> *jrakāro dhṛgiti khyāto vijñānaṃ vajradhṛṅmanaḥ ||*
>
> 'Vajra' is defined as 'Va', namely the five prongs, and as 'Jra', explained as holding. 'Vijñāna' is the mind which holds the *vajra*.

The lady also has two aspects, YO, the automatic union taking place through 'recollection'; and ṢID, the otherworldliness of the act.

The first or destructive meaning of *vajra* is that found in Alaṃkakalaśa's commentary on the *Śrī-Vajramālā* (PTT, Vol. 61, p. 182-4), while expounding the 'unshared sense' of the Tantra: "So as to explain the word '*vajra*', it is said 'The *vajra* and also the *vikalpas*,' because it destroys the set of natures, (*prakṛti*) amounting to one-hundred-sixty (= twice 80 *vikalpas*)" (rdo rjeḥi sgra bśad paḥi phyir / / rdo rje de yaṅ rnam rtog rnams źes gsuṅs te / raṅ bźin gyi tshogs brgya drug cu po rnams bcom pa ñid kyi phyir ro). Tsoṅ-kha-pa's *Rdor bzlas* (Lhasa Collected Works, Cha, f. 24b-4, 5, 6)starts with the first meaning and then passes to the second or positive meaning of *vajra* : "When the 'wind-mind' dissolves there untying the knot of the heart *nāḍī*, it is the sublime place with cessation of the 160 (= twice 80) *vikalpas*. Because it is not perturbed by discursive thought (*vikalpa*), it is explained as field of the (Buddha) Akṣobhya (the imperturbable)'; therefore, one may also understand it as the narrow space laid in the heart of Akṣobhya. That essential place is also called Sukhāvatī, since it is the supreme place for generating great ecstasy' (*mahāsukha*). The *bodhicitta* (there), through cessation of death, is (the Buddha) Amitāyus; and because the infinite light of *prajñā* arises therefrom, it is also called 'field of Amitābha'." ( / sñiṅ gaḥi rtsa mdud grol baḥi gnas der rluṅ sems thim pa ni rnam rtog brgya rtsa daṅ brgya cu [*sic.* for drug cu] ḥgog paḥi gnas dam pa yin pas / rnam rtog gis mi bskyod pas mi bskyod paḥi źiṅ du bśad de mi bskyod pa thug kar ḥgod paḥi dog paḥaṅ des śes par byaḥo / gnad de bde ba can gyi źiṅ duḥaṅ brjod de bde ba chen po skye baḥi gnas kyi mchog daṅ / byaṅ chub kyi sems ni ḥchi ba ḥgog pas tshe dpag med yin la / de las byuṅ baḥi śes rab kyi ḥod mthaḥ yas paḥi phyir ro / / ḥod dpag med kyi źiṅ duḥaṅ gsuṅs so / ). The positive meaning of *vajra* is involved in the frequent discussions of the Jñānapāda school about the 'inviolable drop' (**akṣata-bindu*; T. *mi śigs paḥi thig le*) of the heart, for example, in Vitapāda's commentary on the *Muktitilaka* (PTT, Vol. 65, p. 135-2), where the form of the 'inviolable drop' in the heart is said to be, for example, like a grain of mustard seed; and to be the non-*prapañca* of any *dharma* (*chos thams cad kyi ma spros pa*). Vitapāda also mentions in the same place a theory about the three kinds of *bindu* that they are identified with the three kinds of masters (*ācārya*), the 'causal master' (**hetu-ācārya*), the 'conditional master' (**pratyaya-ācārya*), and 'co-natal master' (**sahaja-ācārya*); and that the 'inviolable drop' is the 'co-natal master'. (Vitapāda's passage is given in full and explained in A. Wayman, *The Buddhist Tantras*, pp. 49-50).

The 'recollection' (*anusmṛti*) takes place through the goddess (*yoṣit*) or 'perfection of insight' (*prajñā-pāramitā*). The *Guhyasamājatantra*, Chapter VII, treats this 'recollection' with various examples. Perhaps the most important illustration involves verse 34 (translated in *Pradīpoddyotana* and *Mchan ḥgrel* context):

*tatra kathaṃ prajñāpāramitāsamayānusmṛtibhāvanā /*
*prakṛtiprabhāsvarāḥ sarve anutpannā nirāśravāḥ /*
*na bodhir nābhisamayo na dhātuḥ na ca sambhavaḥ //*

And what is the contemplation with recollection of the Perfection-of-Insight pledge?

All those with (entrance into, *praveśa*) the Clear Light and its (accompanying) *prakṛtis* (numbering 160 by day and night), are unborn (because the body taken is illusory) and without flux (because not mere appearance, *nirābhāsatvāt*) when there is no (i.e. no attention to) enlightenment, no understanding, no realm (i.e. receptacle, *ādhāra*), and no emergence (of phenomenal abodes).

The *Pradīpoddyotana* at this point cites the *Vajroṣṇīṣatantra* (translated here with help of *Mchan ḥgrel*, p. 60-2):

*| mṛtyunā *tv avikalpena prajñāpāramitā nayā |*
*| prajñāpāramitā jātiḥ prajñāpāramitā smṛtiḥ ||*
*| prajñāpāramitā bodhiḥ prajñāpāramitā layā |*
*| prajñāpāramitā muktiḥ sarvāśāparipūrakā ||*

The Perfection of Insight has the method (=the means, *upāya*) by reason of non-discursive death (=the Clear Light of Death). The Perfection of Insight has the birth (=the Illusory Body emerging from the Clear Light) and the recollection (*smṛti=anusmṛti-aṅga*; for becoming a Buddha in the Intermediate State). The Perfection of Insight has the enlightenment (=yuganaddha) and the merger (with the Clear Light). The Perfection of Insight has the liberation (from the two hindrances, of defilement and the knowable). (For those reasons) it fulfills all hopes.

*||HṚ|| hṛdi kṛtvārthācaryāṃ vai laukikīṃ sa tathāgataḥ |*
*nirmāya saṃvṛtaṃ kāyaṃ kāmāṃś cared yathāyathaṃ ||27||*

The worldling praxis of aim having been formed in the heart, he the Tathāgata, creating a conventional body, practises desires exactly as he cares.

*Mchan*: The praxis of aim on behalf of worldly beings having been posited in the heart of the *sādhaka*—the Tathāgata, namely Vairocana, etc., transforming himself in appearance, i.e. creating a conventional body, practises in desire fields (=the five sense objects) exactly in Tathāgata correspondence (i.e. Vairocana in forms, etc.). The verse shows the engagement in the time of praxis.

*Prakāśikā* on Hṛ: 'Creating a conventional body' means emanating the *maṇḍala-cakra* with the nature of Tathāgatas, goddesses, Bodhisattvas, and krodhas.

Bu-ston (*Bśad sbyar*, Vol. Ta, f. 57a-b) on Hṛ cites Āryadeva: "The one dwelling in the circle of yoṣits, with a single *mudrā*, or with four *mudrās*, should recollect the Svādhiṣṭhāna. Even after the yogin has dwelt on the level of highest bliss, he should always enjoy pleasant forms, sounds, odors, tastes, and tangibles" (/ phyag rgya gcig daṅ ldan paḥam // yaṅ na phyag rgya bźi daṅ ldan / /btsun moḥi ḥkhor na bźugs pas kyaṅ / / bdag byin brlab pa rjes dran bya / / gzugs daṅ sgra daṅ de bźin dri / /ro daṅ reg bya sdug pa rnams / /bde mchog go ḥphaṅ gnas nas kyaṅ / / rnal ḥbyor pa yis rtag tu myaṅ / źes so /).

Concerning those four *mudrās*, i.e. the four goddesses, Locanā, etc., they are referred to as 'his enjoyments' in *Guhyasamājatantra*, Chap. XVIII, p. 157 :

> *tasya bhogāś catur jñeyāḥ svādhiṣṭhānādibhis tathā /*
> *vīrāṇām ekavaktrāṇāṃ ekaikaṃ mūrdhni secanam //*
>
> His four enjoyments are to be known by means of the Svādhiṣṭhāna, etc. Accordingly there is the anointment one-by-one on the head(s) of the one-faced heroes.

In partial explanation of the passage just cited, Nāgārjuna's *Aṣṭādaśa-paṭala-vistara-vyākhyā* (PTT, Vol. 60, p. 10-2) states: " 'His four enjoyments' are the four goddesses, Locanā etc." (loṅs spyod bzi ni spyan la sogs pa bzi ste). Furthermore, we read in *Guhyasamājatantra*, Chap, XVIII, p. 166 (translation aided by Nāgārjuna's *vyākhyā*, p. 16-4-6):

> *vidyārājñīti vikhyātā caturbhogā mahārdhikā /*
> *sarvakāmeti vijñeyā vajrādhipatayas tathā //*
>
> When the four enjoyments (= four goddesses, Locanā, etc.) have the great magical powers (= five Tathāgatas), they are called 'Queen of Vidyā' (= Rūpavajrā, etc.). In the same circumstances, the Diamond Lords (= the Bodhisattvas) are known as 'All desire' (= Yamāntaka, etc.).

The maṇḍala which the *Prakāśikā* refers to has an alternate form according to Tsoṅ-kha-pa's *Pañcakrama* commentary (PTT, Vol. 159, p. 74-5 to 75-1) called a '*gaṇa-cakra*' (tshogs kyi dkyil ḥkhor). In its middle is the yogin skilled in the praxis. The first series is the four yosits which he places in the sequence of E, S, W, N, namely Bde mchog sgyu ma, E-ma-ho bde ba, Sgron ma, and Śaśi. Those are consorts (*sahacarī*, 'wives') (lhan cig spyod paḥi bud med), presumably to be identified with the four goddesses, Locanā, etc. Other sets of four goddesses, totalling sixteen, are disposed in outer circles and called 'female attendants' (*anucarī*; T. rjes su spyod paḥi bud med). The names of those deities belong to Mother Tantra rather than *Guhyasamāja* tradition.

Furthermore, the phrase 'creating a conventional body' can be illustrated in the case of Śākyamuni with tantric reinterpretation (see the theory of the 'Way' ornament in the introductory treatment of 'The seven ornaments and subdivisions'). The *Pradīpoddyotana* (*Mchan ḥgrel*, p. 12-5 to 13-1) has this passage:

/ uktam evaitad bhagavatā / asādhāraṇaguhyamahāyogatantre / athāparaṃ sarvajñāparivārasaṃpatti(ṃ) pravakṣyāmi / tadyathā śuddhodanamahārājo mañjuśrī bhavati / mahāmāyādevī lokeśvaro bhavati / yaśodharā śrīdevī rāhulo vajrasattvaḥ sāradvatīputraḥ sarvanivaraṇaviṣkambhī bhavati / āryānandaḥ sthaviras samantabhadro bhavati / devadattas sthaviro devendras śrīśākyamunis samyaksambuddho mahāvairocano bhavati / anena nyāyena saṅgītikāra iti / parṣad iti / ādikarmikasattvāvatāraṇāya buddhanāṭako 'yaṃ pradarśitaḥ /

This was said by the Lord in the 'unshared' *Guhyamahāyogatantra* [possibly the Yoga-tantra catalogued as the *Vajraśekhara-mahāguhyayogatantra*]: "Now I shall also reveal the perfection of the retinue of omniscience, as follows: Mañjuśrī became the great king Śuddhodana. Lokeśvara became the queen Mahāmāyā. Śrīdevī became Yaśodharā; Vajrasattva, Rāhula; Sarvanivaraṇaviṣkambhin, Śāriputra; Samantabhadra became the 'elder' Āryānanda. Devendra (i.e. Indra) became the 'elder' Devadatta, and Mahāvairocana, the Perfected Buddha Śrī-Śākyamuni". According to that interpretation, what is called the 'compiler' and what is called the 'retinue' is revealed as this drama of the Buddha for introducing the beginner sentient beings (into the Doctrine).

*//DA// dadāti prārthitaṃ sarvaṃ cintāmaṇir ivāparam /*
*haṭha(ś) cāhṛtya kurute buddhānām api saṃpadam //28//*

Like the best wish-granting jewel, *haṭha* grants everything desired, and seizing (by force) enacts even the success of the Buddhas.

*Mchan*: 'Grants everything desired' means :—grants all mundane *siddhis*. 'And even the success of the Buddhas' means :— even grants the supramundane *siddhi*, which is Buddhahood. *Mchan ḥgrel*, Vol. 158, p. 144-5 : 'the wish-granting jewel' (*cintāmaṇi*) grants youth, health, and happiness.

The term *haṭha* (fierce yoga) occurs in the *Guhyasamājatantra*, Chap. XVIII, verse 162:

> *darśanaṃ tu kṛte 'py evaṃ sādhakasya na jāyate |*
> *yadā na sidhyate bodhir haṭhayogena sādhayet ||*
> When one has performed that way and still the *sādhaka's* vision does not occur, nor is *bodhi* achieved, then by *haṭhayoga* it is achieved.

According to Nāgārjuna's *Aṣṭādaśa-paṭala-vistara-vyākhyā* (PTT,. Vol. 60, p. 15-4, 5 and p. 16-1, 2), this involves a fiercer practice with success in fewer days. Explaining the 'six months' (*ṣaṇmāsa*) of verse 161, he says (p. 16-1-5) "If it is not achieved in six months, two months, one, or a half month, then one should try to achieve it in seven days" (gaṅ gi tshe zla ba drug daṅ zla ba gñis daṅ gcig daṅ zla ba phyed kyis ḥgrub par mi ḥgyur ni / deḥi tshe źag bdun gyis bsgrub pa brtsam par bya ste /). The comments show that if success is not reached through the usual procedure of the three *sattvas* (*samaya-sattva*, *jñāna-sattva*, and *samādhi-sattva*) in 'six months', then one applies the procedure through the *jñāna-sattva* with evocation of the *krodha* deity Sumbharāja for success in 'seven days'. The explanation of *haṭhayoga* in Nāropā's *Sekoddeśaṭikā*, p. 45 involves drawing the *prāṇa* into the 'middle vein' (*haṭhena prāṇaṃ madhyamāyāṃ vāhayitvā*).

The general procedure of obtaining *siddhis* is through the 'burnt offering', as in the *Guhyasamājatantra*, XVI, p. 117 (*Mchan ḥgrel*, p. 139-2):

> *homaṃ kurvīta mantrajñāḥ sarvasiddhiphalārthinaḥ |*
> *viṇmūtramāṃsatailādyair āhutiṃ pratipādayet ||*
> The knower of mantras desiring as fruit all (mundane and supramundane) *siddhis*, should perform a burnt offering (*homa*). He should accomplish the evocation by (an inner burnt offering, to wit:—) excrement, urine, flesh, oil, and so forth.

*Pradīpoddyotana* and *Mchan ḥgrel* (Vol. 158, p. 141-5): (The offerings of) 'excrement and urine' mean the five ambrosias (*amṛta*); (of) 'flesh' mean the five kinds. (*Ibid.*, p. 142-1): 'Great flesh' means the five kinds of lamps. (*Ibid.*, p. 142-1): 'All *siddhis*' means of mundane ones, the minor ones of *śāntika*, etc., and the eight great ones of *ri-lu*, etc., called *mahāsamaya* (*Guhyasamāja*, XVI, p. 117, line 17). The reference to 'five ambrosias' is based on a passage in the *Mahāmudrātilaka*, cited in my essay, "Totemic beliefs in the Buddhist Tantras," p. 91: "Ratnasambhava is blood, Amitābha is semen; Amoghasiddhi is human flesh, Akṣobhya is urine; Vairocana is excrement. These are the five best ambrosias." For the five kinds of flesh, Dharmakīrti's commentary on the *Hevajra-tantra* called *Spyan ḥbyed* (PTT, Vol. 54, p. 135-3) contains the Sanskrit words in Tibetan transcription : *Na* means human flesh (*nara*); *Ga* means ox flesh (*gaura*); *Ha* means elephant flesh (*hasti*); final *Śva* means horse flesh (*aśva*); initial *Śva* means dog flesh (*śvan*).

The list 'appeasing' (*śāntika*), etc. is the four previously described (nidāna verse 15) as the jurisdictional activity of the four goddesses, Locanā, etc.; and they yield inferior mundane *siddhis*. The great mundane *siddhis* are eight in number, referred to as '*ri-lu*' etc., where *ri-lu* '('little ball') is a contraction of *ril-bu*. The list of eight *siddhis* is somewhat explained in the annotation to *Mkhas grub rje's Fundamentals of the Buddhist Tantras*. Here we need only list them : 1. "To walk in the sky" (*khecāra*), 2. "To be swift of foot" (*janghākāri*), 3. "To be invisible" (*antardhāna*), 4. "To shape into a little ball" (*piṇḍarūpa*, T. *ril-bu*), 5. "To remove blindness" (T. *mig sman*), 6. "To have the elixir of youth" (*rasana*), 7. "To be invincible in battle" (*khaḍga*), 8. "To have dominion over the entities of the underworld" (*pātāla*).

The following passage of the *Guhyasamājatantra*, XVI, p. 124 (*Pradīpoddyotana* and *Mchan ḥgrel*, p. 146-4, ff.) differentiates between superior and inferior mundane *siddhi*:

> *kāyavākcittasaṃsiddhā buddharūpadharaprabhā* |
> *jāmbūnadaprabhākārā hīnasiddhisamāśritāḥ* ||
> *antardhānādisaṃsiddhau bhavet vajradharaḥ prabhuḥ* |
> *yakṣarājādisaṃsiddhau bhavet vidyādharaḥ prabhuḥ* ||
>
> She (= Vajraḍākinī) who shines with a form like the (respective) Buddha is the (superior) occult success of body (grasping various forms), speech (grasping various sounds), and mind (gaining as desired). They (= mundane fairies, *ḍākinī*) who glisten on the Jāmbu river are the resorts of inferior *siddhi*. The lord Vajradhara would be in the (superior) occult success of 'invisibility' (= united with the Vajraḍākinī, a 'together-born female'). The lord Vidyādhara would be in the (inferior) occult success

of Yakṣarāja, etc. (=united with the mundane fairies, the 'field-born females').

Besides the distinction of inferior and superior kinds among the mundane *siddhis*, these siddhis themselves contrast with the supramundane *siddhi*, as differentiated in the *Guhyasamājatantra*, XVI, p. 117 (*Mchan ḥgrel*, Vol. 15, p. 142-1):

*antardhānaṃ balaṃ vīryaṃ vajrākarṣaṇam uttamam |*
*siddhyate maṇḍale sarvaṃ kāyavajravaco yathā ||*

Everything is brought to success in the *maṇḍala*, as from the word of the 'diamond of body' (=Vairocana), namely: 'disappearance', 'strength', 'striving', and the 'ultimate diamond attraction'.

*Mchan ḥgrel*: 'Strength (*bala*)' means mastery of *vidyādhara*; 'striving (*vīrya*)' means the power of the five *abhijñā*-s; 'in the *maṇḍala*' means initiation, guarding of vows, and contemplation of the path in the *maṇḍala*; 'diamond attraction' means attraction of things difficult to attract. The last named can be compared with the supramundane *siddhi* of *Guhyasamāja*, XII, verse 37 ('Documents'): 'the supreme Buddha attraction' (*buddhākarṣaṇam uttamam*). The five *abhijñā*-s of this tradition were previously detailed under nidāna verse 20.

See also Chaps. VI and XII ('Documents').

Finally, supramundane *siddhi*, here called 'supreme' can be given interpretive levels through Candrakīrti's classifying terminology. Thus, *Guhyasamājatantra*, XIII, p. 62 (*Pradīpoddyotana* in Derge Tanjur, Rgyud, Vol. Ha, f. 104a-4, ff.; *Mchan ḥgrel*, PTT, Vol. 158, p. 94-4, ff.):

*mohasamayasambhūtā vidyārājāno vajriṇaḥ |*
*napuṃsakapade siddhān dadanti siddhim uttamām ||*

A. Translation with 'invariant sense' (*akṣarārtha*):

The vidyārājas and diamond-possessors, arisen from the Delusion-Symbol (*moha-samaya*) confer the supreme *siddhi* upon the adepts (*siddha*) at the place of androgynes.

B. Translation with 'hinted meaning' (*neyārtha*):

The (*krodhas*) Uṣṇīṣacakravartin, etc. (cf. nidāna verse 17) and (Bodhisattvas) Kṣitigarbha, etc. (cf. nidāna verse 16) arisen from (the Buddha) Vairocana (as progenitor of the Moha family), confer Englightenment upon the adepts at (their reciting) the three syllables Oṃ, Āḥ, Hūṃ (in the Clear Light and in *yuganaddha*).

C. Translation with 'evident meaning' (*nītārtha*):

The 'men' and 'women' who have taken an 'aggregate of indulgence' (*upādāna-skandha*) (=a body), arisen from nescience (*avidyā*), confer the extraordinary *siddhi* of *mahāmudrā* upon the adepts realizing at the Clear Light and at the Culmination-of-Light (having attained the Clear Light and *yuganaddha*).

*//YA// yad yad icchati yogendras tat tat kuryād anāvṛtaḥ /*
*asamāhitayogena nityam eva samāhitaḥ //29//*

Whatever the powerful one of yoga wishes, just that he would do without hindrance; and by means of the yoga of 'after'-stability, is continually stabilized.

*Mchan* : The powerful one of yoga—the practitioner of the Saṃpannakrama—whatever he may wish to practise of his own 'strand of desire' (*kāmaguṇa*)—just that he would enjoy unhindered; and by the yoga of such sporting in a 'strand of desire' in the time of after-attainment—the 'after'-stability, he is continually stabilized in the sense of inseparable ecstasy-void.

*Guhyasamājatantra*, XVIII, p. 156:

*asamāhitayogena nityam eva samāhitaḥ /*
*sarvacitteṣu yā caryā mantracaryeti kathyate //*

By the yoga of 'after-stability' one is ever stabilized. That practice in all thoughts is called 'practice of mantras'.

*Pañcakrama*, 3rd krama, verse 36 (with emendations):

*yad yad indriyamārgatvaṃ āyas tat tat svabhāvataḥ /*
*asamāhitayogena sarvaṃ buddhasamaṃ vahet //*

Whatever the sense basis and whatever its path (=sense object), precisely that approach in its own-being leads to all Buddha-equality by the yoga of 'after'-stability.

Śrī Lakṣmī's *Pañcakrama* comm., Vol. 63, p. 50-5: "Among them, the *samāhita* is the contemplation of as many as 38 *samādhis* starting from 'initial training' and going up to the division into the hundred lineages. Accordingly, the *asamāhita* is the place in the intervals by means of 'divine pride' (*devatā-garva*). The two of them do not exist separately in the *yuganaddha-krama* because there is a single own-being of 'profound concentration' (*samādhi*) and 'straying of mind' (*vikṣepa*)" ( / de la mñam par bźag pa ni daṅ po sbyor ba la sogs pa nas / rig brgyaḥi dbye baḥi bar du ji srid tiṅ ṅeḥdzin sum cu rtsa brgyad sgom paḥo/ de bźin du mñam par ma bźag pa ni lhaḥi ṅa rgyal gyis bar mtshams rnams la gnas pa ste / gñis po ḥdi dag zuṅ ḥjug gi rim pa la yod pa ma yin te / tiṅ ṅe ḥdzin daṅ / rnam par gYeṅ ba dag raṅ bźin gcig yin paḥi phyir ro / ).

The *Śri-Paramādya-tantra*'s last chapter has some relevant verses (PTT, Vol. 5, p. 172-4):

*| dbaṅ po gaṅ daṅ gaṅ lam gyur |*
*| de daṅ de yi ṅo bor bya |*
*| mñam par gźag nas rnal ḥbyor gyis |*
*| raṅ gi lhag paḥi lha sbyor bya ||*
*| de ñid rnal ḥbyor ḥdi yis ni |*
*| thams cad ñid ni bsgrub par bya |*
*| saṅs rgyas kun dṅos thams cad ni |*
*| rtag tu mthoṅ źiṅ grub par ḥgyur ||*

Whatever the sense basis and whatever its path, he should act in the own-being of the former and the latter. By yoga after stability, he will unite with his own presiding lord (*adhideva*). By this very yoga he will accomplish everything. He will always see and perfect all the Buddha natures.

*||VA|| vajrapadmasamāyogāj jñānatrayavibhāgavit |*
*liptāliptamatis tatra sukhena viharet sadā ||* 30||

Knowing the portions of the three knowledges, through union of thunderbolt and lotus,—the defiled and the undefiled intelligence would dwell therein with bliss for ever.

*Mchan*: Knowing well the portions of three knowledges—the three (Lights called) Light, Spread-of-Light, and Culmination-of-Light arising through the (sequential) dissolution of the winds, by the *sādhaka*'s taking recourse to union of *vajra* and *padma*—both the defiled and the undefiled intelligence would for ever be stabilized therein with ecstasy combined with void. This refers to what is done by the possessor of discriminative intelligence distinguishing between (a) the stream of consciousness defiled by the trouble of defilement (*kleśa*) when uniting with a partner (*mudrā*) and acting that way, and (b) the stream of consciousness undefiled by the trouble of operating in the defiled path (in like circumstances).

The *Vajramālā* has a brief chapter, no. 14 (PTT, Vol. 3, pp. 209 and 210), entitled, "Chapter Relating the Marriage of the Diamond and the Lotus" (rdo rje padma yaṅ dag par sbyor ba bśad paḥi leḥu). This contains two verses cited here and translated with the help of Alaṃkakalaśa's comments (PTT, Vol. 61, p. 210-4, 5 and 211-1). The first verse at Vol. 3, p. 209-5, brings in the non-tantric terminology of calming (*śamatha*) and discerning (*vipaśyanā*), the two which should be combined in Buddhist non-tantric *yuganaddha*:

> / *pad-ma de yi gnas de la* /
> / *de yi sbyor baḥaṅ mchog tu gsal* /
> / *źi gnas pad-ma źes gsuṅs la* /
> / *de la lhag mthoṅ rdo rjeḥo* //
>
> And his union in that place of the *padma* is most clear when (the master) explains that the *padma* is calming and that the *vajra* there is discerning.

The next verse at Vol. 3, p. 210-1, introduces the tantric terminology of male organ (*liṅga*) and female organ (*bhaga*):

> / *blo ldan rnam rtog bral ba yi* /
> / *rdo rje liṅ-ga źes ni bśad* /
> / *rnam rtog bral baḥi blo ldan gyis* /
> / *bha-ga pad-ma źes ni brjod* //
>
> The *liṅga* possessing intelligence (*mati*) and lacking discursive thought (*vitarka*) is called *vajra*. The *bhaga* lacking intelligence and possessing discursive thought is called *padma*.

On the latter, Alaṃkakalaśa comments (PTT, Vol. 61, p. 211-1): " 'Possessing intelligence' means: has the perfection of distinguished insight (*prajñā*); 'lacking discursive thought' means free from all (eighty) *vikalpas*." (blo ldan źes bya ba la sogs pas gsuṅs te / khyad par can gyi śes rab phun sum tshogs pa daṅ ldan pa laḥo / /rnam rtog bral baḥi źes bya ba ni / rnam par rtog pa thams cad daṅ bral baḥo). When we add to this his comments on the former verse (PTT, Vol. 61, p. 210-4, 5), it becomes possible to explain the two verses this way: Śamatha, or one-pointedness of mind, temporarily clears the mind of defilements but does not destroy them, since they remain in the periphery of consciousness. So it is like the lotus (*padma*) which is not adhered to by the muddy water but is still surrounded by the muddy water (here the 80 vikalpas). Vipaśyanā, or discriminative analysis, is free from the defilements but is without location. So it is like the vajra which is the intelligence free from the 80 vikalpas, but not localized in a particular mind.

The lotus and the diamond intuit that they complement each other: the lotus will prepare the pure spot such as the maṇḍala of residence, and the diamond will introduce the divine intelligence such as the maṇḍala of the residents. Their nuptials are celebrated; otherwise stated, the yogin (whether male or female)brings about their inseparable union with bliss for ever.

> *//JRA// jṛmbhate sarvabhāvātmā māyopamasamādhinā /*
> *karoti buddhakṛtyāni sampradāyapadasthitaḥ //31//*
>
> The universal self of entities sports by means of the illusory *samādhi*. It performs the deeds of a Buddha while stationed at the traditional post.

*Mchan* : The universal self of inner-and-outer entities sports by means of itself staying in the Illusory Samādhi: — Former teachers opined this to be the application to generating the gnosis (*jñāna*) of 'arcane mind' (*cittaviveka*) in meditative attainment (*samāpatti*) through reliance on a partner (*mudrā*); but that is not all it is ! One should understand it also to be the generating of 'arcane mind' in meditative attainment through continuous line by 'arcane body' (*lus dben gyis rgyud nas*) and concretely by 'arcane speech' (*ṅag dben gyis dṅos su*); and we have already explained the method of contemplation at the time of emerging from the meditative attainment. By this is to be understood the pregnant exposition of the doctrine of lust, not only in the phase of the two *caryā*-s (i.e. the first two, the *prapañca-caryā* and the *niṣprapañca-caryā*, explained under nidāna verse 26), but also the reliance on a partner (*mudrā*). In their phase the multiple occurrence of the three *jñānas* is numerous in these phases of the Clear Light of the Supreme Entity and is the way of incorporating the universal void of the Symbolic Clear Light into the third void, the Culmination (-of-Light); hence, if one counts separately the Symbolic Clear Light, there are four voids. // One sees like that, itself appearing in the Illusory Body, as stated in the *Pañcakrama* (3rd, 20b): "Stationed in the Illusory Samādhi one sees everything that way." // It performs the deeds of a Buddha, i.e. performing the aim of sentient beings by various means, and so doing by means of this Illusory Body; while stationed in the Clear Light which is the 'traditional post', i.e. the Supreme Entity. *Prakāśikā* on Jra (PTT, Vol. 60, p. 296-1) : 'Deeds of a Buddha' means that he performs teaching, maturation, and liberation (of the sentient beings); 'the traditional post' is the *siddhānta* (consummate end), the post because it does not shift; 'stationed' means resting there. (saṅs rgyas kyi bya ba ni bstan pa daṅ / / yoṅs su smin pa daṅ /rnam par grol ba la sogs pa byed pa ni mdzad paḥo / / gtan la dbab paḥi gźi ni grub paḥi mthaḥ ste / de ñid mi ḥpho baḥi phyir gnas paḥo / / de las gnas pa ni ṅal so baḥo).

*Pañcakrama*, 1st krama, 2B :

*māyopamasamādhistho bhūtakoṭyāṃ samāviśet* /

Stationed in the Illusory Samādhi he enters the true limit.

*Ibid.*, 1st krama, 58 :

*anena vajrajāpena sevāṃ kṛtvā yathāvidhi* /
*sādhayet sarvakāryāṇi māyopamasamādhinā* //

Having done the service by that diamond muttering according to the rite, he would accomplish all deeds by the Illusory Samādhi.

*Ibid.*, 3rd krama, 20 :

*tasmād eva jagat sarvaṃ māyopamam ihocyate* /
*māyopamasamādhiṣṭhaḥ sarvaṃ paśyati tādṛśaṃ* //

Accordingly, all the world is here said to be illusory. Stationed in the Illusory Samādhi one sees everything that way.

*Ibid.*, 3rd krama (Svādhiṣṭhāna), 29-30 :

*mantramudrāprayogaṃ ca maṇḍalādivikalpanam* /
*balihomakriyāṃ sarvāṃ kuryān māyopamāṃ sadā* //
*śāntikaṃ pauṣṭikaṃ cāpi tathā vaśyābhicārakam* /
*ākarṣaṇādi yat sarvaṃ kuryād indrāyudhopamam* //

He should engage in the training of *mantra* and *mudrā*, in the imagining of *maṇḍala*, etc., in the rites of *bali* and *homa*; and in each case, ever 'illusory-like'. He should engage in appeasing (deities), increasing (prosperity), dominating (the elementary spiritis), overcoming (inimical elements), and in whatever attracting (of *ḍākini*-s), and in each case, 'rainbow-like'.

Tsoṅ-kha-pa, Comm. on *Pañcakrama*, p. 71-1, 2, in illustration of 'non-*prapañca* praxis' (*niṣprapañca-caryā*) cites Anaṅgavajra's *Prajñopāyaviniścayasiddhi* (V, last line of verse 45, and verses 46-47) :

*cittaṃ cāropya bodhau viṣayasukharataḥ sidhyatihaiva janmani* //
*anāspadāḥ kalpanayā vimuktāḥ svabhāvataḥ śuddhatamāḥ samastāḥ* /

*anātmasaṃjñāviṣayāḥ prakṛtyā svapnendrajālapratibhāsatulyāḥ*/46//
*yadāvabuddhā niravagraheṇa cittena sadbhir vipulāśayais tu* /
*tadābhibhūtāḥ sahajāvagatyā na bādhanājālamalibhavanti* //47//
Having elevated the mind to enlightenment, he, enjoying ecstasy in sense objects, is successful in the present life. The sense objects, called 'non-self', by nature like dreams, rainbows, and reflected images, are all intrinsically immaculate, free from discursive thought and without abode. When illustrious persons of wide aspiration fully understand them with a non-apprehending mind, then those (sense objects) are overcome by together-born comprehension and no longer trap (those persons) in their net.

// *YO*// *yogaś caivātiyogaś ca mahāyogaḥ svayaṃ bhavet* /
*vajrī ca ḍākinī caiva tayor yogaś ca yaḥ svayam* // 32 //
Yoga, atiyoga, and mahāyoga occur by themselves; also vajrin, ḍākinī, as well as any union (*yoga*) of both, by themselves.

*Mchan* : 'Yoga' implies both *yoga* and *anuyoga*, and they plus *atiyoga* and *mahāyoga*—the *prathama-prayoga* of four *yogas*—occur by themselves for *māyādehin*. Also *vajrin*, who is chief of the *vijaya-maṇḍala*, plus the *ḍākinī*, plus any *yoga* (of both) occur themselves for *māyādehin*. The two lines refer to the two *samādhis* of *māyādehin* (possessor of Illusory Body).

*Prakāśikā* on Yo (Vol. 60, p. 295-2): Those are the four *yogas* of the 'Stage of Generation', whereby one accomplishes the *samādhis* of 'Initial Praxis', etc. In the present case, *yoga* is 'means' (*upāya*), *anuyoga* is 'insight' (*prajñā*), *atiyoga* is entrance into their union; *mahāyoga* is the attainment of great bliss (*mahāsukha*) from their union. (bskyed paḥi rim paḥi rnal ḥbyor bźi ste / gaṅ gis daṅ poḥi sbyor ba źes bya ba la sogs paḥi tiṅ ṅe ḥdzin ḥgrub par ḥgyur ro / / ḥdir rnal ḥbyor ni thabs so // rjes su rnal ḥbyor ni śes rab bo / / śin tu rnal ḥbyor ni de dag gi sñoms par śugs paḥo / /rnal ḥbyor chen po ni sñoms par śugs pa las bde ba chen po thob paḥo).

Besides, we may interpret that the terms 'yoga', 'atiyoga', and 'mahāyoga' of nidāna verse 32, refer to the yoga mastery of the three lights, as is suggested by the synonyms of the lights in verse 25, śūnya, atiśūnya, and mahāśūnya. Thus the yogin with such mastery can evoke automatically the ḍākinī of śūnya (=prajñā), the vajrin of atiśūnya (=upāya), or their androgynous union. Notice also the series of terms in the full title of the *Guhyasamājatantra* : rahasya, atirahasya, mahāguhya, in which mahāguhya is understood to include both rahasya and atirahasya.

The *Guhyasamājatantra*, Chap. XVIII, verse 32, defines *yoga* as follows :

*prajñopāyasamāpattir yoga ity abhidhīyate |*
*yo ni(ḥ) svabhāva(s) taḥ prajñā upāyo bhāvalakṣaṇam ||*
'Yoga' is defined as the equipoise of insight and means.
Whatever is devoid of intrinsic nature, is 'insight'.
'Means' is the characteristic of modes.

Nāgārjuna's commentary, p. 5-2, 3, 4, 5, illustrates insight, means, and their equipoise, first for each of his five stages (the *pañcakrama*); then for the terms cause, action, and fruit; next, for each of the six members of the *ṣaḍaṅga-yoga*. In the case of the six members, the explanations go as follows :

1. Insight is the sense organs and means is the sense objects. The yoga of their equipoise and enjoyment, is *pratyāhāra*.
2. Insight is the sense organs and means is the Tathāgatas. The yoga as their equipoise, is *dhyāna*.
3. Insight is *paramārtha-bodhicitta* and means is *saṃvṛti-bodhicitta*. The yoga as their equipoise, involving the emanation and reunification of them in upper and lower sequence, is *prāṇa-āyāma*.
4. When insight and means are as previous, the yoga of their equipoise, holding the *bindu* the size of a mustard grain in (*or* at) the three 'tips of nose', is *dhāraṇā*.
5. When insight and means are the Tathāgatas embraced by the goddesses, the yoga of emanating into the sky, as their equipoise, is *anusmṛti*.
6. When insight and means are the Dharmakāya and the Saṃbhogakāya, the yoga of joining them with the Nirmāṇakāya as their equipoise, is samādhi.

Now, although the nidāna verse speaks of those yoga states as occurring by themselves for the possessor of the Illusory Body, the *Guhyasamājatantra*, Chap. XVII, pp. 145-6, employs mythological language representing the four goddesses as imploring the lord in the Clear Light to come forth and make love to them. The order of the goddesses is that in which they superintend the four rites (of appeasing, etc.). The translation is somewhat expanded by the *Pradīpoddyotana* and *Mchan ḥgrel* (p. 162):

*atha te sarve bodhisattvāḥ tūṣṇīṃ vyavasthitā abhūvan |*
*atha bhagavantaḥ sarvatathāgatāḥ sarvatathāgatakāya-vākcittavajrayoṣidbhageṣu vijahāra |*

Then all those Bodhisattvas (their doubts dispelled) became completely silent. Thereupon the Bhagavat who is all (five) Tathāgata (families) took abode in the *bhaga*-s (the Buddhadharmodaya = the Clear Light) of the (four) diamond ladies belonging to (Vajradhara, who is) the *vajra* of the Body, Speech, and Mind of all the Tathāgatas.

Then Māmakī, the wife of the 'mind of all the Tathāgatas' (= Akṣobhya), implored Mahāvajradhara in these passionate terms :

*'Tvaṃ vajracitta bhuvaneśvara sattvadhāto trāyāhi māṃ*
*ratimanojña mahārthakāmaiḥ | kāmāhi māṃ janaka*
*sattvamahāgrabandho yadīcchase jīvitaṃ mañjunāthaḥ ||'*

'May you of adamantine mind, lord of the world, realm of sentient beings, save me with love of great purpose, O thou the gratifier of passion! O father, may the great supreme kin of sentient beings love me, if you, the mild lord, wish that I live.'

Then Buddhalocanā, the wife of the 'body of all the Tathāgatas' (= Vairocana), implored Mahāvajradhara endearingly :

*'Tvaṃ vajrakāya bahusattvapriyāṅkacakra*
*buddhārthabodhiparamārthahitānudarśī |*
*rāgeṇa rāgasamayaṃ mama kāmayasva*
*yadicchase jīvitaṃ mañjunātha ||'*

'May you, the diamond body, the revolving wheel (*aṅka-cakra*) that delights many beings, the revealer of the benefit of the Buddha aim and the supreme-enlightenment aim, love me with passion at the time for passion, if you, the mild lord, wish that I live.'

Then the 'diamond eye of body, speech, and mind' (= Pāṇḍarā), the wife of Lokeśvara (= Amitābha), suffused with passion toward Mahāvajradhara, pleaded with him :

*'Tvaṃ vajravāca sakalasya hitānukampī*
*lokārthakāryakaraṇe sadā saṃpravṛttaḥ |*
*kāmāhi māṃ suratacarya samantabhadra*
*yadicchase jīvitaṃ mañjunātha ||*

'You, O diamond speech, have compassion for everyone's benefit, are always engaged in doing the needful for the world's aim. Love me, O entirely good one (Samantabhadra) with the praxis of ecstasy, if you, the mild lord, wish that I live.'

Then the wife (=Ārya-Tārā) of the Samayavajra (=Amoghasiddhi) of the Body, Speech, and Mind of all the Tathāgatas, exhorted Mahāvajradhara to make love to her:

*'Tvaṃ vajrakāma samayāgra mahāhitārtha*
*saṃbuddhavaṃśatilakaḥ samatānukampi* /
*kāmāhi māṃ guṇanidhiṃ bahuratnabhūtaṃ*
*yadīcchase jīvitaṃ mañjunātha* //'

'O Diamond love, the pinnacle of the Samaya (family), whose aim is the great benefit; you have the mark of the Complete Buddha's family and are compassionate with equality. Love me who is the treasure of virtues made of many jewels, if you, the mild lord, wish that I live.'

Thereupon, the Bhagavat, Vajrapāṇi Tathāgata, immersing himself in the *samādhi* called 'diamond glory partaking of all desires', remained silent, while making love to the wives of all the Tathāgatas by means of the *samayacakra* (atha bhagavān vajrapāṇis tathāgataḥ sarvakāmo-pabhogavajraśriyaṃ nāma samādhiṃ samāpannas tāṃ sarvatathāgatadayitāṃ samayacakreṇa kāmayan tūṣṇīmabhūt / ).

The *Pradīpoddyotana* (PTT, Vol. 158, p. 163-4, 5) explains that the four goddesses, respectively representing the four Brahmāvihāras, which are friendliness (*maitri*), compassion (*karuṇā*), sympathetic joy (*anumodanā*), impartiality (*upekṣā*), succeeded in their love petitions because the Bhagavat, by virtue of the continuity of his previous vow (sṅon gyi smon lam gyi rgyun gi śugs kyis) emerged from the voidness-*yoga* (=the Clear Light) and entering the above-named *samādhi*, engaged in love with those goddesses by means of the *samaya-cakra*, which is the $8 \times 8 = 64$ *kāma-kalā*, or love techniques.

The rich symbolism of the *Guhyasamāja* account emphasizes the exhorting by the female element, the winds, elements, Nature herself, for the Lord to emerge from the absolute plane as the compassionate teacher to show the path to others. For this he must embrace Nature, the wife of others. And yet this takes place by itself.

> || *ṢID* || *niṣiddham api kṛtvā vai kṛtyākṛtya-vivarjitaḥ* |
> *na lipyate svabhāvajñaḥ padmapatram ivāmbhasā* || 33 ||
> Having done even the prohibited, he renounces both the proper and the improper act. The one knowing the intrinsic nature is not adhered to (by sin), any more than is a lotus leaf by water.

*Mchan* : If one practises in the 'strands of desire' (*kāmaguṇa*= the five sensory objects) of the *vidyā* (*rig ma*), is this in conflict with the saying, "Desires are like poisonous leaves" ? (The verse) disputes this. 'Prohibited' :—this is the label which the other vehicle applies to desire for the 'strands of desire'. 'Having done even the prohibited' with the skilful means (*upāyakauśalya*) of this (our) vehicle, 'he renounces' the discursive thinking (*vikalpa*) of 'both the proper and the improper act.' He 'is not adhered to' in his stream of consciousness by the trouble of committed desires, etc., which lead to an evil destiny (*durgati*), because he is 'one knowing the intrinsic nature' of the *dharmas*. According to the texts of 'Ḥphags pa yab sras' (i.e. the tantrics Nāgārjuna and Āryadeva) there is also such a viewpoint in the lower vehicle (Hīnayāna), hence in both (vehicles) it reduces to the greatest absurdity that there is (unethical) permissiveness to take recourse to the 'strands of desire' (form, sound, etc.) of the *vidyā*. But, while the comprehension of reality is the main thing, it is necessary to fulfill the frequently-mentioned characteristic of both firmness in '*yoga* of the deity' (*devatā-yoga*) and non-regression (*avaivartika*) of the Bodhisattva (on the 8th to 10th stages, or Stage of Completion). Because, while the lack of fault refutes the 'permissiveness', there is a difference in the respective candidates of the two (vehicles).

The scriptural citation "Desires are like poisonous leaves" is presumably taken by Tsoṅ-kha-pa from Bu-ston's *Bśad sbyar* on Ṣid (Ta, f. 57b-4) : "Mdo las / ḥdod pa rnams ni dug gi lo ma lta buḥo źes ḥdod yon la sogs spyod bkag paḥo / źe na /". So far I only find a reference to the poisonous flowers, as in the passage "like the flower on the poison tree" (*viṣavṛkṣe yathā puṣpaṃ*), in *Dharma-Samuccaya*, 2º Partie (Chap. IX), p. 280. Also, in the *Udayanavatsarājaparipṛcchā* of the Ratnakūṭa collection (Derge, Kanjur, Dkon brtsegs, Ca, f. 215a-4) there is the half-verse. / ha la ha laḥi dug ḥdra baḥi / ḥdod chags kyis ni de yaṅ ḥkhrugs / "He is agitated by passion which is like the *halāhala* poison." But this poison is produced from the roots of the plant of that name, and is also the poison churned from the ocean according to the Purāṇa legend.

*Prakāśikā* on Ṣid (Vol. 60. p. 295-2): 'Prohibited' means action in violation of the world. For example, to harm those who do injury to the Three Jewels (Buddha, Doctrine, and Congregation); to steal the goods of the miser; to deprive the lustful person of a family; to cut the pride of the proud; to speak harshly to the envious. When one does such acts as those in violation of the world, and under control of 'skill in the means', he is not defiled, for by doing it under control of great compassion (*mahākaruṇā*), there is no obscuration (*āvaraṇa*). (dgag pa ni ḥjig rten daṅ baḥi las so / / dper na dkon mchog gsum la gnod pa can rnams la rnam par ḥtshe ba daṅ / ser sna can la rdzas ḥphrogs pa daṅ / ḥdod chags can bu smad ḥphrog pa daṅ / ṅa rgyal can la ṅa rgyal gcod pa daṅ / phrag dog can la rtsub mo smra ba daṅ / de la sogs pahi ḥjig rten daṅ ḥgal baḥi las rnams thabs la mkhas paḥi dbaṅ gis byas te gos par mi ḥgyur te / sñiṅ rje chen poḥi dbaṅ gis byas par gyur na sgrib par mi ḥgyur ro/).

In accord with the second half of the nidāna verse, Āryadeva writes in his *Cittaviśuddhiprakaraṇa*, verse 115 :

> *paṅkajātaṃ yathā padmaṃ paṅkadoṣair na lipyate /*
> *vikalpavāsanādoṣais tathā yogī na lipyate //*
>
> Just as a lotus sprung from mud is not adhered to by the faults of mud, so is the yogi not adhered to by the faults of discursive thought and habit energy.

The phrase 'knowing the intrinsic nature', or a similar expression, especially occurs in the commentarial interpretations of *Guhyasamāja* passages. Let us begin with the lady (*yoṣit*) as portrayed in the last three verses (emended) of *Guhyasamājatantra*, Chap. IV:

> *ṣoḍaśābdikāṃ samprāpya yoṣitaṃ kāntisuprabhām /*
> *gandhapuṣpaṁ alaṃkṛtvā tasya madhye tu kāmayet //*
> *adhiṣṭhāpya ca tāṃ prājñaḥ māmakīṃ guṇamekhalāṃ /*
> *sṛjed buddhapadaṃ saumyam ākāśadhātvalaṃkṛtam //*
> *viṇmūtraśukraraktādīn devatānāṃ nivedayet /*
> *evaṃtuṣyanti sambuddhāḥ bodhisattvā mahāyaśāḥ //*

Having obtained a lady, 16-yeared, lovely in appearance, having prepared a fragrant flower, one should love (her) in its center. The wise man, empowering that Māmakī girdled with merits, goes out to the calm Buddha plane adorned with the realm of space. He should offer to the gods excrement, urine, semen, and blood. In that way, the Complete Buddhas and the renowned Bodhisattvas are pleased.

The *Pradīpoddyotana* quotes the *Saṃdhivyākaraṇa* expansion of those verses (*Mchan ḥgrel*, p. 41-2, 3, 4) :

*kṣaṇādikālabhedena saṃjñā syāt ṣoḍaśābdikā |*
*anutpādoṣitā śānti(r) yoṣitā iti niścitā ||*
*śāntadharmānapetākhyā kāntisuprabhoditā |*
*pratītyavāsanāgandhaṃ puṣpaṃ jñānavikāsanam ||*
*niḥsvabhāvakule jñeyaṃ sarvajñājñānamadhyamam |*
*kāmayed īdṛśīṃ prājño yoṣitaṃ dharmadhātukāṃ ||*
*na cādhyātmaṃ na bāhyāntaṃ nobhaye 'nyatra saṃsthitā |*
*asthānasthitiyogaḥ syād ato māmakī matā ||*
*tat svabhāvaikayogaṃ tv adhiṣṭhānaṃ tad ucyate |*
*ākāśaikatvasaṃvāsaḥ saumyaṃ buddhapadaṃ bhavet ||*
*ataḥ saṃharaṇān viṭ syād viṣayāḥ parikalpitāḥ |*
*mūtraṃ jñānendriyaṃ saṃsthaṃ śukraṃ viśuddhidharmatā ||*
*raktaṃ sarvajñatājñānaṃ ye dharmāḥ parikalpitāḥ |*
*ta eva devatāḥ khyātā niḥsvabhāvo nivedanam ||*
*evaṃ tuṣyanti te buddhā jinaurasā viśeṣataḥ |*
*laukikī kalpanā yeṣāṃ teṣāṃ eva yathoditam ||*

The peace abiding in the unborn, whose name would be 16-yeared by differentiation of time starting with a moment, is determined as the 'lady' (*yoṣit*). Possessing a calm nature, she is said to be lovely in appearance. The flower has the perfume of habit-energy in dependence and is full-blown with gnosis.

The knowable in the family devoid of intrinsic nature is centered in omniscient knowledge. (There) the wise man should love such a lady belonging to the Dharmadhātu.

She who dwells neither within nor without, nor in both or elsewhere, would be the *yoga* whose station is without location. Accordingly is Māmakī understood.

The singleness of intrinsic nature is what is referred to

as the empowerment. The cohabitation of oneness with space is the calm Buddha plane.

Thus, the excrement is the amassings as the imagined sense objects. The urine is the formation with sense organs (*jñānendriya*). The semen is the true nature of purity. (Menstrual) blood is the knowledge of all knowables. Those imagined natures (personality aggregates, and so on) are the deities. The offering is the lack of intrinsic nature.

In that way, those Buddhas and their spiritual sons are especially pleased. Whoever have mundane imagination, for them it has been told as (above).

The expression 'who knows the intrinsic nature' occurs in the interesting comment by *Pradīpoddyotana* on *Guhyasamājatantra*, Chap. V, verses 7-8:

*mātṛbhaginīputrīṃś ca kāmayed yas tu sādhakaḥ |*
*sa siddhiṃ vipulāṃ gacchet mahāyānāgradharmatām ||*
*mātaraṃ buddhasya vibhoḥ kāmayan na ca lipyate |*
*sidhyate tasya buddhatvaṃ nirvikalpasya dhīmataḥ ||*

The performer who loves the 'mother', 'sister', and 'daughter—achieves the extensive *siddhi* at the true nature of the Mahāyāna summit. Loving the Mother of the Buddha, who is the pervading lord, one is not adhered to (by sin). Buddhahood is accomplished for that wise man, devoid of discursive thought.

The *Pradīpoddyotana* (*Mchan ḥgrel*, pp. 43-44) comments : buddhasya mātāṃ prajñāpāramitāṃ svahṛdisthitāṃ niścārya tayā sahasamāpattiṃ kuryāt / hṛdayasthā mahādevī yogino yogavāhinī / jananī sarvabuddhānāṃ vajradhātvīśvarī smṛteti vacanāt / kāmayann iti mātṛbhaginīduhitṛvaddhitaiṣiṇībhiḥ / samayajñābhiḥ / jñānamudrayā ca paramānandasukham anubhavaḥ/ na ca lipyata iti rāgādikleśair naiva spṛśyate / na kevalam rāgādidoṣair na lipyate / api tu sarvasampattim āpadyata ity āha / sidhyata ityādi / tasya sādhakasya dhīḥ suśikṣitā mudrā / yasya tasya dhīmataḥ / nirvikalpasya svabhāvajñasya / buddhatvaṃ mahāvajradharatvaṃ sidhyate svayam eva niṣpadyate / neyārthaḥ // punar ārya-vyākhyānam ucyate / prajñāpāramitāṃ prajñāṃ dharmakāyaikamātṛkām / kāmaye(n) ni(ḥ)svabhāvākhyāṃ tathatādvayayogataḥ // sambhogatulyatāṃ jātāṃ tāṃ eva bhaginīṃ matām / kāmayen mantramūrtyā tu svādhidaivatāyogavān // sādhako bhāvayet tāṃ tu putrīṃ nirmāṇarūpiṇīṃ / kāmayann īdṛśaḥ yogī bhaginīmātṛputrīkāṃ / sa siddhiṃ vipulāṃ gacchen mahāyānāgradharma(tā)m//nītārthaḥ//

Having drawn forth the (lady) Prajñāpāramitā (from the Clear Light) dwelling in his own heart who is the mother of the Buddha, he should engage in union with her, because it is said (in the *Sarvarahasyatantra*, verse 46):

The great goddess dwelling in the heart, causing the *yoga* of the yogin, the mother of all the Buddhas, is called "Queen of the Diamond Realm'.

'Loving' means by those aware of the pledge, well-wishing, for such as mother, sister, daughter. Experiencing the ecstasy of supreme bliss with the 'knowledge seal', one is 'not adhered to (by sin)', i.e. is not contacted by the defilements of lust and so on. Not only is one not adhered to by the faults (bad destiny) of lust and so on, but also one attains ali perfection, for which reason (the verse) says '(Buddhahood) is accomplished' and so on. The wisdom (*dhī*=*prajñā*) of that performer is the well-trained *mudrā*. For that wise man, who is 'devoid of discursive thought', i.e. knows the intrinsic nature, Buddhahood, i.e, the state of Mahāvajradhara, is accomplished just by itself, i.e. completed. *Hinted meaning*. Also, it is said in the '*Ārya-vyākhyāna*' (the *Saṃdhivyākaraṇa*):

He should love by the non-dual *yoga* of thusness the Prajñā-woman, who is the Perfection of Insight called 'devoid of intrinsic nature', the 'Mother' (the Clear Light) identical to the Dharmakāya. He, equipped with the *yoga* of his own presiding divinity (of the Stage of Completion) should love just that one referred to as 'sister', engendred equal to the Sambhogakāya (which has emerged as the yuganaddha-deha from the wind and mind-only of the Clear Light). But, by (his) incantation body (which has repeatedly contemplated the Clear Light), the performer should contemplate that 'daughter' with the form of the Nirmāṇa(kāya) (of the various Tathāgatas).

The yogin of this kind, loving the 'mother,' 'sister,' 'daughter,' attains the extensive *siddhi,* i.e. the supreme dharma-nature of Mahāyāna.

*Evident meaning.*

It should be mentioned that the *Mchan ḥgrel* identified both the *Sarvarahasyatantra* (the verses of which I have numbered) and the *Saṃdhivyākaraṇa* citations. Besides, the translation has been influenced by the expression '*idṛśa*' applied to the yogin. In order that he be 'of this kind' there should be a relevant statement in each of the three cases, i.e. for the 'mother' "by the non-dual *yoga* of thusness"; for the 'sister' "equipped with the *yoga* of his own presiding divinity"; and for the 'daughter' "by (his) incantation body". This consideration justifies taking the Sanskrit expression *mantramūrtyā* ('by his incantation body') with the suggestion of *tu . . . tu,* to apply to the 'daughter' of the next verse. Otherwise, the yogin would be of two 'such kinds' for the 'sister' and of no 'such kind' for the 'daughter'. This also suggests the solution that the consort of the yogin in the Mahāsādhana phase of the Stage of Generation is the 'daughter'; while his consorts during the Stage of Completion are the 'sister' and the 'mother'. (Much information about this daughter, etc. symbolism is in my article "Female Energy..." reprinted with corrections in *The Buddhist Tantras*).

But also, the *Guhyasamājatantra,* Chap. V, after those verses 7-8, portrayed the astonishment of the Bodhisattvas. So the Lord pronounced verse 9 :

*iyaṃ sā dharmatā śuddhā buddhānāṃ sārajñāninām |*
*sāradharmārthasambhūtā eṣā bodhicaripadam ||*

This is the pure true nature of the Buddhas who know the essential (the Nirvāṇa of no fixed abode). That, having arisen from the nature of the essential (supreme truth) and the entity (conventional truth), is the plane of enlightenment-coursing (Mahāvajradhara).

Thereupon, according to Chapter V, the Bodhisattvas fainted. The *Pradīpoddyotana* (*Mchan ḥgrel,* p. 44-4, 5 to p. 45-1) quotes again the *Saṃdhivyākaraṇa* on this chapter:

*punar āryavyākhyānam ucyate |*
*aspan(d)akam idaṃ guhyaṃ śāntaikaṃ sukham uttamam |*
*sandhyāya kathitaṃ cedaṃ samyaksambodhiprāpakaḥ ||...*
*ākāśānantatāyogād rūpādīnām anantatā |*

*te vai tathāgatāḥ proktā bodhisattvās tathaiva ca* //...
*tat tu saṃgraham ivedaṃ maṇḍalaṃ yat svakāyataḥ* /
*kalpayantīha satkāyāḥ bodhisattvā hi mūrchitāḥ* //
*na jānanti tadityante sukhenonmādacoditāḥ* /
*bodhisattvān mahāsattvān uktān te mūrchitān* //

Further, the 'Ārya-Vyākhyāna' is cited (for the 'evident meaning'): Motionless is this secret (place), peaceful, unique, the supreme ecstasy. And this attainer of perfect enlightenment is stated in the manner of twilight. By the *yoga* (the two dhyānas) of space (=śūnya) and infinity (=mahāśūnya), there is infinity of form, etc. (the skandhas, the elements, the sense bases). Those are indeed the Tathāgatas as well as the Bodhisattvas. Now, that is this comprisal, which is the *maṇḍala* as the (yogin's) body. The Bodhisattvas imagine it in this world as their transitory bodies, so they swoon. Since they do not know that (truth, the intrinsic nature), when exhorted by ecstasy's frenzy, the Bodhisattva Great Beings are said to 'swoon'.

Some other explanations of the seemingly immoral injunctions are made without resort to such interpretations, as above, of knowing the intrinsic nature. For example, the *Guhyasamājatantra*. Chap. XVI, p. 120, has a verse which stipulates conduct precisely the reverse of the Buddhist layman's vows:

*prāṇinaś ca tvayā ghātyā vaktavyaṃ ca mṛṣā vacaḥ* /
*adattaṃ ca tvayā grāhyaṃ sevanaṃ yoṣitām api* //

You should kill living beings, speak lying words, take things not given, and resort to the ladies.

The *Pradipoddyotana* (*Mchan ḥgrel* edition) does not comment on this verse, presumably because the subject already was treated in Chapter IX's commentary. So, *Guhyasamāja*, IX, p. 35: "He should kill all sentient beings with this secret thunderbolt: (anena guhyavajreṇa sarvasattvaṃ vighātayet); *Pradipoddyotana*, PTT, Vol. 158, p. 66-5: "He should destroy all sentient beings by rendering them into the Void (*śūnya*)" (sems can thams cad bsad ciṅ stoṅ par byas pas rnam par gźig par byaḥo). *Tantra* p. 36: "He should contemplate the stealing of all materials with the triple thunderbolt' (haraṇaṃ sarvadravyāṇāṃ trivajreṇa vibhāvayet); PTT, Vol. 158, p. 67-2:

" 'stealing' means he summons the substance of all the Tathāgatas" (phrogs pa ni de bźin gśegs pa thams cad kyi rdzas dgug Paḥo) *Tantra*, p. 36 : "There he should contemplate the conjunction of all of them to the aspect of a lady" (yoṣidākāra-saṃyogaṃ sarveṣāṃ tatra bhāvayet); PTT, Vol. 158, p. 67-4, 5: " 'there', in that *maṇḍala*, he should contemplate the conjunction with i.e. the transformation (of all other male deities) into, the appearance of goddesses" (dkyil ḥkhor der... bud med kyi rnam pa lta bur yoṅs su gyur paḥo). *Tantra*, p. 36 : "He should contemplate all forms as the diamond expressions which are lying words" (mṛṣāvādaṃ vajrapadaṃ sarvabimbān vibhāvayet); PTT, Vol. 158, p. 68-2: "He should contemplate all forms of sentient beings as lying words, since all *dharmas* are like illusions" (thams cad gzugs te sems can thams cad...rdo rjoḥi tshig gi rdzun smra bas zes bya ba ni / chos thams cad sgyu ma lta bu yin pas). Of course, it is not such a terrible doctrine after all, if killing of living beings means only seeing them as void; telling lies, the working with *dharmas* that are seen as illusions; stealing, the drawing into oneself of the divine substance of the Tathāgatas; and uniting freely with the ladies, the imaginative transformation of *maṇḍala* deities into goddesses.

The *Guhyasamāja* in one place suggests that this 'renouncing the proper and the improper act' of the nidāna verse is from the absolute standpoint while in conventional terms we must still make these value judgments. Thus, Chapter IX, p. 38:

*mahādbhuteṣu dharmeṣu ākāśasadṛśeṣu ca* /
*nirvikalpeṣu śuddheṣu saṃvṛtis tu pragīyate* //

While the *dharmas* are marvellous and like the sky, are free from imagination and pure—a convention is expressed.

Another solution is to take 'sin as merit', according to *Pañcakrama*, V, 34-35 :

*yathā saukhyaṃ tathā duḥkhaṃ yathā duṣṭas tathā sutaḥ* /
*yathāvīcis tathā svargas tathā puṇyaṃ tu pāpakam* //
*evaṃ jñātvā cared yogi nirviśaṅkas tu sarvakṛt* /
*pracchannavratam āsādya sidhyante sarvasampadaḥ* //

Having known suffering to be as happiness, the son as the despised person, heaven as the Avīci hell, sin as merit, the yogin should do all deeds without fear. By his recourse to the private asceticism, all perfections are fulfilled.

G. *Bhage-ṣu vijahāra* (*Was dwelling in the bhagas*)

In the six-membered yoga, this is the last member, Samādhi; and in the *Pañcakrama* system, it is the last krama, Yuganaddha, in fact continuing the *śaikṣa-yuganaddha* and ending with *aśaikṣa-yuganaddha*. BHA portrays the yogin as a Buddha in one or another of the five Buddha families; while GE portrays his 'home', where he is, being the female element of the world. The syllable ṢU is understood as the locative indication governed by the verb Vijahāra. Therefore, the author of these verses starts his final *aśaikṣa* topic with ṢU. The Vajrasattva yogin continues by dwelling anywhere (ṢU VI-JA-HĀ-RA) to instruct the advanced Bodhisattvas.

What is the meaning of the word '*bhaga*'? The *Vajramālā* Explanatory Tantra, Chap. 41 (PTT, Vol. 3, p. 219-3) states :

> / *chos dbyiṅs bha-ga źes ni brjod* /
> / *bha-ga rin chen za ma tog* /
> / *gaṅ phyir dbaṅ phyug sogs yon tan* /
> / *ldan pa de phyir bha-ga brjod* //
> / *bha-ga chos rnams su yaṅ bśad* /
> / *dbyiṅs ni byaṅ chub sems su gsuṅs* /
> / *khams gsum pa yi ḥgro ba yi* /
> / *rgyu ni bha-ga źes byar bśad* //

> The Dharmadhātu is called '*bhaga*'.
> The *bhaga* is a jewelled basket (*karaṇḍa*).
> Because it possesses the merits of 'lordliness' and so on, it is called '*bhaga*'. The *bhaga* is also explained as the *dharmas*. The *dhātu* is said to be the *bodhicitta*. The cause of movement of the three realms is explained as '*bhaga*'.

The explanation by the *Sandhivyākaraṇa* Explanatory Tantra is cited by the *Pradīpoddyotana* (*Mchan ḥgrel*, p. 21-2) :

> *yathoktaṃ bhagavatā sandhyāvyākaraṇa-tantre* /
> *sarvabuddhoṣitā yā vā bhūmiḥ syāt sā trayodaśī* /
> *sā ca yoṣit samākhyātā saddharmo bhaga ucyate* //

As it was said by the Lord in the *Sandhivyākaraṇatantra* :

> The Stage resorted to by all the Buddhas is the Thirteenth, and it is called the 'lady'. The Dharma of illustrious persons is said to be the *bhaga*.

(*Mchan ḥgrel* explains that the Tenth Stage has the three lights. The Illusory Body is the Eleventh Stage. The Clear Light is the Twelfth Stage. The Thirteenth Stage is the *Adhimukti-caryā-bhūmi (*mos spyod kyi sa*) [hence Anusmṛti in the six-membered *yoga* or Abhisaṃbodhi of the *Pañcakrama*]. Accordingly, a Fourteenth Stage is allotted to Yuganaddha.)

Candrakīrti's *Pradīpoddyotana* on Chapter Seven, verse 21, devoted to 'remembrance of the Buddha' (*buddhānusmṛti*), comments on the words 'dvayendriyasamāpattyā buddhabimbaṃ vibhāvayet' ("With union of the two organs one should contemplate an image of the Buddha"), as follows : / bhagaḥ paramārthasatyaṃ / tasmin līyata iti liṅgaṃ / kiṃ tat saṃvṛti-satyaṃ / pratiṣṭhāpya prabhāsvare praveśya buddhabimbaṃ mahāvajradharaṃ vibhāvayet / paramārthasatyād vyutthā-payed ity arthaḥ / "The *bhaga* is supreme truth. About the *liṅga*, it is said, 'It lies therein'. And what is it ? Conventional truth. 'Placing it', i.e. introducing it into the Clear Light, one should contemplate an image of the Buddha, i.e. Mahā-vajradhara. One should make it emerge from Supreme truth. That is the meaning." *Mchan ḥgrel* (p. 58-1, 2) comments on the *liṅga* in the sense of Conventional truth that it is the Illusory Body (*sgyu maḥi sku*), which (*ibid*, p. 21-1-7) is golden . Earlier, in *Pradīpoddyotana's* comments on Chapter One (*Mchan ḥgrel*, p. 21-3, 4), the same topic was set forth as follows: / atha prabhā-svarapraveśād anantaraṃ bhagavān mahāvajradharaḥ sarva-tathāgatakāyavākcittādhipatiḥ / sarvakulâtmakam ātmānaṃ paramārthasatyād vyutthāya bhavanirvāṇaikarasasvabhāvena sarvatathāgatamahāsamayamaṇḍalamadhye pratiṣṭhāpayām āsa/ "Immediately after the entrance (of the Illusory Body) in to the Clear Light, the Lord Mahāvajradhara, master of the Body, Speech, and Mind of all the Tathāgatas, arousing himself, who is all the families, from Absolute Truth (*paramārthasatya*), by the intrinsic nature of 'single essence' (inseparability) of the phenomenal world (the Illusory Body as *saṃvṛti-satya*) and Nirvāṇa (the Clear Light gnosis as *paramārtha-satya*) established himself in the center of the 'Great Pledge *maṇḍala* of all the Tathāgatas." This is the four-cornered dustless *maṇḍala*.

Those passages clarify the usage of the word '*bhaga*' as Supreme Truth, the Clear Light, in the sense of what is entered. Hence, mystically, the word for 'female organ' is employed for this arcanum, which therefore can represent any *cakra* of the body with the stipulation that the yogin enters (with a subtle body) that *cakra* and realizes the Clear Light. The comment on '*bhaga*' as 'destruction of defilement' (cf. the introductory section on the *nidāna*) refers to the purifying function of the Clear Light, which is credited with converting the impure Illusory Body into the pure gnostic body as the Saṃbhogakāya.

The explanation of Yuganaddha consistent with the above remarks is treated as follows in the *Pañcakrama*, 5th (Yuganaddha), verse 18 (Śrī Lakṣmī, Vol. 63, p. 51-1, 2) :

*rāgārāgavinirmuktaḥ paramānandamūrtimān* /
*āsaṃsāraṃ sthitiṃ kuryād yuganaddhavibhāvakaḥ* //

Possessing the (Illusory) Body in supreme ecstasy (= the Clear Light), which is free from 'desire' and 'aversion' (= the *prakṛtis* associated with Spread-of-Light and Light), he should remain as long as does *saṃsāra*, contemplating *yuganaddha*.

Śrī Lakṣmī further explains that this verse portrays the state called 'Nirvāṇa without fixed abode' (*apratiṣṭhita-nirvāṇa*). This is referred to in *Pañcakrama*, 5th krama, verses 2, 25 :

*saṃsāro nirvṛtiś ceti kalpanādvayavarjanāt* /
*ekībhāvo bhaved yatra yuganaddhaṃ tad ucyate* //
*etad evādvayajñānam apratiṣṭhitanirvṛtiḥ* /
*buddhatvaṃ vajrasattvatvaṃ sarvaiśvaryaṃ tathaiva ca* //

Having eliminated the two imaginations '*saṃsāra*' and '*nirvāṇa*'—then wherein unification occurs, is called '*yuganaddha*' (the pair united). Just that is the non-dual knowledge, the Nirvāṇa without fixed abode, Buddhahood, the state of Vajrasattva, as well as universal sovereignty.

But the human mind prefers that a dwelling be localized somewhere. The *Guhyasamājatantra*, Chap. XVII, p. 139, has the passage :

/ atha te sarve mahābodhisattvāḥ tān sarvatathāgatān evam āhuḥ / sarvatathāgatakāyavākcittasiddhīni bhagavantaḥ kutra sthitāni kva vā saṃbhūtāni / sarvatathāgatāḥ prāhuḥ / trikāyaguhyaṃ sarvatathāgatakāyavākcittaṃ vajrācāryasya kāyavākcittavajre sthitam / mahābodhisattvā āhuḥ / kāyavākcittaguhyavajraṃ kutra sthitam / sarvatathāgatāḥ prāhuḥ / ākāśe sthitam / mahābodhisattvāḥ prāhuḥ / ākāśaṃ kutra sthitam / sarvatathāgatāḥ prāhuḥ / na kvacit / atha te mahābodhisattvā āścaryaprāptā adbhutaprāptāḥ tūṣnīṃ sthitā abhūvan / Then all those great Bodhisattvas spoke as follows to all the Tathāgatas : "Lords, where dwell the occult powers (*siddhi*) of the Body, Speech, and Mind of all the Tathāgatas ? Where have they arisen ?" All the Tathāgatas replied : "The secret of three bodies—the Body, Speech, and Mind of all the Tathāgatas dwells in the diamond of Body, Speech, and Mind of the diamond hierophant." The great Bodhisattvas asked : "Where dwells the secret diamond of his Body, Speech, and Mind ?" All the Tathāgatas replied: "It dwells in the sky." The great Bodhisattvas asked: "Where dwells the sky ?" All the Tathāgatas replied: "Nowhere." Then those great Bodhisattvas in wonderment and amazement became silent.

Another interpretation of the word 'bhaga' is found in Celupā's *Ratnavṛkṣa-nāma-rahasya-samāja-vṛtti* (PTT., Vol. 63, p. 174-1) "It is said : 'Because it makes known everything, the mind(citta) is called "*bhaga* of the lady". From that is born the Teacher.' " ( / ji skad du / thams cad śes par byed paḥi phyir / thugs ni bud med bha-gaḥo źes so / / de las byuṅ ba ni ston paḥo / ). However, the *citta* to which Celu-pa refers is actually the *bodhicitta*. There is a celebrated verse about this, which was pronounced by Vairocana in the *Guhyasamāja*, Chap. Two :

*sarvabhāvavigataṃ skandhadhātvāyatanagrāhyagrāhakavarjitam / dharmanairātmyasamatayā svacittam ādyanutpannaṃ śūnyatābhāvam //*

"My *citta* is free from all modes-of-being; avoids the personality aggregates, realms, and sense bases, as well as subject and object; is primordially unborn, the intrinsic nature of voidness—through the sameness of *dharmanairātmya*."

There are also some other explanations of *yuganaddha*. Thus, *Pañcakrama*, 5th krama, verse 12, associates *yuganaddha* with the 'central vein' of the body :

*piṇḍagrāhānubhedābhyāṃ praveśas tathatālaye /*
*utthānaṃ ca tato yatra samatād yuganaddhakam //*

By means of contraction (*piṇḍagrāha*) and expansion (*anubheda*)—the entrance, so in the abiding, and then wherein the rising—through equality (of the two), there is '*yuganaddha*'.

The *Subhāṣita-saṃgraha* (Part II, p. 42) quotes the *Saṃvaratantra* about *yuganaddha*:

*eṣa svābhāvikaḥ kāyaḥ śūnyatākaruṇādvayaḥ /*
*napuṃsaka iti khyāto yuganaddha iti kvacit //*

This Svābhāvika Body, the non-duality of voidness and compassion, called the Androgyne, is sometimes said to be *yuganaddha*.

Finally, *Pañcakrama*, 5th krama, verse 26 (Śrī Lakṣmī. p. 52-2,3) defines *yuganaddha* in terms of *samādhi*:

*vajropamasamādhis tu niṣpannakrama eva ca /*
*māyopamasamādhiś cāpy advayaṃ tac ca kathyate //*

For the Diamond-like Samādhi is precisely the *niṣpannakrama*; and the Illusory Samādhi is the non-dual (knowledge).

At this point, Śrī Lakṣmī quotes a verse without naming the source : "With insight (*prajñā*) one does not stay in *saṃsāra*; with compassion (*karuṇā*) one does not stay in (the quiescent) *nirvāṇa*:—For a long time with not the means (*upāya*) and for the same long time with the means" ( / śes rab kyis ni srid mi gnas / / sñiṅ rjes mya ṅan ḥdas mi gnas / / thabs med pa yis yun riṅ daṅ / / thabs kyis kyaṅ ni yun riṅ ñid / ). Here 'insight' is not the 'means' and 'compassion' is.

*//BHA// bhavaty aṣṭaguṇaiś caryair upetaḥ sarvavit svayam /*
*vicarej jñānadehena lokadhātor aśeṣataḥ //34//*

Equipped with the eight *guṇas* to be practised, an omniscient being arises, and by himself wanders all over the worldly realm by means of the knowledge body.

*Mchan* : 'Eight guṇas' are subtle form, etc. (*sūkṣmarūpādi*); 'himself'—the yogin.

*Pradipoddyotana* on *Guhyasamāja*, Chap. XV, verse 51; *Mchn ḥgrel* edition, p. 124-4 : "Because he has the eight *guṇa-aiśvarya* he has glory (*śrimat*)" ( / yon tan gyi dbaṅ phyug brgyad daṅ ldan pas na / de ni dpal ldan paḥo / ). On this remark, *Mchan ḥgrel* comments in part that it is the *śaikṣa-yuganaddha*. *Prakāśikā* on Bha (Vol. 60, p. 295-2): 'Equipped with the *guṇas*' means he has the lordliness of eight *guṇas* of the subtle, etc. or has the lordliness of body, etc.; 'an omniscient being arises' means that he knows the mental make-up of all sentient beings of past, present, and future, and knows their death, transmigration, and rebirth; also, for the sake of sentient beings he 'by himself wanders by means of the *jñāna-deha*', that is to say, he wanders 'all over the *lokadhātu*' by the illusory aspect as well as through all the Buddha fields (yon tan źes bya ba la sogs pa smos te / phra ba la sogs pa yon tan brgyad kyi dbaṅ phyug gam skuḥi dbaṅ phyug la sogs pa de daṅ ldan paḥo / / sems can thams cad rig ḥgyur / źes pa ni ḥdas pa la sogs paḥi dus gsum gyi naṅ na gnas pahi sems can thams cad kyi sems kyi spyod pa daṅ ḥchi ḥpho ba daṅ skye ba la sogs pa śes par ḥgyur re / / de bźin du yaṅ sems can gyi don bya ba phyir bdag ñid ye śes lus kyi spyod / ces pa ni sgyu ma lta buḥi rnam pas ḥjig rten gyi khams ma lus pa ste / saṅs rgyas kyi źiṅ rnams yoṅs su spyod do / ).

*Pradipoddyotana* on *Guhyasamāja*, Chap. XVII, p. 135 and verse 39; *Mchan ḥgrel* edition, p. 154-3:—

(a) *Pradipoddyotana* comment on the words *trivajraḥ parameśvaraḥ* : "The three *vajras* are the diamond Body, Speech, and Mind; and he is 'supreme' (*parama*) among them." "Furthermore, the eight are : (1) lordliness (*aiśvarya*) of body, (2) lordliness of speech, (3) lordliness of mind, (4) of magical prowess (*ṛddhi*), (5) omnipresent lordliness (*sarvagataiśvarya*) (6) of wish (*icchā*), (7) of creating (*kartṛ*), (8) lordliness of the *guṇas* (*guṇa*)."

(b) *Mchan ḥgrel* : (The eight are :)

(1) ability to simultaneously display innumerable corporeal manifestations.

(2) ability to simultaneously teach the *dharma* to the different classes of sentient beings in their own language.

(3) unsullied omniscience.

(4) display of innumerable magical feats.

(5) omnipresence in all realms (*viṣaya*), times (*kāla*), and states (*avasthā*).

(6) ability to fulfil wishes as soon as wished.

(7) creation of various forms, stationary or moving, exactly as desired.

(8) having the *guṇas* of the ten powers, etc.

By 'ten powers, etc.' the reference is made to the ten powers (*daśa-bala*) and other attributes of the Tathāgata, such as the four confidences. According to the *Mahāvyutpatti*, Nos. 120-129, the ten powers are : 1. power to know the possible and the impossible (*sthānāsthāna*), 2. power to know the maturation of *karma*, 3. power to know the various convictions (*adhimukti*), 4. power to know the various elements (*dhātu*), 5. power to distinguish between a superior and inferior sensory power (*indriya*), 6. power to know the paths going everywhere (*sarvatra-gāminī-pratipad*), 7. power to know all accompaniment of meditation (*dhyāna*), liberation (*vimokṣa*), profound concentration (*samādhi*), meditative attainment (*samāpatti*), defilement (*saṃkleśa*) and purification (*vyavadāna*), 8. power to recollect former lives (*pūrvanivāsa*), 9. power to know transmigration and rebirth (*cyuty-utpatti*), 10. power to know the destruction of the fluxes (*āsrava-kṣaya*).

Also, the *yogin* who 'wanders by himself' in verse 'BHA'—despite the mysterious maidens (*kanyā*) mentioned under 'GE' and in *Guhyasamāja*, Chap. XV—is in that chapter classified by different families, according to *Pradīpoddyotana* (*Mchan ḥgrel*, p. 120-4, 5 and 122-2). So, in the Sanskrit text, p. 94, the phrase, 'He would shine like a Buddha' (*bhaved buddhasamaprabhaḥ*) refers to the *yogin* belonging to Vairocana. 'The king who holds all *dharmas*' (*sarvadharmadharo rājā*) is the *yogin* of Amitābha. 'By the praxis of Vajrasattva' (*vajrasattvaprayogataḥ*) means Akṣobhya's *yogin*. 'Shining like Vajrasattva' (*vajrasattvasamaprabhaḥ*) refers to Ratnasambhava's *yogin*. And 'the one accomplishing the desire and the liberation' (*kāmamokṣaprasādhakaḥ*) is the *yogin* of Amoghasiddhi's family. Besides, text, p. 95, the 'one of diamond nature' (*vajradharmātman*) is the superior *yogin* belonging to Amitābha.

*Guhyasamājatantra*, XV, 11, places this attainment on the Tenth Stage : "He would be Vajradharmātman, dwelling on the Tenth Stage, the king who holds the Vāksamaya, the Parameśvara who is supreme." (sa bhaved vajradharmātmā daśabhūmipratiṣṭhitaḥ / vāksamayadharo rājā sarvāgraḥ parameśvaraḥ).

*//GE// gehaṃ tasyāmbaraś caiva yatra sa carati prabhuḥ /*
*tatraiva ramate nityaṃ mahāsukhasamādhinā //35//*

His home is the sky wherever he the Lord does roam. By the samādhi of great ecstasy he forever rejoices in that very place.

*Mchan* : '*samādhi* of great ecstasy' means the consubstantial bliss (*sahajānanda*). 'That very place' is the sky and is explained as *paramārtha-satya.*

Saraha's *Dohā-koṣa* (verses 93, 96 in Shahidullah's numbering) as I translate from the Prakrit (given here) and the Tibetan texts reproduced in M. Shahidullah, *Les Chants Mystiques de Kāṇha et de Saraha*, was suggested for inclusion here by the citation in Tsoṅ-kha-pa's (*Gsal baḥi sgron me* commentary on the *Pañcakrama* (PTT, Vol. 159, p. 70-5 to p. 71-1):

93. rūaṇe saala bi jo ṇaü gāhaī,
kunduru-khaṇaī mahāsuha sāhaī ?
jima tisia tisittaṇe dhābaī
mara sose nabhajjalu kahi pābaī.
96. kamala-kuliśa bebi majjha ṭhiu jo so suraa-bilāsa,
ko tahī ramaī ṇa tihuaṇe kassa ṇa pūria āsa ?

At the moment of 'resin' (*kunduru* is twilight language for indefinable 'union'), does he gain the great ecstasy (*mahāsukha*) who does not know completely the true nature (*rūaṇa*, **rūpaṇa*, taken equivalent to *svarūpa*) ? As one with avid thirst races for the water of a mirage and dies of thirst—how can he obtain the water of the sky ? That sport by pleasure located between the lotus and the diamond, if anyone could not take pleasure there, in the three worlds, whose hope could he fulfil ?

*Prakāśikā* on Ge (Vol. 60, p. 295-3,4) : 'The sky' means the realm of space (*ākāśa-dhātu* or *kha-dhātu*); 'the Lord who roams wherever' is Śrī Vajrasattva, the Lord of the five who are Akṣobhya, etc.;... 'By the *mahāsukhasamādhi* he forever rejoices in that very place' has as external meaning that by producing in immediacy the reality of the Clear Light he rejoices by rejoicing in emanating and reunification; ... as to 'wherever the Lord does roam', he roams in whatever lotus of *mudrā* by the form of upper and lower *bodhicitta* of Śri Vajradhara, because the Tantra says, 'Whatever the sky within the *bhaga*, it is ornamented with five skies';... this abiding in his own form of introspection is the inner meaning.

Those remarks of the *Prakāśikā* introduce a number of difficulties, but also suggest the research to be brought up now. The nidāna verse has the phrase 'his home is the sky'. *Guhyasamāja*, XII, verse 2 ('Documents') speaks of a spot of a great forest and in a secluded mountain. The *Pradipoddyotana* on this verse first explains the verse according to its literal form in terms of a beautiful place for meditation, labelling this explanation the 'hinted meaning' (*neyārtha*). Then, to show the 'evident meaning' (*nitārtha*), it cites some verses from the '*Ārya-Vyākhyāna*', in fact from the *Saṃdhivyākaraṇa* (PTT, Vol. 3, p. 242), translated with some remarks from *Mchan ḥgrel*, p. 83-2, 3 :

> *ākāśakalpanāyogaiḥ skandhā mahāṭavi matāḥ* ||
> *asthānasthitiyogena pradeśe mahadālaye* |
> *sambhogakalpavṛkṣe 'smin vividhe siddhipuṣpite* ||
> *nirmāṇaphalasaṃśobhe samyaksambodhiparvate* |
> *abhāvavijane ramye sādhyaṃ tad vajrasaṃjñakam* ||
>
> By procedures of considering their sky (=the Clear Light), the personality aggregates are claimed to be the 'great forest'.
>
> By the *yoga* of the place of no location (*apratiṣṭhitanirvāṇa*), there are those 'flowers' of the various (supramundane) *siddhis* on the wishing tree of Sambhoga (the illusory body) in a 'spot' which is a great place.
>
> When there is the decoration of Nirmāṇa 'fruit' on the joyous 'mountain' (Dharmakāya) of right completed enlightenment that is 'secluded' by lack of states, what is to be accomplished has the name 'vajra' (i.e. Vajradhara).

Ratnākaraśānti's *Piṇḍikṛta-sādhanopāyikā-vṛtti-ratnāvali-nāma* PTT, Vol. 62, pp. 69-5 to 70-1) concerns itself with the same verse of Chap. XII, and adds further levels of interpretation following Candrakīrti's classifying terms. Here, his 'Yathāruta' interpretation is most helpful :

> The 'great forest' is the sky of 'she who is love's umbrella'. The 'spot' is the sky of *Devadattā. 'Adorned with flowers, fruit, and so on' is the sky of the Moon Lady. The 'mountain' is the sky of the Tortoise Lady. 'Secluded' is the sky of *Dhanavijayā (Nor rgyal ma). Because it is said : "Whatever the sky within the *bhaga*, it is ornamented with five skies, beautified with eight petals and a nave with filaments. The ambrosia with the form of *śukra*, there located, ever drips."

The description of eight petals indicates either the heart-*cakra*, or the *cakra* which in the male is at the root of the penis; the latter seems meant here. Previously we took note that the latter *cakra* constitutes the *yogin's* 'woman'. On the other hand, the remark in the *Prakāśikā* on Ge, "by the form of upper and lower *bodhicitta*" suggests both *cakras*.

The *Prakāśikā* on Ge also says, "whatever lotus of *mudrā*," which refers to the families of goddesses respectively going with the five yogins mentioned under 'BHA', who, according to the *Prakāśika*, abide in their own form of introspection. According to Kloṅ-rdol-bla-ma, as cited in my "Female Energy ...", p. 94, the butcher maiden belongs to Akṣobhya's family; the washerman maiden to Vairocana's; the necklace-stringer maiden to Ratnasambhava's; the dancer maiden to Amitābha's; the artisan maiden to Amoghasiddhi's.

Also, there are 'ages' ascribed to various ones of those maidens. According to the *Guhyasamājatantra*, Chapter Four, verse 19 (*Mchan ḥgrel*, p. 40), and Chapter Sixteen verse 91 (*Mchan ḥgrel*, p. 147), the maiden belonging to Akṣobhya's family is aged 12; the one of Vairocana's 16. The article "Female Energy... " shows that this is consistent with the sizes ascribed to maṇḍalas of Body, Speech and Mind in the *Guhyasamājatantra*. Its Chapter Four mentions (Akṣobhya's) maṇḍala of Mind to have twelve *hastas*; its Chapter Sixteen mentions Vairocana's maṇḍala of Body to have sixteen *hastas*, and Amitābha's maṇḍala of Speech to have twenty *hastas*. On this principle, the maiden of Amitābha's family is aged 20. In that article, p. 105, I cited a passage from Saraha setting forth five ages, the eight-yeared Kumārī, the twelve-year-old Śālikā, the sixteen-yeared one called Siddhā, the twenty-year-old *Bālikā, and the twenty-five-yeared *Bhadra-kapālinī. By implication, Ratnasambhava's and Amogha-siddhi's maidens, in whatever order, have the ages of 8 and 25. The *Guhyasamājatantra* (Chap. 8, verse 7) mentions the age 25, but no age 8. Since this Tantra regularly has a four-fold correspondence in terms of the four goddesses, and hence to four Tathāgatas, the basic three plus Amoghasiddhi (the '*karmanātha*'), it follows that Amoghasiddhi's maiden is aged 25, but so far I find no passage to confirm this. In that article, p. 108, I included a quotation from the *Mahāmudrātilaka* : "If one does not obtain a twelve-yeared, or sixteen-yeared female, adorned with good features, long eyes, attractive figure and youth, then a twenty-yeared one is proper. Other 'seals' (*mudrā*) above twenty put the occult power far off. One should offer his sister, daughter, or wife to the 'master' (*guru*)." This passage is one evidence that the 'ages' refer to the length of time it takes the yogin to reach the *siddhi*. Other interpretations of the 'ages' presented in that article were, for the sixteen-yeared maiden, the sixteen voidnesses as well as sixteen vowels, the sixteen transits of winds and the sixteen digits of the moon. The twelve-yeared maiden can be interpreted as the twelve vowels by leaving out the 'two neuters' (ṛ, ṝ, ḷ, and ḹ) from the 16-vowel group, or as twelve transits by leaving out the last four transits.

Besides, according to *Guhyasamājatantra*, Chap.XV, verse 51, the maidens can belong to eithert he realm of desire (*kāmadhātu*) or the realm of form (*rūpadhātu*). According to the *Pradipoddyotana* on this, the ones in the realm of desire can be the daughters of the six passion families (the Tuṣita gods, etc., a standard category of non-tantric Buddhism), the ones called '*surabhogā*' are the daughters of the Cakravartins; and the '*kulavratā*' means they can belong to the families of gods, asuras, and so on. The ones in the realm of form have superior capacity (for siddhi).

|| ṢU || *eṣv evābhāsabhedeṣu sandhyā-rātri-dineṣu ca* |
*vyavahāraḥ kṛto loke jñānatrayanidarśanāt* || 36 ||

A conventional illustration is made in the world regarding just these distinctions of lights as the twilight, the night, and the day—so as to see the three gnoses (*jñāna*).

Both *Mchan* and the *Prakāśikā* have little to add here.

These illustrations are made to the disciple by a revered *guru* by way of Initiation (*abhiṣeka*). The *Maṇi-mālā* commentary on the *Pañcakrama* states (PTT, Vol. 62, p. 208-4): "The exalted *ācārya*, by removal of the eye-veil (*timira*), reveals to the disciple the outer *abhisaṃbodhis*" (slob dpon mchog ni rab rib spaṅs pas slob ma la ni phyi rol byaṅ chub bstan). Therefore, in his Abhisaṃbodhi-krama of the *Pañcakrama*, Nāgārjuna precedes the actual delineation of the *abhisaṃbodhis* with verses showing the disciple's exhortation to the *guru* to reveal those *abhisaṃbodhis*.

*tatsamārādhanaṃ kṛtvā varṣaṃ māsaṃ athāpi vā* |
*tasmai tuṣṭāya gurave pūjāṃ kuryāt tu śaktitaḥ* || 3 ||
*tatas tuṣṭo mahāyogī pañcakāmopabhogataḥ* |
*ālokasyodayaṃ kuryāt samāpattividhānataḥ* || 5 ||

*kalaśādau susaṃsthāpya bodhicittaṃ prayatnataḥ* /
*ardharātre cābhisiñcet suśiṣyaṃ kṛpayā guruḥ* // 6 //
*abhiṣekaṃ tu samprāpya pratyūṣasamaye punaḥ* /
*sampūjyārādhayet stotrair guruṃ śiṣyaḥ kṛtāñjaliḥ* // 7 //
*draṣṭukāmo 'bhisambodhiṃ sarvaśūnyasvabhāvikām* /
*stutvā kṛtāñjaliḥ śiṣyo guruṃ saṃcodayet punaḥ* // 12 //
*prayaccha me mahānātha abhisambodhidarśanam* /
*karmajanmavinirmuktam ābhāsatrayavarjitam* // 13 //
*evam ārādhito yogī sadbhūtaguṇakīrtanaiḥ* /
*śiṣye kāruṇyam utpādya kramam evam athārabhet* // 16 //

Having propitiated (the hierophant) for a month or even for a year, he should make offering as he is able to that pleased *guru* .... Then the *mahāyogī*, delighted through enjoyment of the five pleasures, should arouse light by a rite of equipoise (*samāpatti*). By engaging the 'mind of enlightenment' he well disposes the flask and so on; and at midnight the *guru* kindly initiates the good disciple. Having received initiation, the disciple at the time of dawn respectfully bows to the *guru* and pleases him with worshipful verses of praise .... When that disciple, desirous of seeing the *abhisaṃbodhi* which is the intrinsic nature of universal void, had praised, then respectfully bowing to the *guru*, he should exhort him further : 'Oh, great lord, pray offer me the glimpse of *abhisaṃbodhi*, liberated from *karma* and rebirth, and free of the three lights !' ....The *yogī*, thus gratified by the recital of holy qualities, feeling compassion toward the disciple, then begins the steps this way :

*Pañcakrama*, 2nd krama, verse 30 :

*saṃvittimātrakaṃ jñānam ākāśavad alakṣaṇam* /
*kiṃ tu tasya prabhedo 'sti saṃdhyārātridivātmanaḥ* //

The gnosis (*jñāna*) which is purely introspective is characterless like the sky. But it has a division going with the twilight, the night, the day.

*Pañcakrama*, 4th krama, 17 :

*āloko rātribhāgaḥ sphuṭaravikiraṇaḥ syād aivālokābhāsaḥ*
*saṃdhyālokopalabdhaḥ prakṛtibhir asakṛd yujyate svābhir etat* /

'Light' is the (moon-rise) part of night. The day with its spreading rays of the bright sun is 'Spread-of-Light'.

Twilight is 'Culmination-of-Light'. They work again and again by their own prakṛtis.

Therefore, the Clear Light, or universal void, is free of day, night, and twilight. These conventional illustrations also involve the distinction of inner and outer Abhisaṃbodhis, as are explained by Āryadeva in his *Caryā-melāpaka-pradipa* (PTT, Vol. 61, p. 308-2), where we should observe that he employs the word 'nescience' (*avidyā*) as in nidāna verse 3 :

/ de la mṅon par byaṅ chub paḥi rim pa ni rnam pa gñis te / ḥdi lta ste phyi daṅ naṅ giḥo / / de la daṅ por phyiḥi bstan par bya ste / tho raṅs kyi thun mtshams su ma rig paḥi snaṅ ba ḥdas na ji srid ñi ma gsal bar ma gyur pa ste / ḥdi la ni ḥod gsal ba dri ma med paḥi rnam pa gsal źiṅ lus daṅ ṅag daṅ yid daṅ bral ba thams cad stoṅ paḥi mtshan ñid can no / / ñi ma śar ba ni snaṅ ba mched paḥo / / ñi ma nub paḥi thun mtshams su ma rig paḥo / / zla ba śar baḥi tshe ni snaṅ baḥo / / de ltar stoṅ pa ñid rnam pa bźi phyi rol ṅes par bstan pa bśad nas / da ni naṅ gi mṅon par byaṅ chub pa so so raṅ gis rig paḥi mtshan ñid can rim pa ḥdis bstan par bya ste / daṅ por smig rgyu lta bu la ḥod zer lṅaḥi tshogs daṅ ldan par mthoṅ ṅo / / gñis pa snaṅ ba ste / zla baḥi ḥod zer lta buḥo / / gsum pa ni snaṅ ba mched pa ste / ñi maḥi ḥod zer lta buḥo / / bźi pa ni snaṅ ba thob pa ste / mun pa lta buḥo / / de nas mun pa daṅ bral baḥi skad cig la ḥod gsal ba ste śin tu gsal brtag tu snaṅ baḥi mtshan ñid can don dam paḥi bden paḥi raṅ gi mtshan ñid ye śes kyi mig gis mthoṅ ṅo /

Here, there are two kinds of Abhisambodhi sequences, namely, outer and inner. Of those, I shall first explain the outer kind. In the morning twilight, when the nescience light has passed away but still the sun is not bright—this characterizes the Clear Light, clear, of immaculate aspect, the universal void free from body, speech, and mind. The rising of the sun is Spread-of-Light. The twilight of sunset is nescience. The time of moonrise is Light. Having in that way related the external illustrations of the four kinds of voidness, I shall teach the inner Abhisambodhis by this sequence characterized by introspection : One sees first a mirage appearance with a

> mass of five light rays. Second is Light, like moon-rays. Third is Spread-of-Light, like sun-rays. Fourth is Culmination-of-Light like darkness. Then, in an instant free from darkness, there is Clear Light, characterized by a very bright lasting light, the individual characteristic of Paramārtha-satya, which one sees with the Eye of Knowledge.

In that passage, Āryadeva presents four outer *abhisaṃbodhis* (revelations), namely, natural phenomena revealing the voids or lights; and five inner *abhisaṃbodhis* (also, revelations), namely, psychological states that are actually the voids or lights.

The 'revealed' source for the Abhisambodhi illustrations is *Guhyasamājatantra*, Chap. XV p. 95 :

> *astamite tu vajrārke sādhanaṃ tu samārabhet* |
> *aruṇodgamavelāyāṃ sidhyate bhāvanottamaiḥ* ||
> When the diamond sun is setting, he should begin the *sādhana*. At the initial appearance of dawn he will succeed with the supreme contemplation.

The *Pradīpoddyotana*, *Mchan ḥgrel* edition, on this (PTT, Vol. 158, p. 121-2), explains that the 'diamond sun' (*vajrārka*) is characterized by the attainment of the 'means' gnosis (*upāya* kind of *jñāna*), hence Spread-of-Light. When this sets, there is the form of 'insight' (*prajñā*), hence Light. Then before the Clear Light can emerge, that Light must pass into Culmination-of-Light, which is the initial appearance of dawn, or nescience (*avidyā*). Then, on the basis of the three gnoses, namely, voidness, further voidness, and great voidness (Light, Spread-of-Light, and Culmination-of-Light), riding on the winds, the *yogin* soars to the Clear Light and perfects the *mahāmudrā* ('great seal').

The success in the practice is indicated in the *Guhyasamājatantra*, Chap. XVIII, p. 162 :

> *vajrapadmasamāyogāj jvālya santāpya yoginā* |
> *udyate sphaṭikākāraṃ jñānasūryam ivāparam* ||
> Through union of *vajra* and *padma* by the yogin, blazing, burning,——
> The incomparable sun of knowledge rises with crystalline appearance.

That description clearly points to the mystical experiences of Gautama Buddha under the Tree of Enlightenment during the night inaugurated by defeat of the Māra host at dusk, and finally Full Enlightenment at the flush of dawn—in the joy-faced night (*nandimukhāyām rajanyām*), or night becoming rosy-colored, quoted from the *Mahāvastu* in my "Notes on the Sanskrit Term *Jñāna*," p. 265. The follow-up to that early study is that the color of the sky represented the three lights by three natural features, the blackness of night (Culmination-of-Light), the red glow of the sun wishing to rise (Spread-of-Light), the setting full moon (Light), a sort of "three-in-one", the revelation of the Clear Light—in Āryadeva's language : "free from body, speech, and mind".

> *|| VI || vicitravyavahārāś ca laukikaiḥ parikalpitāḥ |*
> *pathatrayavibhāgena jñānatrayasamudbhavāḥ || 37 ||*
>
> Worldlings imagine the multiform conventions, which divided into three paths, originate the three knowledges.

*Mchan* : 'The multiform conventions' are : male, female, neuter; right, left, middle; harsh, mild, medium; etc. 'Three paths' means those leading to the Clear Light.

The 'three paths' are probably the Body, Speech, and Mind referred to in the *Prakāśikā* on Vi.

I collected a number of these 'multiform conventions' in the article "Female Energy...," from which its Table 2 headed "The Great Time" is here reproduced :

IX. THE GREAT TIME

| *Oṃ* | *Āḥ* | *Hūṃ* |
|---|---|---|
| Prajñā, the form of woman | Upāya, the form of man | Androgyne |
| 8-petalled lotus | 5-pronged thunderbolt | |
| Moonlight | Sunlight | Fire |
| Night | Day | Juncture of day and night |
| Left | Right | Middle |
| Waking | Dream | Dreamless sleep |
| Void | Further Void | Great Void |
| Light | Spread-of-Light | Culmination-of-light |
| Body | Speech | Mind |
| Vairocana | Amitābha | Akṣobhya |
| Birth | Intermediate State | Death |
| Nirmāṇakāya | Saṃbhogakāya | Dharmakāya |
| *Tamas* | *Rajas* | *Sattva* |
| Head | Neck | Heart |
| Inspiration | Retention | Expiration |

Indrabhūti presents another list of synonyms and correspondences in his commentary on the *Śrī-saṃpuṭa-tilaka* called *Ṭīkā-smṛti-saṃdarśanāloka* (PTT, Vol. 55, p. 77-2):

/ sñiṅ stobs daṅ snaṅ ba daṅ lus daṅ sems daṅ. stoṅ pa daṅ zla ba daṅ śes rab daṅ mtshan mo daṅ gźan dbaṅ daṅ oṃ daṅ āḥ ḥo / / de bźin du rdul daṅ snaṅ ba mched pa daṅ ṅag daṅ sems las byuṅ ba daṅ / śin tu stoṅ pa daṅ / ñi ma daṅ / thabs daṅ / ñin mo daṅ / kun brtags daṅ / a daṅ hrī ḥo / de bźin du mun pa daṅ snaṅ ba thob pa daṅ / / yid daṅ ma rig pa daṅ stoṅ pa chen po daṅ sgra gcan daṅ yaṅ dag par sbyor ba daṅ mtshams daṅ yoṅs su grub pa daṅ / hūṃ daṅ phaṭ ṅo /

Sattva (-guṇa), Light, Body, citta, Void, Moon, Insight (*prajñā*), Night, paratantra, Oṃ and Āḥ. Likewise, rajas (-guṇa), Spread-of-Light, Speech, caitta, Further Void, Sun, Means (*upāya*), Day, parikalpita, A and Hrī. Likewise, tamas (-guṇa), Culmination-of-Light, Mind, avidyā, Great Void, Rāhu, saṃyoga (marriage), twilight, pariniṣpanna, Hūṃ and Phaṭ.

A little further in the same work, Indrabhūti says (p. 77-5): Here, 'inferior' (*hīna*) means that by Oṃ = entrance (of the wind), he generates the fairies located in *pātāla*. Likewise, 'medium' (*madhya*) means that by Āḥ = staying (of ditto), he generates those located over *bhūmi*. And, 'best' (*praṇīta*) means that by Hūṃ—rising (of ditto), he generates those ranging in the sky (*khecarī*). Likewise, in respective order, there are innumerable sets, including three *maṇḍalas*, three paths, three eyes, three bodies (*kāya*), three liberations (*vimokṣa*), three worlds (*loka*), three gestations (*bhava*), three realities (*tattva*), three times, three *saṃdhyā* (dawn, noon, and dusk), three firmaments (? *gagana*), three creature worlds (*jagat*), the triple fortificaton (*tripura*), three germ syllables (*bīja*), triangle (*trikoṇa*), three places (possibly = three seats, *pīṭha*), three *guṇas*, three letters (*akṣara*). three lights (*āloka*). three characters (*svabhāva*), three realms (*dhātu*), three faces (*mukha*), three hearths, three kinds of form (*rūpa*).

*//JA// janma ca sthitibhaṅgena antarābhavasaṃsthitiḥ /*
*yāvantyaḥ kalpanā loke cittavāyu-vijṛmbhitaḥ //38//*

(Namely) birth, and by loss of abode—formation of the

intermediate state. To the extent there is discursive thought in the world, so is there phenomenal projection of mind and (its vehicular) winds.

*Mchan*: The verse refers to birth, death, and the state between those two (the *antarābhava*). Just as in the case of the two preceding verses, this one presents synonyms of the three gnoses. So also earlier (nidāna verse 25) *citta*, *caitta*, *avidyā*; and so on. The synonyms are collected in the 2nd krama (*sems dmigs kyi rim pa*) of the *Pañcakrama*. In the case of the intermediate state, this generates the Illusory Body (*māyā-deha*). The ultimate root is the extremely subtle wind and the mind mounted upon it. Discursive thinking (*kalpanā*) phenomenalizes that wind and its mounted consciousness. *Prakāśikā* on Ja (PTT, Vol. 60, p. 295-4, 5) : 'To the extent there is discursive thought in the world' means the discursive thought going with the twelve-membered Dependent Origination (ji sñed ḥjig rten gyis brtags pa / źes pa ni rten ciṅ ḥbrel bar ḥbyuṅ ba yan lag bcu gñis la sogs pahi rnam par rtog paḥo).

In my article "Buddhist Genesis and the Tantric Tradition", there are various passages from the works of Tsoṅ-kha-pa to show that he laid great stress upon the concordance with the three things, birth, death and the intermediate state. According to Tsoṅ-kha-pa, contemplation of the Dharmakāya purifies death; of the Sambhogakāya, the intermediate state; of the Nirmāṇakāya, birth. Such contemplation takes place both in the Stage of Generation and in the Stage of Completion.

*//HĀ// hāsyalāsyakriyāś caiva navanāṭyarasānvitāḥ /*
*mudrāmantravikalpaś ca vajrasattvaviceṣṭitam //39//*

Both the acts of laughter and accompanied dance with the nine sentiments of dramatic art, as well as mudrā, mantra, and mental formation, are enacted by Vajrasattva (the tantric hierophant).

*Mchan* : 'Laughter' and the mutual gaze at the time of the *caryā* (i.e. steps in divine courtship). 'Accompanied dance': a dance (*lāsya*) accompanied with singing and instrumental music. 'The nine sentiments of dramatic art' : this refers to accomplishing the Illusory Body from the wind-and-mind-only belonging to the *sādhaka*'s innate body (*nija-deha*). 'Mudrā' of body; 'mantra' of speech; 'mental formation' of binding (*ḥchiṅ ba*). 'Enacted by Vajrasattva' : this furnishes the reason for the earlier statement that the one who knows the intrinsic nature is not adhered to by sin.

*Prakāśikā* on Hā (Vol. 60, p. 295-5): 'Mental formation' means the various mentals, such as one-pointedness; 'enacted by Vajrasattva' means that all those (acts) are enacted through the Illusory Samādhi (*māyopama-samādhi*) (rnam par rtog pa ni sems las byuṅ ba rtse gcig pa la sogs paḥo // rdo rje sems dpaḥi rnam ḥphrul źes pa ni de dag thams cad sgyu ma lta buḥi tiṅ ṅe ḥdzin las rnam par ḥphrul pa ste).

Mudrā, mantra, and mental formation (in *samādhi*) are coordinated respectively with the three mysteries of the Buddha his Body, Speech, and Mind. The first two are especially, credited with attracting the deities (the mental formation is also required for 'binding' them), as in the *Guhyasamājatantra*, Chap. XIV, p. 87 (*Mchan ḥgrel*, p. 115-5):

*mudrābhedena sarveṣāṃ mantrabhedena sarvathā /*
*ākarṣaṇapadaṃ proktaṃ na cen nāśam avāpnuyāt //*
*vajrasattvo mahārājo codaniyo muhur muhuḥ //*
*sa eva sarvamantrāṇāṃ rājā paramaśāśvataḥ //*

By division of (mahā-) mudrā (into *mantra-deha* and *jñāna-deha* ) of all (the gods), and by division of (diamond-) incantation (into two kinds) in every case— the way of attracting is explained. If it were not so, that (way of attracting) would be unsuccessful. Vajrasattva (the latter, the sixth, as the basis of the former five) is the Great King to be exhorted (kept in mind) again and again. (For,) just he is the ever-supreme king of all incantations.

Vajrasattva's activities are summarized in *Pañckrama*, 3rd krama, verse 31; Śrī Lakṣmī, Vol 63, p. 39-2, 3:

*śṛṅgārādyupabhogaṃ ca gitavādyādisevanam /*
*kalāsu ca pravṛttiṃ ca kuryād udakacandravat //*

He should practise the experience of the 'erotic', etc. (the nine sentiments), the recourse to (the three adamantine) songs and instrumental music (the four beginning with vīṇā), and so on, as well as engagement in the (sixty-four) *kalā* (or *kāmakalā*) (in each case) in the manner of the 'moon in the water' (i.e. while in the Illusory-like Samādhi (*māyopama-samādhi*).

In Indian dramatic theory, *lāsya* is the sweet, graceful, and feminine dance. The nine sentiments are : erotic (*śṛṅgāra*), heroic (*vira*), furious (*raudra*), humorous (*hāsya*), wonderful (*adbhuta*), compassionate (*kāruṇya*), disgusting (*bibhatsa*), frightful (*bhayānaka*); plus the ninth, tranquil (*śānta*) with indifference to worldly objects and pleasures. Two passages should clarify their tantric interpretation. The first is from Śrī Rāhuguptapāda's *Prakāśa-nāma-śrihevajrasādhana* (PTT, Vol, 56, p. 132-1):

> Among those (nine sentiments), the 'single taste' (*ekarasa*) together with (the goddess) Nairātmyā is the 'erotic'; the staying at the burning ground is the 'heroic'; the furried brow and bared fangs is the 'disgusting'; the blazing light is the 'furious'; the enhancement (exaggeration) of face is the 'humorous'; the garland of dripping heads is the 'frightful'; the consciousness of assisting sentient beings is the 'compassionate'; the illusory form is the 'wonderful'; the defilement of lust, etc. is the 'tranquil'.

The second is from Śrī Lakṣmī, Vol. 63, p. 39-2 :

> (They are) union with the partner (*mudrā*) ('erotic'), staying in the burning ground, etc. ('heroic')., enjoying the ambrosia ('furious'), rite of revived corpse (*vetāla-vidhi*) ('disgusting'), holding of various emblems ('humorous'), drastic rites (*abhicāra*) ('frightful'), empathy with the great suffering of all sentient beings ('compassionate'), accomplishing enlightenment by the five great pledges, (*samaya*) in conflict with the world (i.e. the five that oppose the five layman vows) ('tranquil'), and the characteristic of having the Clear Light in immediacy ('wonderful').

The goddess Nairātmyā of the former passage belongs to the Mother Tantra tradition; outside of this fact, the passage is appropriate and helps explain Śrī Lakṣmī's text, since she leaves out the titles 'erotic', etc.

The three adamantine songs are very likely the group of three songs discussed in the *Sṅags rim chen mo* (f. 242b2, ff.): "The three songs are the 'song of reality' (*tattvagita*), 'song of true nature' (*dharmatāgita*), and 'song of mudrā' (*mudrāgita*)" (glu gsum ni de kho na ñid kyi glu daṅ chos ñid kyi glu daṅ phyag rgyaḥi gluḥo). By 'songs' are meant verses that are sung, namely, 'song of reality' means a verse for 'reality of intrinsic nature' (*svabhāva-tattva, T. raṅ bźin gyi de kho na ñid), one for 'reality of mystic attainment' (*vibhūti-tattva, ḥkhor baḥi de kho na ñid), and one for 'reality of purity' (viśuddhi-tattva, rnam par dag paḥi de kho na ñid). Then, a verse each for 'song of true nature'—referring to the pure *dharmadhātu*, and 'song of *mudrā*'—referring to the pride (*garva*) of body, make five verses in all, as presented and explained in *Sṅags rim chen mo*.

The four kinds of musical instruments are personified as goddesses in the maṇḍalas of the Mother Tantras *Saṃpuṭatantra* and *Hevajratantra* (Raghu Vira and Lokesh Chandra, *A New Tibeto-Mongol Pantheon*, Part 12), to wit: Vaṃśā, Vīṇā, Mukundā, Murajā. Jālandharipāda's *Hevajrasādhanasya-ṭippaṇi-śuddhi-vajrapradīpa* (PTT, Vol. 56, p. 121-5) assigns colors to these goddesses as follows: the yellow goddess Vīṇā, the red goddess Vaṃśā (bamboo flute), the smoky-colored goddess Murajā (barrel drum), the white goddess Mukundā (round drum) (/pi waṅ ma ser mo // gliṅ bu ma dmar mo / / rdza rṅa ma du baḥi mdog can ma / / rṅa zlum ma dkar mo /).

For the sixty-four *kalā*, it should be observed that the list of *Kāmasūtra* begins with *gita-vādya*, so *gitavādyādi* in the above *Pañcakrama* verse III, 31, can refer to the *kalās* in the ordinary meaning of the sixty-four worldly arts. However, Śrī Lakṣmī's commentary also permits the interpretation of *kalā* as *kāmakalā*. On p. 39-3, she states this particular list as beginning with 'embracing' (*āliṅganam, ḥkhyud pa*) and 'kissing' (*cumbana, ḥo byed*), expressions which occur among the forty 'male natures (cf. under nidāna verse 2), but here obviously relate to *kāma-śāstra* terminology of *catuḥṣaṣṭi*. Kloṅ rdol Bla ma, Vol. I, Section Ma, presents two versions of arriving at the number sixty-four (*catuḥṣoṣṭi*): the kiss (*ḥo byed pa*), the embrace (*ḥkhyud pa*), the bite (*so ḥdebs pa*), the fore-play (*yaṅ dag par bskyed pa*), erotic cries (*sid kyi sgra sgrogs pa*), the male posture in coitus (*skyes paḥi bya ba*), (the woman's) getting on top (*steṅ na ḥdug pa*), (the eighth one not printed somehow, perhaps the 'oral intercourse' of *Kāmasūtra*); each one divided into eight varieties, yielding sixty-four. The alternate list amounts to eight varieties of the embrace, eight of the kiss, eight of the male posture in coitus, eight of the bite, eight of the scratch, eight of the foreplay, eight of erotic cries, (and again, the eight of an omitted eighth one, perhaps the 'oral intercourse'), making sixty-four in all. Neither solution actually names the respective eightfold subdivisions, so this *kāma-kalā* terminology remains lexical as far as these tantric texts are concerned, but creates mythologically salacious reading out of the four respective movements of the goddesses as elements (upwards, at acute angles, forward, and downward).

*||RA|| ratnam anyam na cāstiha svādhiṣṭhānād ṛte mahat |*
*prabhāsvaraviśuddhaṃ ced vahniśuddho maṇir yathā ||40||*

There is no jewel in this world so great as the Svādhiṣṭhāna, if purified by the Clear Light like a gem cleansed by fire.

*Mchan* : Svādhiṣṭhāna = Illusory Body. 'No jewel in this world so great' because it can confer in this very life the goal of Buddhahood. 'No jewel' : no secret state. 'Purified by the Clear Light' : by entering the Clear Light. *Prakāśikā* on Ra (Vol. 60, p. 296-1): 'By fire', etc. means : if the Svādhiṣṭhāna-body is purified by the Clear Light attained by the fourth stage, then, like gold cleansed by fire, it becomes immaculate and devoid of phenomenalization. Therefore, it is only known through contemplation of the fourth stage (mes źes bya ba la sogs pa smos te / rim pa bźi pas thob paḥi ḥod gsal bas gal te / bdag byin gyis rlob paḥi sku dag par ḥgyur na / deḥi tshe mes sbyaṅs paḥi gser bzin du rnam par dag pa dri ma med ciṅ spros pa med par ḥgyur ro / / deḥi phyir rim pa bźi pa yaṅ sgom par byed par rig pa kho naḥo).

Following are some passages about the Svādhiṣṭhāna'.

*Pañcakrama*, 3rd krama, 12 :

*svādhiṣṭhānakramaṃ labdhvā sarvabuddhamayaḥ prabhuḥ |*
*janmanīhaiva buddhatvam niḥsaṃdehaṃ prapadyate ||*

He the lord, composed of all the Buddhas, having arrived at the stage of Svādhiṣṭhāna, without doubt attains Buddhahood in this very life.

*Pañcakrama*, 3rd krama, 25 :

*sarvākārāvaropeto asecanakavigrahaḥ |*
*darśayet taṃ suśiṣyāya svādhiṣṭhānaṃ tad ucyate ||*

Endowed with the best of all aspects is the body which one never tires of seeing. (He) reveals that to the good disciple. That is called 'Svādhiṣṭhāna'.

Finally, Śrī Lakṣmī, Vol. 63, p. 10-5 to 11-1, has this to say :

/ yaṅ dag paḥi mthaḥ don dam pahi bden pa de yis rnam par sbyaṅ ba ni sgyu ma lta buḥi tiṅ ṅe ḥdzin mi snaṅ bar byaḥo / / de la dper na phyiḥi mṅon par byaṅ chub paḥi rim pa ḥam / naṅ gi mṅon par byaṅ chub paḥi rim pa ḥam / ril por ḥdzin paḥi tiṅ ṅe ḥdzin nam / rjes su gźig paḥi tiṅ ṅe ḥdzin gyis sgyu maḥi sku ḥod gsal baḥi bskal paḥi me yis mi snaṅ bar byas na rnam par dag par ḥgyur ro / / ji skad du / bdag la byin rlabs ma gtogs paḥi / / rin chen gźan ni yod pa min / /gal te ḥod gsal dag ḥgyur na / /me yis dag paḥi nor bu bźin / /źes bya ba ḥbyuṅ baḥi phyir ro /.

The purification by that Paramārtha-satya which is the true end (*bhūtakoṭi*), would make disappear the Illusory Samādhi. Now, for example, the Illusory Body becomes purified when made to disappear by the 'fire of the aeon' of the Clear Light through the sequence of outer abhisambodhis, the sequence of inner abhisambodhis, the *samādhi* of 'contraction' (*piṇḍagrāha*), or the *samādhi* of 'expansion' (*anubheda*);—because the text states : "There is no jewel in this world so great as the Svādhiṣṭhāna, if purified by the Clear Light like a gem cleansed by fire."

## APPENDIX I

# THE LAṄKĀVATĀRA-SŪTRA AND THE GUHYASAMĀJATANTRA

Here we shall treat some remarkable transitional yoga experiences that even promise to clarify the Buddhist "non-self" theory.

The learned author Ratnākaraśānti makes a fascinating tie-up between the *Laṅkāvatāra* and the *Guhyasamāja* in his *Prajñāpāramitopadeśa* (PTT, Vol. 114, p. 249-3, 4, 5 to p. 250-1). In illustration of his preceding exposition of yoga in four stages, he cites the *Laṅkāvatāra* (Sagathakam, verses 256-258), but the verses in Tibetan reflect some minor variants (indicated here by underlining) of the Sanskrit text as presently edited by Bunyiu Nanjio :

*cittamātraṃ samāruhya bāhyam arthaṃ na kalpayet |*
*tathatālambane sthitvā cittamātram atikramet ||*
*cittamātram atikramya nirābhāsam atikramet |*
*nirābhāsasthito yogi mahāyānaṃ sa paśyati ||*
*anābhogagatiḥ śāntā praṇidhānair viśodhitā |*
*jñānam anātmakaṃ śreṣṭhaṃ mahāyānena paśyati ||*

The following translation incorporates some of Ratnākaraśānti's comments :

256. When he relies on 'mind-only' he does not imagine the external entity [2nd stage of yoga]. Being stationed in the meditative support of thusness, he goes beyond 'mind-only' [3rd stage of yoga].

257. Going beyond 'mind-only,' he goes beyond the non-appearance [of the sign-sources (*nimitta*) of the external entity] Stationed in the non-appearance [of the sign-sources of both dharmas and dharmatā] [4th stage of yoga] the yogin sees by the Mahāyāna.

258. His effortless going (*anābhogagati*) [the effortless revelation of the supramundane stages] is peaceful [because these stages are undefiled and non-discursive] and purified by his vows [that are not not aimed at the lower enlightenments, i.e.of śrāvaka and pratyekabuddha].

By means of the Mahāyāna, he sees the knowledge that is selfless [because utterly nonmanifest] and best [because free from defilements and habit-energy].

The author claims that the same is stated by the *Guhyasamāja* in one verse (in Chap. XV, p. 109 in Bhattacharyya's edition):

*svacittaṃ cittanidhyaptau sarvadharmāḥ pratiṣṭhitāḥ |*
*khavajrasthā hy amī dharmā na dharmā na ca dharmatā ||*

When one examines the mind [with insight], [one concludes] that all *dharmas* are located in one's own mind. [2nd stage of yoga]. These *dharmas* are located in the diamond of sky [3rd stage of yoga]. There is no *dharma* and no *dharmatā* [4th stage of yoga].

Ratnākaraśānti's discussion of the four stages can be summarized as follows:

1st stage of yoga: The meditative object on the phenomenal limit of the entity. This is a kind of waking state.

2nd stage of yoga : All dharmas are 'mind-only'; still the phenomenal limit. This is a kind of dream state, because if all dharmas are 'mind-only' they are all in the mind and not outside, a feature of the dream state.

3rd stage of yoga : Goes beyond 'mind-only'; the thusness end of the entity, or the non-appearance of phenomenal dharmas. This is a kind of dreamless sleep.

4th stage of yoga : Having gone beyond the sign-sources of natures (*dharma*), now goes beyond those of underlying nature (*dharmatā*). This ushers in the Mahāyāna, i.e. the first *bhūmi* called Pramuditā.

In further explanation, the four stages are referred to elsewhere as the four parts of *nirvedha-bhāgīya* constituting in the Prajñāpāramitā scriptures and *Abhisamayālaṃkāra* digest, the Stage of Action in Faith (*adhimukti-caryā-bhūmi*) of the Bodhisattva. Obermiller, who so far has the best description,* points out that the four are given in the *Mahāyāna-Sūtrālaṃkāra*, within XIV, 23-26 and the Sanskrit commentary thereon. In summary :

*E. Obermiller, "The Doctrine of Prajñā-paramitā as exposed in the *Abhisamayā-laṃkāra* of Maitreya," *Acta Orientalia*, Vol. XI, 1932. At p. 37, he cites Haribhadra's *Āloka* commentary, including the term *tattvārtha-ekadeśapraviṣṭa*.

1. The state of warmth — light (*āloka*)
2. The state of summits — spread of light (*āloka-vivṛddhi*)
3. The state of forbearance — [directed only to the meaning of reality (*tattvārtha-ekadeśapraviṣṭa*)]
4. The state of supreme mundane natures (*laukikāgradharma-avasthā*) — samādhi without interval (*ānantarya-samādhi*)

The expression 'samādhi without interval' means that this state, while still mundane, leads directly to the supramundane state, namely the first Bodhisattva Stage of the Mahāyāna.

Now, it is striking that non-tantric Mahāyāna Buddhism allots to these states the terminology 'light' etc. that reminds us of the tantric vocabulary so important to the Guhyasamāja tradition about the three lights that lead up to the Clear Light. In our earlier section on the two stages (Stage of Generation and Stage of Completion) the *Pañcakrama* was cited with translation, "By *yoga* of a beginner, he attains the Eighth Stage, and seeing the three lights he is settled in the Tenth Stage." This shows that the tantric theory of the mysterious lights leading up to Buddhahood should not be confused with this Prajñāpāramitā theory of lights leading up to the Bodhisattva career. However, there may have been an intention to establish a parallel of mystical experiences; and such parallels are consistent with my tentative dating of the *Guhyasamājatantra* and Explanatory Tantras in the 4th and 5th centuries, A.D. Besides, my discussion earlier in this book shows that the 'lights' also occur in mundane conditions.

Now, returning to that verse of the *Guhyasamāja*, Chap. XV, the basic tantra already shows the context as 'dream examination.' Besides, we may consult the *Pradīpoddyotana* commentary and its annotation (the *Mchan-ḥgrel*) for further information about the verse in question. In the *Pradīpoddyotana* (PTT, Vol. 158, p. 132-2, 3, 4), the parts of the verse can be understood as answering questions.

Question 1: Where are the *dharmas* ? The verse, alluding to the dream state, replies : 'all dharmas' are located within one's mind.

Question 2: Where is that mind ? The verse, alluding to

dreamless sleep, replies: It is in the diamond of sky, to wit, the Clear Light. [Recall in this connection Table III of this book, "The Clear Lights," indicating the Clear Light of dreamless sleep.]

Questions 3 and 4: Suppose it be asked if there is a presence separate from the mind. The verse replies : There is no *dharma*, to wit : there is no self-nature of the entities. Suppose it be asked if there is sometimes (*kadā cit*) an underlying nature (*dharmatā*). The verse replies : There is no underlying nature.

Here the *Pradīpoddyotana* cites two verses without identifying the source (which the *Mchan-ḥgrel* traces to a citation in *Spyod bsdus*, i.e. the *Caryāmelāpakapradīpa*, and states to be consistent with the *Vajramālā*) :

> *tathaiva dhātvāyatanendriyādau jñānadvaye tatra susaṃhate tasmin* |
> *śūnye mahad-viśati yaḥ prasuptaḥ svapnaṃ prapaśyet khalu vātaṃ saṃśrayāt* ||
> *supte prabuddhe cana ca nānyatedaṃ saṃkalpayet svapna-phalābhilāṣī* |
> *svapnopamās te sarvadharmā mṛṣāmṛṣāś cāpi tayor abhāvaḥ* ||

> In like manner, one is in deep sleep when he enters great in that void (Culmination of Light) wherein the pair of gnoses (Light and Spread-of-Light) are gathered, in the elements (four, i.e. earth, etc.), the sense bases (four objects), the sense organs (four, eye, etc.), and so on (the personality aggregates, i.e. the first four). Should one take recourse to the winds, surely he will see a dream.
> The one wishing the fruit of dream (i.e. good fruit from a good dream), should examine this non-difference, not even in sleeping and waking. All dharmas are like a dream. Moreover, falsehood and truth are not present in the two (sleeping and waking).

Apparently, the first verse is intended to amplify the answers to the first two questions, referring to the states of dream and dreamless sleep. The second verse should therefore be construed to amplify the answers to the third and fourth questions, explaining the denial of a *dharma* or *dharmatā*. The logical distinction of truth and falsehood is not present. And yet there is no denial of the fruit of dream.

If one compares this *Pradīpoddyotana* explanation of the

*Guhyasamāja* verse with what Ratnākaraśānti said about it, there does not appear any essential disagreement, even though the discussion proceeds somewhat differently. Indeed, there is no disagreement as yet with those verses cited from the *Laṅkāvatāra-sūtra*, where in the fourth stage the yogin sees the Mahāyāna; because in the second of the two verses edited and translated above, one realizes that "all *dharmas* are like a dream," which is a frequent teaching of the Mahāyāna.

Now, it is a striking feature of those stages of yoga, as Ratnākaraśānti understands the *Laṅkāvatāra* verses, with the further corresponding statements drawn out above, that certain statements seem to conflict with others. That is to say, in the 2nd stage, it is said that all *dharmas* are mind-only. If that is what they are, then why in the 3rd stage does one go beyond mind-only to reach reality? And if one has reached reality, why should he go to a further state said to deny both the *dharma* and the *dharmatā*? It seems to be the case that the individual statements constitute the mottos for a given level of yoga experience and for the yogins with that experience. But if this be granted, it denies that the same precept is given to all yogins.

Now, it appears that this is the identical procedure of statement found in the old Buddhist classic, the *Dhammapada* (XX, 5, 6, 7), "All constructions are impermanent" (*sabbe saṅkhārā aniccā*), "All constructions are suffering" (*sabbe saṅkhārā, dukkhā*), "All *dhammas* are non-self" (*sabbe dhammā anattā*). In illustration, the first statement, "All constructions are impermanent," is convincing on the intellectual level, and so is addressed to laymen, monks, and anyone else who will listen. But, having said this, the Buddha said something else about the constructed things, "All constructions are suffering," and this statement is not convincing on the intellectual level; it turns out to be the precept to the *āryas*, or *śrāvakas*, the disciples of the Buddha who are told to look upon suffering as suffering and upon happiness as suffering because it entails suffering or will lead to suffering. Furthermore, the Buddha said, "All *dhammas* (S. *dharmāḥ*) are non-self," bringing into the discussion the celebrated teaching of Buddhism, the non-self (*an-ātman*) theory that has always been characteristic of Buddhism. This statement is not convincing on the intellectual level, because *dharmas* such as love and hate are understood by the intellect to require a self that loves and hates. Therefore, the statement cannot be made intelligently to everyone, but also it is not just the way the disciples should look upon constructed things, because in Buddhism the *dharmas* are not only in the constructed category but also there is the unconstructed kind, for example, Nirvāṇa. Nirvāṇa is the goal of the path, for which it is necessary to follow the procedures of Meditation as a yogin. Therefore, it may be concluded along the same lines that the statement, "All *dhammas* are non-self," is the precept for the yogins.

Then the question naturally arises, if the statement, "All *dhammas* are non-self," is a yoga precept, can it be placed among the stages of yoga that have been set forth above on the basis of the *Laṅkāvatāra* verses and *Guhyasamāja* verse ? This precept is immediately identifiable with the 2nd yoga stage, which is the stage that takes the 'self' out of "all *dharmas*." In explanation, the statement, "All *dharmas* are mind-only" refers to the dream state. In this state, the object (the world of *dharmas*) is paramount and the self is in abeyance; hence, "All *dharmas* are non-self" (cf. the quotation of Anaṅgavajra under the Nidāna verse JRA). Accordingly, one may also conclude that the *Dhammapada* precept, "All constructions are suffering," applies to the 1st stage of yoga, the meditative object on the phenomenal limit of the entity, involving the phenomenal self that suffers. In agreement the Buddha said (*Dhammapada*, XXI, 7-12), "The disciples of Gautama are always well awake (*pabujjhanti*)." Certainly yoga begins in the waking state.

The above helps us regarding the 3rd stage of yoga. This is said to go beyond mind-only (the dream state) and to refer to dreamless sleep, with the non-appearance of phenomenal *dharmas*. It follows that this is the stage when the subject is paramount and the object is in abeyance, and so one sees no dream. This conclusion forces the word *dharmatā* (underlying nature) to apply to the subject.

Having concluded that much, it is also possible to appreciate the meaning of the 4th stage, when there is no *dharma* but also no *dharmatā*. In short, "there is no *dharma*" denies a dream; and "there is no *dharmatā*" denies a dreamless sleep—thus denying both subject and object. This turns out, according to the foregoing treatments, to be a climactic transitional state—in one case, leading immediately to the onset of the Mahāyāna; and in another case, to complete Buddhahood.

Since this comparison of the *Laṅkāvatāra* verses with the single *Guhyasamāja* verse has been sufficiently exposed on its own terminological side, it should be of interest to see to what extent this dovetails with *Guhyasamāja* yoga stages previously presented in this work. My subsection "The six members of yoga and the five *kramas* in the Stage of Completion" presented the commentarial exegesis of certain verses in the *Guhyasamāja*, Chap. VI, including verse 4:

> He should accomplish the selflessness of *citta* being visualized (*cittanidhyaptinairātmyaṃ*), (then) the contemplation of speech (*vācā*) and body, (then) the triple conjunction, (finally) the abode equal to space.

If one wishes to match these up with the stages already discussed in this appendix, it follows immediately that the "selflessness of *citta* being visualized" is the 2nd stage of yoga: "all *dharmas* are located within one's mind" and this is the non-self of *dharmas*. Tnerefore, the preceding contemplation ('body as the mantra visualized') corresponds to the 1st stage of yoga. It follows, that this treatment does not allow the more generalized interpretation of yoga stages, as previously, to lead up to either the beginning of the bodhisattva path (Mahāyāna) or to Complete Buddhahood. Indeed, the context shows that the interpretation is fully within the Mahāyāna scope, just as the four *nirvedha-bhāgiya* were within the pre-Mahāyāna scope. In the present case, the "body as the mantra visualized" is the accomplishment of the Stage of Generation (=the first seven Bodhisattva stages), and "selflessness of *citta* being visualized" is the beginning of the Stage of Complction (=the last three Bodhisattva stages). Then, the comparison continues along the same lines, that the "contemplation of speech and body" is the Mahāyāna version of the 3rd stage of yoga, the Svādhiṣṭhāna, or initial Mahāmudrā, as the thusness end, or the non-appearance of phenomenal dharmas. Finally the "triple conjunction," or "divine body made of mind," is equivalent to the transitional 4th stage of yoga, which goes beyond the sign-sources of *dharmas* and *dharmatā* presumably to be "purified by the Clear Light like a gem cleansed by fire" (Nidāna verse RA).

Finally, the "abode equal to space" which generates the body of Mahāvajradhara has no equivalent in the four stages of yoga. Nevertheless, it is analogous to the further statement in the *Laṅkāvatāra* verses : "His effortless going is peaceful and purified by his vows," except that now it applies to the Buddha stage rather than to the Bodhisattva stages.

The foregoing rather neatly demonstrates a tie-up between the *Laṅkāvatārasūtra* and the *Guhyasamājatantra*; and in the latter case, the consistency between the stages of yoga in its Chapter VI and the stages in that verse of Chapter XV. Besides, the material in this appendix will serve as an introduction to both the second and third appendixes.

## APPENDIX II

# THE ARCANE-BODY CONTROVERSY

My use of the word "arcane" and solution of the forty verses into two groups going with the Stage of Generation and Stage of Completion can be finally justified by consideration of what I term the "Arcane-Body Controversy."

It is true that I have already presented some material about this matter in my Introduction to the Yoga of the Guhyasamājatantra. But this is an exciting topic about a Tibetan controversy that reaches back to important Indian theories of the fruits of *yoga*; as such it deserves a special treatment. Various forms of Indian philosophy take account of a subtle body (*sūkṣma-śarīra*). However, it is only in such Tantric currents as the one presented in the foregoing work that a whole upward career is worked out for this subtle body. This kind of body is of course denied immediately by the materialistic person. Here I am not arguing for the existence of such a mysterious body, but simply reporting the facts of the *Guhyasamāja* system, which speaks of an "arcane body" which on the Stage of Completion is called the "illusory body" or "impure illusory body," that can emerge from the ordinary body.

In fact, the theory is by no means original with the *Guhyasamājatantra* because ancient Buddhism already referred to it with the terminology of "mental body" or "body made of mind" (*manomaya-kāya*), to which I have previously alluded. Here I should add that the *Laṅkāvatārasūtra* mentions three kinds of mental body, which combine well with the theory in the Ārya school of the tantric Nāgārjuna and Āryadeva that the Stage of Completion begins with the Eighth Bodhisattva Stage. The first mental body, with stabilization in the pleasure of *samādhi* (*samādhisukhasamāpatti-manomaya*), which according to that scripture is developed in the course of the first seven Bodhisattva stages, therefore, belongs to the Stage of Generation. The second kind, which completely comprehends the intrinsic nature of the *dharmas* (*dharmasvabhāvāvabodha-manomaya*) and which is said to proceed to all the Buddha realms necessarily would be placed in the Stage of Completion as the "arcane body" of that Stage. According to the *Guhyasamāja* tradition, that "arcane body" is succeeded by, or next subjected to, the "arcane speech" and then the "arcane mind." It is only at the phase of "arcane mind" that this mental or spiritual body "completely comprehends the intrinsic nature of the *dharmas*," which means in *Pañcakrama* terminology that it completely understands the eighty *prakṛtis* associated with the three Light stages, as experienced on the Tenth Bodhisattva Stage. The third kind of mental body, which performs the instigations natural to its class (*nikāyasahajasaṃskārakriyā-manomaya*), i.e. natural to the class of Buddhas, is the *yuganaddha-deha* of this Tantric tradition.

At first glance, a certain verse of the *Guhyasamājatantra* does not seem related to the above, but I shall demonstrate the relevance of Chapter XV, verse 22, of that Tantra, as follows, which is almost the same as the last verse of Chapter XII ("Documents"):

> *buddho dharmadharo vāpi vajrasattvo 'pi vā yadi /*
> *atikramed yadi mohātmā tad antaṃ tasya jīvitam //*
> If someone would go beyond whether as a Buddha, a holder of Dharma, or as a Vajrasattva; and if he is deluded, he would lose his life.

Candrakīrti's *Pradīpoddyotana* (Mchan ed., p. 122-2, 3) repeats substantially its comment on the Chapter XII verse, to wit, that the expression "Buddha" means "yogin of Vairocana," and so on. In this case, Celu-pā's *Ratnavṛkṣa* commentary on Chapter XV (PTT, Vol. 63, p. 211-5) is more helpful. It explains that "Buddha" is the Diamond of Body ; "holder of Dharma" is the Diamond of Speech; and "Vajrasattva" is the Diamond of Mind (saṅs rgyas ni sku rdo rjeḥo / chos ḥdzin pa ni gsuṅ rdo rjeḥo / rdo rje sems dpaḥ ni thugs rdo rjeḥo /). This comment immediately associates this verse with the expressions Body, Speech, and Mind that have such an important role throughout the *Guhyasamājatantra* as well as in certain *nidāna* verses. In consideration that this Chapter XV has previously in its verse 11 referred to the Tenth Stage (of the Bodhisattva), one may recall in this connection the rather remarkable statements about the last three Bodhisattva Stages (Eighth through Tenth) in the manual of the Tathāgatagarbha theory, the *Ratnagotravibhāga* (ed. of Johnston, pp. 3.21-4.6):

/ tatra yato 'ṣṭamyāṃ bodhisattvabhūmau vartamānaḥ

sarvadharma-vaśitaprāpto bhavati tasmāt sa bodhimaṇḍavaragataḥ sarvadharmasamatābhisaṃbuddha ity ucyate / yato navamyāṃ bodhisattvabhūmau vartamāno 'nuttaradharmabhāṇakatvasaṃpannaḥ sarvasattvāśayasuvidhijña indriyaparamapāramitāprāptaḥ sarvasattvakleśavāsanānusaṃdhisamudghātanakuśalo bhavati tasmāt so 'bhisaṃbuddhabodhiḥ supravartitadharmacakra ity ucyate / yato daśamyāṃ bhūmāv anuttaratathāgatadharmayauvarājyābhiṣekaprāptyanantaram anābhogabuddhakāryapratipraśrabdho bhavati tasmāt sa supravartitadharmacakro 'nantaśiṣyagaṇasuvinīta ity ucyate /

Among those, for the reason that his attainment of power over all *dharmas* takes place on the Eighth Bodhisattva Stage, it is said (in the *Dhāraṇīśvararājasūtra*), 'He, having proceeded to the best terrace of Enlightenment (= the Tree of Enlightenment), was enlightened on the equality of all *dharmas*'. For the reason that his endowment of preaching the incomparable Dharma, his knowing of the good rules for the hopes of all sentient beings, his attainment of the highest perfection of faculties, and his virtue of annihilating the continuance of defilement habit-energy in all sentient beings, take place on the Ninth Bodhisattva Stage, it is said, 'He, with enlightenment fully awakened, has well set into motion the Wheel of the Dharma.' For the reason that immediately after receiving, on the Tenth Stage, the Crown-Prince consecration for the incomparable Tathāgata-Dharma he is roused (*apratipraśrabdha*) to the effortless Buddha duties—it is said, 'He who well set into motion the Wheel of the Dharma has well trained the innumerable host of disciples."

That is to say, in this particular tradition, it is the Body of the Buddha sitting under the Bodhi Tree that occurs on the Eighth Stage, his Speech as the Wheel of Doctrine that is on the Ninth, his Mind roused to Buddha duties that is on the Tenth. In Tantrism, this Body, Speech, and Mind are called the "three mysteries of the Buddha."

This plausible explanation of the sequence 'Buddha', 'Dharma holder', and 'Vajrasattva' of the *Guhyasamāja* verse, still leaves unexplained the mysterious remark that the one who would go beyond in such status would lose his life if he be deluded. However, this is a reasonable remark in the light of the *Laṅkāvatāra*'s second kind of "mental body," prevalent on the Eighth through Tenth Bodhisattva Stages, because the *Laṅkāvatāra*'s claim that this body visits all the Buddha realms is a way of saying that it has emerged by yoga praxis from the ordinary body. If the yogin does not have skill in guiding his movements in these Buddha realms—whatever we may think them to be—he could lose his life, because the separation of the "mental body" would be tantamount to death's separation. This points to the importance of the first kind of "mental body," that immersed in *samādhi,* because presumably this is a necessary preparation for the dangerous trips of the subsequent second kind. If this sort of teaching has been derived from the life of the Buddha, one can promptly think of Gautama's celebrated austerities by the Nairañjanā River when his body eventually became so wasted that viewers could not decide whether he was dead or alive. This extreme mortification immediately preceded Gautama's passage to the Bodhi Tree where, according to the tradition of the above Tathāgatagarbha literature, he represented a Bodhisattva of the Eighth Stage.

Indeed, the premise of such a "mental body" or illusory body as the "arcane body" of the Stage of Completion makes it clear why the great commentators on this Tantra, e.g. the Indian tantrics Nāgārjuna and Āryadeva, and Tsoṅ-kha-pa in Tibet, again and again emphasized that the Stage of Generation must precede the Stage of Completion. Any tantric who would try to practise the Stage of Completion without first having the Stage of Generation, would be relying on instruction and precepts which demand that the body be an "arcane body" in the sense of that advanced Stage, while in fact the person enterprising that Stage would only be starting with his ordinary human body that is not even a sanctified body in the worldly sense of withdrawal from certain foods, the opposite sex, and society generally—let alone "arcane" in any way.

All the above is necessary to appreciate Tsoṅ-kha-pa's insistence on an "arcane body" in both the Stage of Generation and Stage of Completion. His solution, as I have come to understand it, is easy to state: the "arcane body" of the Stage of Generation is the "hundred lineages" in the Atiyoga phase; and the "arcane body" of the Stage of Completion is the first two members of the six-membered yoga, namely *pratyāhāra* and *dhyāna*. But while he expressly identified the second kind of "arcane body" in that manner, I never found him stating the first kind in such a simple manner: he always wrapped the matter in complicated discussions, because of the controversy.

In accordance with Tsoṅ-kha-pa's annotation of the Forty Verses and my grouping of those verses, I placed the minute correspondences called the "hundred lineages" (T. *rigs brgya*) in the first group of verses concerning the Stage of Generation, in fact beginning with the set which I associated with the division of *vajra* called Atiyoga. Then, more recently to my surprise, I could find no mention of these "hundred lineages" in a work by Tsoṅ-kha-pa's faithful disciple Mkhas-grub-rje devoted to the topic of the Stage of Generation, namely the latter's work *Rgyud thams cad kyi rgyal po dpal gsaṅ ba ḥdus paḥi bskyed rim dṅos grub rgya mtsho żesb ya ba*. ("The 'Ocean of Siddhis' about the Stage of Generation in the King of all Tantras, the *Śrī-Guhyasamāja*"), wherein I find important points of Tsoṅ-kha-pa's position amplified and defended by Mkhas-grub-rje. His silence on the matter was confirmed when I perused a work by Blo-bzaṅ-chos-kyi-rgyal-mtshan, the First Panchen Lama, namely his *Gsaṅ ḥdus gdams ṅag rim lṅa gsal sgron gyi sñiṅ poḥi gnad kun bsdus pa* ("Concise statement of the essential points, clarifying the *Pañcakrama* precepts of the *Guhyasamāja*"). This work expressly states that the "hundred lineages" belong to the Stage of Completion, with the remark, "The contemplation in which there is the arising as the body of a deity involved with the illustrious 'hundred lineages' and so forth, is the arcane body of the Stage of Completion" (dam pa rigs brgya la sogs paḥi lha skur śar bar bsgom pa ni rdzogs pa rim paḥi lus dben yin te). Accordingly, the author treats these "hundred lineages" in his work devoted to the Stage of Completion.

Of course, I again referred to Tsoṅ-kha-pa's elaborate discussions of the "arcane body" problem to see if, after all I might have misunderstood his position. I could find no reason to change my conclusion. Besides, Tsoṅ-kha-pa, in his *sādhana* of the *Guhyasamāja* entitled *Rnal ḥbyor dag paḥi rim pa* ("the pure stages of yoga") (PTT, Vol. 160, p. 89-4) states: "After generating in that way the thirty-two gods, he should respectively contemplate them in sequence as the nature of the five personality aggregates, the four elements, the eight consisting of eye, etc., the five sense objects starting with form, and the set of ten beginning with right arm; this is Atiyoga" (de/ ltar lha sum cu so gñis po bskyed paḥi ḥog tu re re nas rim pa bźin phuṅ po lṅa daṅ / khams bźi daṅ mig la sogs pa brgyad daṅ / gzugs la sogs pa lṅa daṅ / lag pa gYas pa la sogs pa bcuḥi ṅo bor bsam par bya ste / śin tu rnal ḥbyor ro /) Our earlier discussions show that Atiyoga is the third of the four yogas in the Stage of Generation, called Yoga, Anuyoga, Atiyoga, and Mahāyoga. Tsoṅ-kha-pa's remark further confirms my division of the verses in which I assign Atiyoga to the third group of verses (Bhagavān Sarva), because it is precisely in these verses that Tsoṅ-kha-pa begins his "arcane body" comments, starting with the verse about the five personality aggregates. Besides, Tsoṅ-kha-pa, when explaining the fourteen fundamental falls of the Vajrayāna in his *Dṅos grub kyi sñe ma* and grouping those falls (PTT, Vol. 160, p. 70-1,2) classifies as a fall in the Stage of Generation the fall No. 8, "to abuse the five *skandhas,* for their nature belongs to the five Buddhas." Pursuant to the given reason ("their nature belongs to the five Buddhas"), one could extend this remark about the personality aggregates (*skandha*) to the sense bases and so on, with which deity is identified in the Atiyoga stage. Doubtless, Tsoṅ-kha-pa follows a tradition which places the "hundred lineages" in the Stage of Generation; and I need not speculate on the particular reasons for later luminaries of his school to have understood the matter differently. Still, it is possible to set forth the chief controversial aspect in the following manner.

Tsoṅ-kha-pa has his most complicated discussion of the "arcane body" controversy in his *Pañcakrama* commentary, starting Vol. 158, p. 201 and continuing for a number of pages in the photographic edition (each page with five folio sides). It so happens that Tsoṅ-kha-pa repeats much of the same discussion about the "arcane body" in a later work, his *Mthaḥ gcod* ("Deciding the alternatives") on the individual chapters of the *Guhyasamājatantra*, namely, in his *mthaḥ gcod* of Chapter VI (PTT, Vol. 156, pp. 39 and 40). I have presented this Chapter in "Documents" and also treated the relevant verses (nos. 3-6) in my section "The six members of yoga and the five kramas in the Stage of Completion." Since Tsoṅ-kha-pa's discussion here shows that the argument devolves about the expression in verse 3, "the one who has body as the mantra visualized" (*mantranidhyaptikāyena*), it is well to present Candrakīrti's comment on that verse 3, as I edit from the *Pradīpoddyotana* manuscript and accordingly translate in *Mchan ḥgrel* context:

/ mantranidhyapti ityādi / mantrā ālikālijāḥ / sarpādisvabhāvās teṣāṃ strīpuṃnapuṃsakatvena tryakṣarādhār [abhūt]ā mantrāḥ tryakṣarāṇi / teṣāṃ praveśasthitivyutthānasvabhāvena parijñānaṃ mantranidhyaptiḥ / tatra pūrvakaṃ kāyena vajrajāpasya sādhanabhūtena nirmāṇaśarīreṇa vācā vajrajāpenopalakṣitaḥ / manasi hṛdi hṛdisthito vajrasattvaḥ coditaḥ/yathābhūtaparijñānena viṣayīkṛtaḥ / bhāvayed iti / yogisantānasya vākyamāṇakāṃ catasro 'vasthā niṣpādayet / kās tā ity āha / pravārā ityādi / pravārām utkṛṣṭāṃ cittavivekalakṣaṇāṃ vajrajapād adhikatvāt siddhim iti / svādhiṣṭhānalakṣaṇāṃ mahāmudrā manaḥ saṃtoṣayatīti manaḥsaṃtoṣaṇāṃ mahāmudrāviśuddhikaratvāt / priyām iṣṭāṃ bhavaśama-ekalakṣaṇaṃ mahāvajradharamūrtiṃ niṣpādayet /

As to the verse "The one who has body as the mantra visualized...", 'mantras' arise from the (sixteen) vowels and the (thirty-three or thirty-four) consonants and are constituted by such expressions as SARPA. Among them, when mantras have as basis three syllables by way of female (Āḥ), male (Oṃ), and androgyne (Hūṃ), they are the three syllables. The thorough knowledge of those (three) by way of inhalation (Oṃ), holding of breath (Āḥ), and exhalation (Hūṃ) is the 'mantra visualized'. Here, the one who previously has the (arcane) body, that is, the body of hypostasis (by the five Tathāgatas and so on) which arose through a *sādhana* of diamond muttering, should accomplish, i.e. intensely contemplate, exhorted by speech, i.e. by Diamond Muttering, in the mind, i.e. in (one's own) heart, that is, (exhorted) meaning 'distinguished' while the Vajrasattva dwelling in the heart (within the central 'vein' of the *dharmacakra*) is made the object (of consciousness) by that thorough knowledge (of the three phases of the wind) as they really are, that is (should

> accomplish) four states to be explained of the yogin's stream of consciousness. What are those ? (The text) says: the 'surpassing one', and so on, namely (1) the 'surpassing one', i.e. outstanding one, with the character of 'Arcane Mind', because it outlasts Diamond Muttering; (2) 'successful one', with the character of Personal Blessing, namely the Mahāmudrā; (3) 'one satisfying the mind', that is, "It brings satisfaction to the mind," because it purifies the Mahāmudrā; (4) 'beloved one', i.e. wished for, that is, he accomplishes the body of Mahāvajradhara with the single character of the phenomenal world and the realm of quiescence.

With that passage before us, it is easier to see how those who took Candrakīrti's commentary as the most authoritative one on the *Guhyasamājatantra*, would be troubled to determine by this passage which of the two Stages to assign the "arcane body". Candrakīrti's subsequent commentary on Chapter VI shows that the contemplation of the winds by means of the three syllables can be understood either in the form appropriate to the Stage of Generation or to that appropriate to the Stage of Completion. Some persons could maintain that this verse of the *Guhyasamājatantra* refers to the five stages which Nāgārjuna systematized in his *Pañcakrama*, beginning with Diamond Muttering; for, as well known, the *Pañcakrama* deals only with the Stage of Completion. On the other hand, some persons could point to the word '*pūrvakaṃ*' in Candrakīrti's commentary to suggest that the "body as the mantra visualized" is a prior accomplishment, already at hand when the yogin is exhorted by Diamond Muttering of the Stage of Completion variety. Besides, Candrakīrti did not help matters when, in his commentary on Chapter XII, 60-64 (see "Documents"), he explained the Stage of Completion, not with this terminology from Chapter VI, verse 3, but rather with the terminology of six-membered yoga from Chapter XVIII. In the case of the six members, Diamond Muttering would have to be assigned to prāṇāyāma, the third member, leaving the first two members, *pratyāhāra* and *dhyāna*, to be argued about. No wonder there were disagreements over this "arcane body" !

As I understand Tsoṅ-kha-pa's solution, it allows for both interpretations of the expression "body as the mantra visualized". This amounts to an admission that the two stages called Stage of Generation and Stage of Completion are distinctions imposed upon the basic Tantra. If we decide upon the Stage of Generation, we can consult Candrakīrti's commentary on Chapter XII, 60-64, to see at once that in the case of the four steps, he mentions that the three syllables of Oṃ, etc. are deposited in the body in the second step, Upasādhana =Anuyoga. This agrees with our placing in the second group of verses the material on muttering by means of the three syllables, allotting four seconds to each (*nidāna* verse 12, YE). This is held to generate the primeval lord (*ādinātha*). However, in Tsoṅ-kha-pa's position, this body of the second step is still not the "arcane body". For the latter attainment the yogin must pass to the third step, the Atiyoga, in which there is the hypostasis of divinity into the body by such means as the correspondences established in the "hundred lineages". This body becomes called in the fourth step the "mantra-puruṣa", seen with three heads, etc. Then, if the same line of Chapter VI, verse 3, is understood to refer to the Stage of Completion, the "body as the mantra visualized" is the "arcane body" of the Stage of Completion, namely *pratyāhāra* and *dhyāna*, to which the two *nidāna* verses (KĀ-YA) are devoted. In such a case, the remaining four members, *prāṇāyāma*, etc., of the six-membered yoga, have to be equated with the five steps of the *Pañcakrama*.

Because the above is itself so involved and technical, I have decided to forego any more of Tsoṅ-kha-pa's portrayal of varying positions about this "arcane body". In summary, the "arcane body" of the Stage of Generation becomes that way because imagined to be invested with deities. But according to the theory of steps, the yogin should first pass through a kind of symbolic death through attainment of the void; then imagine himself in an intermediate state by three-syllabled breathing; now he can pass to a symbolic birth wherein his body is inhabited by deities; and finally return to the world with transfigured consciousness. The yogin is now ready to embark upon the dangerous Stage of Completion, with the drawing forth of an advanced "arcane body," the Illusory Body. This Illusory Body—the "arcane body" of the Stage of Completion—is the reenactment of the primeval androgyne.

APPENDIX III

# THE PRAXIS ACCORDING TO ĀRYADEVA

There are many ways of setting forth the indications of practice that were touched upon in the foregoing introductions and annotation of the nidāna verses. Perhaps the clearest statement of the practice in the Stage of Completion is that found in Āryadeva's *Caryāmelāpakapradīpa*, a work which has already contributed considerably (for example, the 'hundred lineages' stem from here). Āryadeva's passage happens to be extant in Sanskrit in Bendall's edition of the *Subhāṣita-saṃgraha*, Part II, pp. 33-35; but Bendall did not trace the Āryadeva work.

The Sanskrit passage is found in the Tibetan translation in bits and snatches, and one section could not be traced at all. Unless the *Subhāṣita* compiler had a completely different recension of the Āryadeva text, he must have skipped around to piece together a running account; and my study of the context shows that he is faithful to Āryadeva's intention. The exact Tibetan equivalent begins in PTT, Vol. 61, p. 312-3, line 7, but the first words of the Āryadeva citation may be a paraphrase of p. 311-2. In the following reproduction of Bendall's edited Sanskrit, I shall insert the places of the Tibetan translation; and follow the text with my English translation and comments.

pustake *Āryadeva*-pādair bhāvanopadeśaḥ spaṣṭākṣareṇoktaḥ / (Possibly paraphrase of p. 311-2 :) udyāne vijane śrāvakādi-uktaṃ śa-rahite (p. 312-3, line 7:) paramārthasatyālambanapūrvakaṃ *svādhiṣṭhāna* krameṇa vajrasattvarūpam ātmānaṃ niṣpādya (p. 312-5, line 4:) prathamarūpādi-trividhaviṣayam āsvādya tad anu śodhanādividhinā sarvāhāram abhisaṃskṛti-siddham adhyātma-kuṇḍam anusmṛtyātmākṛtiṃ samādhisattvasya mukhe triśikhāgniṃ juhomīty ahaṃkāram utpādyābhyavaharati / tataḥ sukhena pariṇāmati rasāyanaṃ ca bhavati / evaṃ kāyavajraṃ saṃtarpya (portion not traced in Tibetan :) yāṃ kāṃcit svābhaprajñārūpeṇa sarvālaṃkṛtagātrā trivali-taraṅgabhaṅgābhirāmā atyantakṛśamadhyaromarajjv (*sic.* for rājy')-antaritavipulagambhīranābhideśā jaghana-ghana-nitamba-stabdhaśṛṅgāra-lalita-kamalagati-sasmita-vadanā saumyadṛṣṭyā mahāsukhānurāgaṇatayā (p. 315-5, line 8:) 'ṅke vyavasthitā / tato "mahāsiddhiṃ niṣpādayāmī" ti dṛḍhāhaṃkāram utpādyāliṅganacumbanacūṣaṇa-(p. 314-4, line 3 :) kucagrahaṇa-pulakatāḍana-daśananakhadānamardana-(p. 313-1, line 1 :) śītkāra-kokila-bhṛṅganādanāḍīsaṃcodanādikaṃ kṛtvā (p. 314-4, line 4:) śūcīkūrparādikaraṇa-pramodanatayā pracalitamuktāhāravalaya-kaṭaka-keyūranūpura-(p. 313-1, line 2:) vajrapadmasaṃgharṣaṇāt prajñopāya-samāpattyā skandhādisvabhāvāt sarvatathāgatānāṃ mūrdhānam ārabhya dvāsaptati-nāḍīsahasrāṇi nirjharadhārākāreṇ-ālikālidra / vibhūya rāga-virāga-madhyarāga-krameṇa tataḥ prajñāpāramitādi-svarūpān pratyātmavedyān karoti / evaṃ śrī-Mahāsukhasamādhim abhyasya prāptotkarṣo yogī tatraiva gaṇamaṇḍale nigrahānugraheṇa sattvān paripācayet / (p. 314-1, line 8 :) evaṃ punaḥ punar bhūtakoṭiṃ praviśya punaḥ punar hy utthāya pañca tathāgatarūpān pañca kāmaguṇān āsvādayati yathā na mlāyate manaḥ / (p. 314-2, line 5:) tato nirvikalpo mahāyogī svātmanaḥ sarvabhāvasvabhāva-pratipādanāya loke garhitaṃ viśodhya pracchanne pradeśe sthitvā 'bhyavaharati / tathā ca mudrābandho na maṇḍalaṃ na caityaṃ na ca pustakavācanaṃ na kāyakleśaṃ na paṭakāṣṭhapāṣāṇapratimāṃ praṇamati na Śrāvaka-Pratyekabuddhaṃ na tithinakṣatramuhūrtakālāpekṣaṇaṃ karoti / sarvam etad adhyātmenaiva sampādayati // (p. 314-5, line 8 :)

*vane bhikṣāṃ bhramen nityaṃ sādhako dṛḍhaniścayaḥ /*
*dada(n)ti bhayasaṃtrastā bhojanaṃ daivyamaṇḍitam //*
*atikramet trivajrātmā nāśaṃ vajrākṣaraṃ bhavet /*
*surīṃ nārīṃ* (sic. *for nāgīṃ*) *mahāyakṣīṃ asurīṃ mānuṣīm api //*
*prāpya vidyāvrataṃ kāryaṃ trivajrajñānasevitam iti //*

(p. 313-4, line 1:) evaṃ laukikadhyānam apanīya manorājyam apahāya sadāpraruditamanā yoginībhiḥ saha ramamāṇo yathā rājā *Indrabhūtis* tadvat kalevaraṃ parivartya vajrakāyo bhūtvā 'ntaḥpureṇa sahāntardhāyāṣṭaguṇaiśvaryaguṇānvito buddhakṣetrād buddhakṣetraṃ gacchati / yathoktaṃ *Mūlasūtre* /

*sarvadevopabhogais tu sevyamāno* (*sic* for-mānair) *yathāsukham* |
*svādhidaivatayogena svam ātmānaṃ* (*sic.* for parātmānau)
*prapūjayet* ||
(Tibetan ends at p. 313-4, line 4).

*Translation*

In a book of Āryadeva the precepts of the contemplation are stated in lucid words:

In a solitary glade, free as well from the words of Śrāvakas, (the *yogin* contemplates this way:—) Having first taken Supreme Truth as the meditative object, by the Stage of Personal Blessing (Svādhiṣṭhāna-krama) he abides with himself as the body of Vajrasattva. First he experiences the three kinds of form and of the other sensory objects. After that, for the rites of purification and so on, upon all food—he recalls the inner hearth, whose shape is real, and arouses the pride, "I make a burnt offering in the three-tongued flame which is the configuration of the self on the face of the Samādhi Being," and partakes of food. Then it blissfully changes and becomes elixir (*rasāyana*). Thus (the performer having satiated the diamond of body (with elixir), (takes) some (consort, *mudrā*), by way of form, a *prajñā* like himself (or: his own light, *svābha*). She has a body with all ornaments, gratifying through the restless breaking of the three folds (at her navel), the place of her wide and deep navel hidden by the streak of hair across her narrow waist her massive hips with firm buttocks; her gait amorous, playful, and sweet; her face with smiles; pleasant to see, and stationed in (the *yogin's*) proximity through the attraction of great ecstasy (*mahāsukha*).

Then he confirms his pride, thinking, "I shall accomplish the *siddhi* of Mahā (mudrā)." Having done the embracing, kissing, sucking, holding of breast, beating with bristling hair; the bite, the scratch, the bruise; erotic cries, cooing, humming of bees, calling through a tubular stalk (*nāḍi*), and so on—because she is thrilled by his (yogī) postures of *śūci*, *kūrpara*, and so on, she shakes her string of pearls, armlet, bracelet of lower and of upper arm, and anklet. Then, through the friction of the diamond and the lotus, by union of *prajñā* and *upāya*, starting at the head since the intrinsic nature of *skandhas* belongs to all Tathāgatas, the 72,000 *nāḍis* become a fluid (*dravībhūya*) of vowels and consonants in the manner of a torrent, in the sequence of 'desire,' 'aversion,' and 'indifference'. Thus he introspects the true forms of Prajñāpāramitā and so on. In this way the *yogin*, practising the glorious Mahāsukhasamādhi, reaches eminence, and matures the sentient beings by hindering and assisting in the (32-deity) group-*maṇḍala*.

In that way, again and again he enters the true limit (*bhūtakoṭi*); and having emerged again and again he experiences the five 'strands of desire' as the five Tathāgata forms, so the (sublime) mind does not fade.

Then, the great *yogin*, discursive thought lacking in himself, so as to teach the intrinsic nature of all entities, cleansing what is forbidden in the world, stays in a private place and enjoys, to wit :— he makes no *mudrās*, *maṇḍalas*, or *caityas*, nor recites texts, nor mortifies the body, nor bows to images of cloth, wood, or stone, nor (takes refuge) in Śrāvakas or Pratyekabuddhas, nor depends on time in terms of lunar days, asterisms, or *muhūrtas*.

> All that fulfils solely the inner nature. (*Guhyasamājā*, XVI, p. 126:) The *sādhaka* with firm resolve, always seeks alms in the glade. Trembling with fear they give food divinely prepared. Should the triple-diamond one go beyond, there would be loss and (then) the diamond syllable. Obtaining either a goddess, a *nāga*-lady, great *yakṣī*, demi-goddess, or human woman, he should engage in *vidyāvrata*, relying on the knowledge of the three diamonds.

In that way dispelling the worldly meditations, and abandoning the realm of fancy, with ever-ecstatic mind he rejoices in the midst of the *yoginīs*, like King Indrabhūti, who transmuted his physical body (*kalevara*) and became a diamond body, whereupon he disappeared from the midst of his queens; and endowed with the merits of the eight *guṇa-aiśvarya*, wandered from Buddha field to Buddha field. As said in the *Mūlasūtra* (i.e. *Guhyasamāja*, VII, 2, with variant readings) :

> By recourses that enjoy all desires (=deities) according to pleasure; and by the praxis of one's presiding lord one (respectively) worships others and oneself.

So ends the *Subhāṣita-saṃgraha* citation of Āryadeva's 'lucid words'. Fortunately, Āryadeva includes two passages from the *Guhyasamāja*, one near the beginning of Chapter Seven and the other near the end of Chapter Sixteen, which enable me to bring in some of the commentarial tradition. Besides, Śākyamitra's *Caryāmelāpakapradipa-ṭikā* in Columbia University's Narthang edition was consulted in the relevant section near the end, but proved of little value.

In order to explain Āryadeva's account in the terminology already drawn from the *Guhyasamājatantra* and associated commentarial literature, it is necessary to observe that he says, "Having first taken Supreme Truth as the meditative object..." and says in the next sentence in further explanation, "First he experiences the three kinds of form. . . ." One can refer to the three kinds of each sense object (as in *Guhyasamāja*, Chap. VII) by desire, aversion, and indifference, as does Āryadeva.

*Yoga Stages 1 and 2*
*Body as the Mantra Visualized*
*Selflessness of the Mind Visualized*

The account begins with the yogin located in a solitary glade. In this connection Āryadeva cites *Guhyasamāja*, XVI, p. 126, "The *sādhaka* with firm resolve, always seeks alms in the glade. Trembling with fear they give food divinely prepared. . . ."* The *Pradipoddyotana* (*Mchan ḥgrel*, p. 148-1) mentions the unshared food but does not clarify who does the giving or why they are frightened. It converts the yogin's glade to the 'great forest' (*vane mahāṭavyāṃ*). Celu-pā's commentary, *Ratnavṛkṣa-nāma-rahasya-samāja-vṛtti* (PTT, Vol, 63, p. 227-2), is more helpful, because it explains, "food not shared with men and having the hundred flavors" (mi daṅ thun moṅ ma yin paḥi ẑal zas ro brgya daṅ ldan pa); and "those tree divinities frightened by the fiery nimbus (*tejas*) of his evocation power, give (it)" (śiṅ la gnas paḥi lha de dag sgrub dbaṅ deḥi gzi brjid kyis skrag nas ster bar ḥgyur ro). This explanation immediately associates those *Guhyasamāja* verses with the episode

*The verse is correctly given in Bhattacharyya's edition to begin with *vane*, the second line to begin with *dadanti*; while Bagchi's edition incorrectly assigns the *vane* line to verse 98B, and starts verse 99 with *dadanti*. The *Pradipoddyotana* manuscript supports Bhattacharyya here with the words *vane-ityādi*.

of the Buddha's enlightenment under the Tree, which is called 'terrace of enlightenment' (*bodhimaṇḍa*) and has four 'divinities of enlightenment' (*bodhidevata*) (cf. my *Buddhist Tantras*, p. 186). It is obviously a development from the early Buddhist legend of the girl Sujātā, who brought food in a golden bowl to the meditating Gautama who, after six years of fruitless austerity, decided on a middle course (cf. Edward J. Thomas, *The Life of Buddha*, pp. 70-71). As to who are those tree divinities, Tsoṅ-kha-pa (commentary on *Pañcakrama*, PTT, Vol. 159, p. 77-3) states the 'companion for accomplishing the food' (kha zas sgrub paḥi grogs) to be the Yakṣī, the Kiṃkarā (servant), etc. (gnod sbyin mo mṅag gźug ma sogs) as the best. This explanation is consistent with the standard explanation of the female figure on the Sānchī gate as a Yakṣī or Yakṣiṇī. Also, earlier in *Guhyasamāja*, Chap. XVI and its commentary, there are several mentions of the Yakṣī lady; for example, *Mchan ḥgrel*, p. 146-2, identifies these yakṣī-s as Vajraḍākinī-s.

Āryadeva's account starts with the yogin tantamount to the Body of the Buddha sitting under the Bodhi tree. Hence the solitary glade is the yogin's own body as the *maṇḍala*. It is the "arcane body" of the Stage of Completion, discussed under the Nidāna verses KĀ-YA, and is equivalent to the Eighth Stage of the Bodhisattva. Now, our earlier discussions have gone into the matter of how this "arcane body" is actually the accomplishment of the previous Stage of Generation and is brought forward into the Stage of Completion. This is now combined with a new stage of yoga; and as the first appendix showed, the new stage has been referred to as "the selflessness of *citta* being visualized," a yoga state of dream.

The two stages are suggested by the two celebrated gestures of the seated Buddha—right hand in the earth-touching gesture ('body as the mantra visualized'), and left hand level at the heart in the equipoise (*samāpatti*) gesture ('selflessness of the mind visualized').

### *Yoga Stage* 3
### *The Svādhiṣṭhāna, or initial Mahāmudrā*

Āryadeva has taken the first two yoga stages for granted and goes immediately to the 3rd stage, saying, "Having first taken Supreme Truth as the meditative object, by the Stage of Personal Blessing (*svādhiṣṭhāna-krama*) he abides with himself as the body of Vajrasattva." Under Nidāna verse CIT, Āryadeva's same work was already cited in a remarkable passage on how to visualize the Supreme Truth, in a process that leads to the yoga condition of deep sleep and the revelation of the Clear Light. In the present passage, observe that Āryadeva's expression *ātmākṛti* (configuration of the self) is consistent with the conclusion in Appendix No. 1 that in the 3rd stage of yoga, referring to dreamless sleep, the subject is paramount and the object is in abeyance—the subject now being indicated as "configuration of the self". Despite this condition of pure subjectivity devoid of dream object, the description emphasizes the extreme bliss, since the yogin dwells in the circle of the goddesses. One may refer to Nidāna verse HṚ (no. 27) for more information; cf. there, Bu-ston's citation of Āryadeva. The present passage continues with the union of the male and female energies, and Āryadeva summarizes, "Thus he introspects the true forms of Prajñāpāramitā and so on." Tsoṅ-kha-pa's commentary on *Pañcakrama* (PTT, Vol. 159, p. 75-5) treats this part of the account as illustrative of *niṣprapañca-caryā*. Concerning the 'inner hearth,' Tsoṅ-kha-pa (*ibid.*, p. 75-3) states that the yogin "eats while contemplating a burnt offering offered to the face of the Samādhi-sattva" (tiṅ ṅe ḥdzin sems dpaḥi źal du sreg rdzas dbul paḥi bsam pas bsaḥ ste). Presumably, what the yogin now eats is the food "divinely prepared" which the tree divinities offered earlier.

Furthermore, it is in this same connection that Āryadeva cites the *Mūlasūtra.** On the verse as identified, the

*There is no doubt that Āryadeva means the *Guhyasamājatantra* (first seventeen chapters) by his citation from the '*Mūlasūtra*'. The verse has some variant readings of Chapter Seven, verse 2, as well as some corruptions; but also the edited Sanskrit of the Tantra has a corrupt reading in this verse. The Bendall verse has the reading 'svam ātmānaṃ' where the published Tantra has 'parāṅgaiś ca'. The *Pradīpoddyotana* manuscript (5B-3-4) expands: 'svātmānaṃ parāṃś ca'. The *Pradīpoddyotana* suggests that the original reading is 'svaṃ parāṃś ca'. However, by my correcting principle of adopting a reading as close as possible to the edited Sanskrit when it is corrupt, I decided to correct the reading 'parāṅgais ca' to 'parātmānau'. The standard form of the verse should therefore read:

*sarvakāmopabhogais tu sevyamānair yathecchataḥ* /
*svādhidaivatayogena parātmānau prapūjayet* //

*Pradīpoddyotana* explains how one worships oneself by the praxis of one's presiding lord, namely by the arduous ascetic practices called the twelve qualities of a purified man (*dhutaguṇa*). However, as the next *Guhyasamāja* verse (VII, 3) clarifies, it is by the worship and satisfaction of others, i.e. by offerings of the five deified sense objects (*kāmaguṇa*), that one speedily attains Buddhahood. Āryadeva thus points to this worship of others as the way in which King Indrabhūti transmuted his physical body. This is also the message of Chapter VI, 2 ('Documents').

About the vowels and the consonants in the *nāḍis* totalling 72,000, the *Sṅags rim chen mo* shows the way of conceiving them in the body. The placement of these vowels and consonants of course is done in the phase called the Stage of Generation, with the achievement of 'mantra body' (*mantramūrti*). The fruition of this letter placement occurs in the Stage of Completion; and this constitutes another reason for requiring the two Stages in the given order. At f. 380b-6, Tsoṅ-kha-pa repeats the citation of some Tanjur authority, and mentions that the *Saṃvarodayatantra* and other Tantras are consistent regarding the placement of the sixteen vowels :

> The Lord said : The wise person should contemplate this way : A at the root of the thumb, Ā at the calf of the leg, I at the thigh joint, Ī at the private part (i.e. genitals), U at the root of the navel, Ū at the stomach, Ṛ at the middle of the breast, Ṝ at the hand, Ḷ at the neck, Ḹ at the lip, E at the cheek, AI at the eye, O at the root of the ear, AU at the head, AM and AḤ in the body at the crown of the head. Such is the disposition on the 'white side' (left), so also on the 'black' (right) in reverse.
>
> This Vajrasattva is in women and also in men at all times.

Notice that the name Vajrasattva is employed for a sexless (or else, androgyne) body that is the same for men and women, and is explained as a *mantra*-body. Hence, when Āryadeva

The Bendall version substitutes *deva* for *kāma*, which in this case amounts to the same meaning, because 'all desires' means 'all sense objects' and these are identified with deities (*deva*). Again the substitution of *yathāsukham* for *yathecchataḥ* hardly departs from the intention. However, the Bendall reading *sevyamāno* ought to be corrected to *sevyamānair*. The verse with these modifications accounts for the translation adopted previously.

said, "he abides with himself as the body of Vajrasattva," the remark can apply to either a yogin or yoginī. So also it is possible to bring in the explanation presented in Appendix II that on the Bodhisattva's Ninth Stage he sets into motion the wheel of the *dharma*; that is to say, in the fruitional Stage of Completion the yogin sets into motion the wheel of *mantras*. To continue with Tsoṅ-kha-pa's exposition of letter placement:— The explanation of 'white side' as left and 'black side' as right (side of body), in the case A at the left thumb or right thumb, stems from the commentary on the *Saṃvarodaya-tantra* according to *Sṅags rim*, f. 381a-4. The *Sṅags rim*, f. 381b-6, mentions that the consonants are grouped under the elements, with certain consonants repeated according to the following breakdown :

| | | |
|---|---|---|
| *ākāśa* : | ka, ṅa, ña, ṇa, na, ma, ha, kṣa | — 8 |
| *wind* : | gha, jha, ḍha, dha (2), bha, ya (2), śa | — 9 |
| *fire* : | ga, ja, ḍa (2), da, ba, ra (2), ṣa | — 9 |
| *water* : | kha, cha, ṭha, tha, pha, va (2) | — 7 |
| *earth* : | ca, ṭa, ta, pa, la (2), sa | — 7 |
| | | 40 |

Those syllables are held in this tantric tradition to give rise to the thirty-two characteristics and eighty minor marks of the Buddha's body (cf. Nidāna verse 23, YA). The *Sṅags rim*, f. 380a-6, cites in this connection Dīpaṅkarabhadra's *Śrīguhyasamājamaṇḍalavidhi* (known in Tibetan tradition as the Four Hundred and Fifty Verses, *Bźi brgya lṅa bcu pa*) for a half-*śloka* translated by indications in the commentary by Ratnākaraśānti, the *Śrīguhyasamājamaṇḍalavidhi-ṭīkā* :

> / *dbyaṅs yig mtshan daṅ yaṅ dag ldan* /
> / *ka sogs dpe byad ḥod zer can* /
>
> The (16) vowels are the source of the (32) characteristics (*lakṣaṇa*). The (34) consonants radiate the (80) minor marks (*anuvyañjana*).

*Sṅags rim*. f. 380b-2, identifies the vowels as white in color, the consonants as red. The white vowels are mystically called 'moon'; the red consonants, 'second moon' or 'sun'. *Ibid*, f. 380b-1, by dividing the vowels into two, one makes a 'right' group (for the male *upāya*) of sixteen, and a 'left' group (for the female *prajñā*), to yield the total of 32 for the characteristics.

Likewise, the consonants, classified as above with series adding up to 40, are divided into two for *upāya* and *prajñā* to yield the total of 80 for the minor marks.

The above data on the vowels requires some further clarification. The statement that the vowels on the 'black' (right) side are in reverse means, according to that above-cited commentary on the *Saṃvarodaya-tantra*, that for that side one contemplates the vowel placement in the reverse order, i.e. starting from the AM and AḤ at the crown of the head. The vowel depositing constitutes the sixteen parts of the *bodhicitta* (*byaṅ chub kyi sems kyi cha bcu drug*). At this point the *Sṅags rim* cites the Hevajra-tantra, Part I, Chap. viii (Snellgrove ed.) : śukrākāro bhaved bhagavān tatsukhaṃ kāminī smṛtaṃ (50A) : "The Lord is the aspect of *śukra*; Kāminī is the ecstasy of that (*bodhicitta*)." Thus, the Lord, or Vajrasattva, who is in both men and women, is the *śukra* ('semen') white aspect, while the Goddess Kāminī, presumably also in both men and women, is the ecstasy (*sukha*) red aspect of the sixteen parts of *bodhicitta*, yielding a total of 32 for the characteristics.

## *Yoga Stage 4*
## *The divine body made of mind*

The next problem is to determine who is 'the triple-diamond one'. The verse just preceding those cited by Āryadeva must be considered (*Guhyasamāja*, XVI, 97 :):

> *svamudrāṃ vā 'thavā cinted dhyānatryakṣaravajriṇām* /
> *pañcabuddhāś ca sarvajñāḥ priṇante nātra saṃśayaḥ* / /
>
> Or he should contemplate his own *mudrā* belonging to the three-syllable vajrins of meditation. The omniscient Buddhas will be pleased; there is no doubt of it.

The *Pradīpoddyotana* comments : / svamudrāṃ ityādinā jñānamudrayā sahacaryāṃ darśayati / svamudrāṃ hṛdayasthām vajradhātvīśvarīṃ tryaksaravajriṇāṃ vairocanādiyogināṃ bāhyāṅganānapekṣiṇāṃ dadyāt / "By the words 'his own *mudrā*' and so on, (the verse) shows the praxis together with the Jñānamudrā. He should give (in marriage) his 'own *mudrā*', the 'Queen of the Diamond Realm' dwelling in the heart, belonging to the 'three-syllable vajrins', i.e. the yogins of Vairocana and so on, who have no eye to external women." Earlier in his commentary on Chapter XII, 76, ("Documents"), Candrakīrti explained the terms 'Buddha', 'Vajradharma', and 'Vajrasattva' as respectively the yogin of Vairocana, yogin of Amitābha, and yogin of Akṣobhya.

Regarding those females or *mudrā*-s of the verse cited by Āryadeva, namely, the goddess, nāga lady, and so on, *Mchan ḥgrel*, p. 148-2, mentions that she is the respective goddess of the three families, thus Locanā for Vairocana's yogin; Pāṇḍarā for Amitābha's yogin; and Māmakī for Akṣobhya's yogin. 'Knowledge of the three diamonds' means knowledge of the diamond of Body, of Speech, and of Mind. But then, why are five females mentioned in the verse? The *Pradīpoddyotana* does not help here. Possibly they stand for the *mudrā*-s of five different ages, usually 16-yeared; that is, I presume that they are pseudonyms of the five, the 'butcher maiden' etc., listed under Nidāna verse GE (no. 35).

What is meant by his going beyond? The *Pradīpoddyotana* manuscript explains: / atikramed ity ādinā caryāphalam āha / trivajrātmā yogī atikramet / mānuṣyabhāvam abhibhavati / naśyati / nāśaṃ prākṛtaṃ śarīraṃ tatparāvṛttyā vajravad abhedyam akṣaram avinaśvaraṃ bhavet / "By the words 'Should he go beyond' (the verse) states the fruit of the praxis. Should the 'triple-diamond' yogin go beyond, he would overpower the human condition. The vulgar body with 'loss' is lost. By its transmutation, the 'syllable' inseparable like a 'diamond' would not be susceptible of destruction." The going beyond of the 'triple-diamond yogin' contrasts with the going beyond of the 'deluded self', which is the topic of the last verse in Chapter XII and with Chapter XV, verse 22 (see Appendix II).

Regarding the *vidyāvrata*, left in the original Sanskrit above as well as previously in my citation of verses from Chapter XVI in the opening material for the set of *nidāna* verses on Kāyavākcitta (Body, Speech, and Mind), the term is well explained by Buddhaguhya in his *Dhyānottara-paṭala-ṭikā* (PTT, Vol. 78, p. 80-4,5 and p. 81-1). '*Viayāvrata*' (rite of the *vidyā*) means *devatā-yoga* (union with divinity), especially at the *saṃdhis*. Therefore, the *Pradīpoddyotana* comments (*Mchan ḥgrel*, p. 147-4) : vidyāvratī tābhiḥ sārdhaṃ guhyapūjāṃ samāpattiṃ catuḥsaṃdhyāṃ kuryāt ("The *vidyāvratin* should engage in the secret-offering kind of equipoise together with those [goddesses] at the four junctures.") These are of course the morning, noon, sunset, and midnight observances.*

It is well to point out one feature of Āryadeva's account that was not brought forward in our previous discussions of the *Guhyasamāja* yoga. He says, "In that way, again and again he enters the true limit (*bhūtakoṭi*); and having emerged again and again he experiences the five 'strands of desire' as the five Tathāgata forms, so the (sublime) mind does not fade." Śākyamitra says (Narthang ed., f. 345b-7) : "The true limit is the Clear Light" (yaṅ dag paḥi mthaḥ ni ḥod gsal ba ste). This shows that the ultimate fruit promised for this yoga is not achieved simply by doing it once; but rather by repetition of entering into the yoga state of artificial dreamless sleep with revelation of the Clear Light, until the "diamond body" or purified "illusory body" achieves the independence to wander "from Buddha field to Buddha field." Then, as *Mkhas grub rje's Fundamentals of the Buddhist Tantras* suggests, the yogin is the Bodhisattva of the Tenth Stage, in the retinue of the Saṃbhoga-kāya. Still, perhaps the most significant finding of this appendix is the clear indication from Āryadeva's account that it is in the yoga artificial dreamless sleep that occurs the reintegration of male and female energies frequently referred to as *yuganaddha*. Hence, this is the intimation of what has been earlier referred to in this work as the Dharmakāya union with the goddess along with the Clear Light (of death). This suggests, as well, that in this theory the ordinary state of dreamless sleep (occurring every night or in each period of normal sleep) is such a reunion of male and female—mystically, death—from which comes the new life, the birth, i.e. the reawakening (see Table III, The Clear Lights). The yogin, by artificially evoking this state, seeks to capture, strengthen, and restore the androgyne.

*Ratnākaraśānti's *Piṇḍīkṛta-sādhopāyikā-vṛtti-ratnāvalī* (PTT, Vol. 62, p. 68-5) mentions three kinds of *vrata*, (1) *vajravrata*, namely of the diamond, the "mind of enlightenment"; (2) *caryāvrata*, namely of three kinds of engagement; and (3) *vidyāvrata*.

APPENDIX IV

# GRADING OF THE FOUR-STAGE YOGA

Previously (p. 163) it was noted from the *Sṅags rim* that for accomplishing the four steps of yoga there is a lesser, a middling and a great. Let us therefore, without introducing new material attempt a grading by way of this suggestion.

## A. *The lesser four steps*

The lesser would certainly be the four-stage yoga pointed out by Ratnākaraśānti (see Appendix I) to be shared between the *Laṅkāvatārasūtra* and the *Guhyasamājatantra*. He referred to a verse of *Guhyasamāja*, chap. XV, and I found it to be consistent with one way of understanding the stages of *Guhyasamāja*, Chap. VI. In this interpretation, the four-stage yoga is equivalent to the four *nirvedhabhāgiyas* that lead to the First Bodhisattva Stage.

## B. *The middling four steps*

The middling would be the four stages that go with the Stage of Generation. These steps are clearly stated in *Guhyasamāja*, Chap. XII, and are well explained in Candrakīrti's commentary (see 'Documents'). The steps of *Guhyasamāja*, Chap. VI, can be understood this way; and the four steps, considered as subjective yoga can be correlated with steps of external ritual, as was shown. Besides, the explanation of the four steps with the terminology of three *samādhis* is used to correlate the class of Yoga Tantra with the Stage of Generation of the Anuttarayogatantra.

## C. *The great four steps*

The great would be the interpretation of four stages as equivalent to the *ṣaḍaṅgayoga* of the Stage of Completion, also expressible in terms of five stages (Nāgārjuna's *Pañcakrama*). This is also one way of understanding the stages of *Guhyasamāja*, Chap. VI in association with the Explanatory Tantra *Vajramālā*.

The basic Tantra itself showed the higher interpretation of the four stages by identifying them, in chap. XV, with the four goddesses, Locanā, etc., who confer enlightenment. On the terminological level, one may further interpret the four steps of yoga of *Guhyasamāja*, chap. XII, as applicable to the Stage of Completion.

Using Candrakīrti's classifying terminology, the lesser is shared with non-tantric Buddhism, the middling is shared by the Anuttarayogatantra with the three lower Tantras, and the great is unshared.

# BIBLIOGRAPHY

A. Abbreviations.

ed.—edited

G.O.S.—Gaekwad's Oriental Series, Oriental Institute, Baroda.

PTT—Peking Tibetan Tripitaka. This is *The Tibetan Tripitaka; Peking Edition.* Reprinted under the Supervision of the Otani University, Kyoto. Tibetan Tripitaka Research Institute, Tokyo-Kyoto, 1956.

Toh. No.—*A Complete Catalogue of the Tibetan Buddhist Canons*, ed. by Hakuju Ui, et al, Tohoku Imperial University, Sendai, Japan, 1934, for numbers 1-4569. *A Catalogue of the Tohoku University Collection of Tibetan Works on Buddhism*, ed. by Yensho Kanakura, et al, Tohoku University, Sendai, 1953, for numbers 5001-7083.

tr.—translated

B. Bibliography.


Abhayākaragupta (pāda). *Āmnāya-mañjari*, commentary on the *Śri-Saṃpuṭa-tantra*, PTT, Vol. 55.

,, *Niṣpannayogāvali*, ed. by B. Bhattacharyya, G.O.S. CIX, 1949.

,, *Upadeśa-mañjari*, PTT, Vol. 87.

,, *Vajrāvali-nāma-maṇḍalasādhana*, Toh. No. 3140.

*Advayasamatāvijaya*, PTT, Vol. 3 (the last work).

Alaṃkakalaśa. *Śri-Vajramālā-mahāyogatantra-ṭikā-gambhirārtha-dipikā-nāma*, PTT, Vol. 61.

*Āmnāya-mañjari*. See Abhayākaragupta.

Ānandagarbha. *Śri-Guhyasamāja-mahātantrarāja-ṭikā*, (PTT, Vol. 84.)

,, *Śri-Paramādya-ṭikā*, (PTT, Vol. 73.)

Anaṅgavajra. *Prajñopāyaviniścayasiddhi*, ed. by B. Bhattacharyya in *Two Vajrayāna Works*, G.O.S. XLIV, 1929.

Āryadeva. *Caryāmelāpaka-pradīpa*, PTT, Vol. 61.

,, *Cittaviśuddhiprakaraṇa*, Sanskrit and Tibetan texts, ed. by Prabhubhai B. Patel, Visvabharati, 1949.

*Ārya-nanda-garbhāvakrānti-nirdeśa*, Ratnakūṭa collection, Toh. No. 57.

Āryaśūra. *Jātakamāla*, ed. by Hendrik Kern, Harvard Oriental Series, Vol. One, 1943.

Asaṅga. *Mahāyāna-Sūtrālaṃkāravṛtti*, ed. by Sylvain Lévi, Paris, 1907.

,, *Śrāvakabhūmi*. See Wayman, Alex.

*Bhagavadgītā*, tr. by S. Radhakrishnan, New York, 1948.

Bhavyakīrti. *Pañcakrama-ṭikā maṇimālā-nāma* (attributed to Nāgabodhi), PTT, Vol. 62.

,, *Pradīpoddyotanābhisaṃdhi-prakāśikā-nāma-vyākhyā-ṭīkā* (the '*Prakāśikā*'), PTT, Vols. 60-61.

*Blue Annals, The.* See Roerich, George N.

*Bṛhadāraṇyaka Upaniṣad*, in S. Radhakrishnan, *The Principal Upaniṣads*, New York, 1953.

Buddhaghoṣa. *Visuddhimagga*, Harvard Oriental Series edition.

Buddhaguhya. *Dhyānottara-paṭala-ṭīkā*, PTT, Vol. 78.

Buddhaśrījñāna. *Mukhāgama*, Toh. No. 1853.

,, *Muktitilaka*, Toh. No. 1859.

,, *Samantabhadra-nāma-sādhana*, Toh. No. 1855.

Bu-ston. *Bśad sbyar*, collected works, Ta; Śata-Piṭaka Series, New Delhi, 1967.

*Candraguhyatilaka-nāma-mahātantrarāja*, Toh. No. 477.

Candrakīrti (non-tantric). *Prasannapadā nāma mādhyamikavṛtti* ed. by Louis de La Vallée Poussin.

Candrakīrti (tantric). *Guhyasamājābhisamayālaṃkāra-vṛtti*, PTT, Vol. 62.

,, *Pradīpoddyotana*, in Derge Tanjur, *Rgyud ḥgrel*, Ha; in PTT, Vol. 158 (with *Mchan ḥgrel*, see Tsoṅ-kha-pa).

*Caryāmelāpaka* (*-pradīpa*) and *ṭikā*. See Āryadeva and Śākyamitra

*Caturdevīparipṛcchā* = *Caturdevatāparipṛcchā*, PTT, Vol. 3. See Smṛtijñānakīrti and Tsoṅ-kha-pa.

Celu-pā (Celuka). *Ratnavṛkṣa-nāma-rahasya-samāja-vṛtti*, PTT, Vol. 63.

Chakravarti, Chintaharan. *Tantra; Studies on their Religion and Literature*, Calcutta, 1963.

*Chāndogya Upaniṣad*, in S. Radhakrishnan, *The Principal Upaniṣads*.

Candra, Lokesh. See Vīra, Raghu.

Chang, Chen chi. *Teachings of Tibetan Yoga*, New York, 1963.

Chou Yi-liang. "Tantrism in China," *Harvard Journal of Asian Studies*, 1944-45.

*Daśabhūmika-sūtra*, ed. by Dr. J. Rahder, Paris, 1926; *Daśabhūmiśvaro nāma Mahāyānasūtra*, ed. by Ryūkō Kondō, Tokyo, 1936.

Dasgupta, Shashibhusan. *An Introduction to Tantric Buddhism*, Calcutta, 1950.

,, *Obscure Religious Cults*, 2nd edition, Calcutta, 1962.

Dasgupta, Surendranath. *A History of Indian Philosophy*, Cambridge, 1932, Vol. I.

*Devendraparipṛcchā-tantra*. As quoted in Candrakīrti's *Pradīpoddyotana*.

Dharmakīrti (tantric). *Hevajra-pañjikā* called *Spyan ḥbyed*, Toh. No. 1191.

*Dharma-samuccaya*, Chaps. VI-XII, ed. and tr. by Lin Lí-kouang (revised by A. Bareau, J.W de-Jong, and P. Demiéville), Paris, 1969.

Dimock, Edward C. "Doctrine and Practice Among the Vaiṣṇavas of Bengal," *History of Religions*, 3:1, Summer 1963.

,, *The Place of the Hidden Moon*, Chicago, 1966.

Ekādaśasvara. *Mahāvajradharapathakramopadeśāmṛtaguhya*, Toh 1823.

Eliade, Mircea. *Yoga: Immortality and Freedom*, New York, 1958.

Falk, Maryla. *Nāma-Rūpa and Dharma-Rūpa*, Calcutta, 1943.

Geiger, Mrs. M. and Prof. W. "Pāli Dhamma, vornehmlich in der kanonischen literatur," Abh. de Bayer, Ak. d. Wiss., Philos.-philol. u. hist. Kl., XXXI, 1, Munich, 1921.

*Guhyasamāja-tantra*, ed. by Benoytosh Bhattacharyya, G.O.S. LIII, 1931; reprint, 1967; also ed. by S. Bagchi, Darbhanga, 1965;* also ed. by Matsunaga, *Journal of Koyasan University*, No. 10, 1975.

*References to Bhattacharyya's edition are shown by page numbers, and to Bagchi's edition by verse numbers in a given chapter.

Hadano, Hakuyū. "Human Existence in Tantric Buddhism," *Tohoku Daigaku Bungaku-bu Kenkyū-nempo*, No. 9, 1958.

*Hevajra-tantra*, ed. and tr. by D.L. Snellgrove, London, 1959, two vols.

Indrabhūti (or Indrabodhi). *Jñānasiddhi*, ed. by B. Bhattacharyya in *Two Vajrayāna Works*, G.O.S. XLIV, 1929.

" *Śri-sampuṭa-tilaka . . . ṭikā-smṛtisaṃdarśanāloka* PTT, Vol. 55.

Jagannatham, Y. *Divine Love and Amorous Sentiment*, publ. by author, Eluru, 1956.

Jālandharipāda. *Hevajrasādhanasya-ṭippaṇiśuddhi-vajrapradīpa*, PTT Vol. 56.

Jinadatta. *Śri-Guhyasamāja-tantra-pañjikā-nāma*, PTT. Vol. 63.

*Jñānavajrasamuccaya*. See *Śri-Vajrajñānasamuccaya*.

*Kālacakra-tantra*, Toh. Nos. 361-365; also its exegesis, the *Vimalaprabhā*, Toh. 845, is tantamount to 'revealed scripture'.

Kamalaśīla. (First) *Bhāvanākrama*, in G. Tucci's *Minor Buddhist Texts*, II (Rome, 1958).

*Kāma-sūtra* of Vātsyāyana, with the commentary *Jayamaṅgala* of Yaśhodhara. Ed. by Śrī Gosvamī Dāmodar Shastri, Benares City, 1929.

Kloṅ-rdol bla-ma. Collected Works, Vol. I, Section Ma, ed. by Ven. Dalama, Mussoori, 1963.

*Kṛṣṇayamāri-tantra*. Probably the *Sarvatathāgatakāyavākcitta-kṛṣṇayamāri-nāma-tantra*, Toh. No. 467.

Kumāra. *Pradipadipa-ṭippaṇīhṛdayādarśa* (commentary on *Pradipoddyotana*), PTT, Vol. 60.

Kun-dgaḥ-don-grub. *Man ṅag rim gñis gter mdzod*. Indian reprint.

Lakṣmīṃkarā. *Pradipoddyotana-viṣamapadapañjikā-nāma*, Toh. No. 1792.

*Lalitavistara*, ed. by S. Lefmann, Halle, 1902; also ed. by P.L. Vaidya, Darbhanga, 1958.

*Laṅkāvatāra-sūtra*. Ed. by B. Nanjio, Kyoto, 1956; tr. by D.T. Suzuki, London, 1932.

Lessing, Ferdinand D. See Mkhas-grub-rje.

Līlavajra. *Guhyasamāja-tantra-nidāna-gurūpaaeśa-bhāṣya*, PTT, Vol. 66
,, *Śrī-guhyagarbha-mahātantrarāja-ṭikā-nāma*, PTT. Vol. 82.
*Madhyāntavibhāga*, and *Madhyāntavibhāga-bhāṣya*, ed. by Gadjin M. Nagao, Tokyo, 1964.
*Mahāmahāyānaratnarājasūtra*. As quoted in Candrakīrti's *Pradī. poddyotana*.
*Mahāmudrātilaka-tantra*, Toh. No. 420.
*Mahāvairocana-sūtra* or *Vairocanābhisaṃbodhi*, Toh. No. 494.
*Mahāvyutpatti*, ed. by R. Sakaki.
*Mahāyāna-Sūtralaṃkāra*. See Asaṅga.
*Maitri Upaniṣad*, in S. Radhakrishnan, *The Principal Upaniṣads*.
*Maṇimālā*. See Bhavyakīrti.
Matsunaga, Yūkei. "A Doubt to Authority of the Guhyasamāja-Ākhyāṇa-tantra," *Journal of Indian and Buddhist Studies*, XII:2, March, 1964.
,, "On the Saptālaṅkāra," *Journal of Indian and Buddhist Studies*, XI:2, March, 1963.
see *Guhyasamāja-tantra*.
Mkhas-grub-rje, *Mkhas grub rje's Fundamentals of the Buddhist Tantras*, tr. by Ferdinand D. Lessing and Alex Wayman, *Indo-Iranian Monographs*, Vol. VIII, The Hague, 1968.
*Mūlasūtra* (as quoted in Āryadeva's *Caryāmelāpaka*). Stands for *Guhyasamāja-tantra*. (as quoted in *Pradīpoddyotana*). Stands for *Tattvasaṃgraha*.
Nāgabodhi. *Śrī-Guhyasamāja-maṇḍalopāyikā-viṃśati-vidhi-nāma*, PTT, Vol. 62.
Nāgabuddhi. *Karmānta-vibhaṅga-nāma*, PTT, Vol. 62.
,, *Samāja-sādhana-vyavasthāli*, PTT, Vol. 62.
Nāgārjuna (tantric). *Aṣṭādaśa-paṭala-vistara-vyākhyā*, PTT, Vol. 60.
,, *Pañcakrama*, ed. by Louis de La Vallée Poussin, Gand, 1896.
,, *Piṇḍikṛta-sādhana* (= *Piṇḍikrama-sādhana*), PTT, Vol. 61, and Sanskrit ed. by Poussin in preceding (Gand, 1896).
,, *Ṣaḍaṅgayoga-nāma*, PTT, Vol. 85.
,, *Seka-catuḥ-prakaraṇa*, PTT, Vol. 61.
,, *Śrī-Guhyasamāja-mahāyogatantrotpattikrama*

*sādhana-sūtramelāpaka-nāma* (the '*Sūtramelāpaka*"), PTT, Vol. 61.

Nāgārjuna (tantric). *Śrī-Guhyasamājatantrasya tantraṭikā-nāma*, PTT, Vol. 59.

Nāropā. *Sekoddeśaṭikā*, ed. by Mario E. Carelli, G.O.S. XC, 1941.

*Nyāya Mañjarī*. Tr. by J. A. Bhattacharyya, *The Calcutta Review*, Oct. 1955.

Obermiller, E. "The Doctrine of Prajñā-pāramitā..." *Acta Orientalia*, 1932.

Padmavajra. *Sakalatantrasambhavasañcodanī-śrīguhyasiddhi-nāma* (the '*Guhyasiddhi*'), Toh. 2217.

" *Śrī-Ḍākārṇavamahāyoginītantrarājavāhikaṭikā-nāma*, Toh. 1419.

Paṇḍit Smṛti. See Smṛtijñānakīrti.

Poussin, L. de La Vallée. See Vasubandhu. See Nāgārjuna (tantric).

" *Vijñaptimātratāsiddhi*. *La Siddhi de Hiuan-Tsang*, two vols., Paris, 1928-1929; *Index*, Paris, 1948.

" (with Cordier, P.), "Les soixante-quinze et les cent dharmas," in *Le Muséon*, Nouvelle Série, Vol. VI, Louvain, 1905.

*Pradīpoddyotana*. See Candrakīrti.

*Prakāśikā*. See Bhavyakīrti.

Praśāntajñāna. *Upadeśa-niścaya-nāma-śrīguhyasamāja-vṛtti*, PTT Vol. 63.

Radhakrishnan, S. *The Dhammapada*, London, 1950.

" " *The Principal Upaniṣads*, New York, 1953.

Ratnākaraśānti (also called Śānti-pā). *Kusumāñjali-guhyasamāja-nibandha-nāma*, PTT, Vol. 64.

" *Piṇḍīkṛta-sādhanopāyikā-vṛtti-ratnāvali*, PTT, Vol. 62.

" *Prajñāpāramitopadeśa*, PTT, Vol. 114.

" *Śrī-Guhyasamāja-maṇḍalavidhi-ṭikā*, PTT, Vol. 65.

Ray, Kamala. "The Ten Incarnations of Viṣṇu in Bengal," *Indian Historical Quarterly*, Vol. XV, 1941.

Rgyal-tshab-rje. *Dpyid thig zin bris*, in Lhasa collected works, Vol. Ka.

Roerich, George N. *The Blue Annals*, Part One, Calcutta, 1949; Part Two, Calcutta, 1953.

*Sādhana-mālā*, ed. by B. Bhattacharyya, two vols., G.O.S. XXVI and XLI, 1925-8.

*Saddharmapuṇḍarīka-sūtra*, ed. by K. Kern and Bunyu Nanjio, *Bibliotheca Buddhica* No. 10, St.-Pét., 1908-12.

Śākyamitra. *Caryāmelāpakapradīpa-ṭīkā*, PTT. Vol. 62, and Narthang edition.

,, *Kosalālaṃkāra* (commentary on the Yoga-tantra *Tattvasaṃgraha*), Toh. No. 2503.

*Saṃdhinirmocana-sūtra*, tr. into French with Tibetan text ed. by Etienne Lamotte, Louvain, 1935.

*Saṃdhivyākaraṇa-nāma-tantra* (an Explanatory Tantra of the *Guhyasamāja*), PTT, Vol. 3.

*Saṃpuṭa* (*-tilaka*) (= *Saṃpuṭa-nāma-mahātantra*), Toh. No. 381.

*Saṃvara-tantra* (= *Tantrarājaśrīlaghusambara-nāma*), Toh. No. 368.

*Saṃvarodaya-tantra* (= *Śrī-Mahāsambarodaya-tantrarāja-nāma*), Toh. No. 373.

Sāṅkṛtyāyana, Rāhula. "Recherches Bouddhiques" *Journal Asiatique*, Oct.-Dec., 1934.

Saraha. *Dohā-koṣa*. See Shahidullah, M.

*Sarvarahasya-nāma-tantrarāja*, PTT, Vol. 5.

*Śatapathabrāhmaṇa*, tr. by J. Eggeling, *Sacred Books of the East*, Vol. 12.

Shahidullah, M. *Les chants mystiques de Kāṇha et de Saraha* Paris, 1928.

Smṛtijñānakīrti. *Caturdevatā-vyākhyāna-upadeśa-pauṣṭika*, PTT, Vol. 66.

*Śrī-Guhyasamāja-tantrarāja-vṛtti*, PTT, Vol. 66.

*Vajravidāraṇa-nāma-dhāraṇī-vṛtti*, Toh. 2684.

Śraddhākaravarman. *Vajrajñānasamuccaya-tantrodbhava-saptālaṃkāra-vimocana*, PTT, Vol. 60.

Śrī-Abhayākaraguptapāda. See Abhayākaragupta.

*Śrīcakrasaṃvara* (= *Saṃvara-tantra*).

Śrī Lakṣmī. *Pañcakrama-ṭīkā-kramārtha-prakāśikā*, PTT, Vol. 63.

*Śrī-Māyājāla-tantra*. As quoted in Candrakīrti's *Pradīpoddyotana*.

*Śrī-Paramādya-tantra*, PTT, Vol. 5.

Śrī Rāhuguptapāda. *Prakāśa-nāma-śrīhevajrasādhana*, PTT, Vol. 56.

*Śrī-Vajrahṛdayālaṃkāra-tantra*, PTT, Vol. 3.

*Śrī-Vajrajñānasamuccaya*, an Explanatory Tantra of the *Guhyasamāja*, PTT, Vol.3.

*Subhāṣita-saṃgraha*, ed. by Cecil Bendall, in *Le Muséon*, Nouvelle Série, Vol. 4-5, 1903-04.

*Tantraṭīkā*. See Nāgārjuna (tantric).

*Tattvasaṃgraha* (= *Sarvatathāgatatattvasaṃgraha-nāma-mahāyāna-, sūtra*), Toh. No. 479.

Thakur, Saraswati Goswāmi, tr., *Shri Brahma-Saṃhitā*, with commentary by Shri Shrila Jeeva Goswāmi Madras, 1958.

Thomas, Edward J. *The Life of Buddha, as Legend and History*, New York, 1952.

Tsoṅ-kha-pa. (A) on the *Guhyasamājatantra*:

,, *Don gsal ba* (= *Dpal gsaṅ ba ḥdus paḥi gnad kyi aon gsal ba*), Toh. No. 5290; PTT, Vol. 160.

,, *Mchan ḥgrel* or *Mchan bu* (= *Sgron ma gsal bar byed pa*), *ṭippani* on the *Pradipoddyotana*, Toh. No. 5282; PTT, Vol. 158.

,, *Mthaḥ gcod* (= *Rin po cheḥi myu gu*), Toh. No. 5284; PTT, Vol. 156.

,, *Dbaṅ gi don gyi de ñid rab tu gsal ba*, PTT, Vol. 160.

,, *Rnal ḥbyor dag paḥi rim pa*, Toh. No. 5303; PTT, Vol. 160.

(B) on Explanatory Tantras of the *Guhyasamājatantra*:

,, *Bźis źus* (= *Srog rtsol gyi de kho na ñid gsal ba*), commentary on *Caturdevīparipṛcchā*, Toh. No. 5285; PTT, Vol. 159.

,, *Rgyud bśad thabs kyi man ṅag gsal bar bstan pa*, commentary on *Vajrajñānasamuccaya*, Toh. No. 5286; PTT, Vol. 160.

(C) on the *Pañcakrama* of the *Guhyasamāja* cycle:

,, *Rim pa lṅa rab tu gsal baḥi sgron me* (frequently referred to in the present work as 'comm. on *Pañcakrama*'), Toh. No. 5302; PTT, Vols. 158-159.

,, *Rim lṅa gdan rdzogs kyi dmar khrid*, PTT, Vol. 159.

,, *Rdo rje bzlas paḥi rim pa zin bris*, Toh. No. 5292 (A).

(D) on other tantric matters:

Tsoṅ-kha-pa. *Dṅos grub kyi sñe ma*, exposition of Vajrayāna morality, PTT, Vol. 160.

,, *Yid ches gsum ldan*, commentary on *Nā-ro ḥi* chos drug, Toh. No. 5317; PTT, Vol. 161.

,, *Sṅags rim chen mo*, on stages of the tantric path, Toh. No. 5281; folio references to the Peking blockprint.

(E) non-tantric:

,, *Lam rim chen mo*, on stages of the path to enlightenment, Tashilunpo blockprint edition.

Tucci, Giuseppe, See Kamalaśīla.

,, *Indo-Tibetica*, 4 volumes, Rome, 1932-41.

,, "Some Glosses upon the Guhyasamāja," *Mélanges chinois et bouddhiques*, III, 1934-5.

,, *The Theory and Practice of the Maṇḍala*, London, 1961.

,, *Tibetan Painted Scrolls*, Rome, 1949; two vols. and portfolio of plates.

*Udayanavatsarājaparipṛcchā-nāma-parivarta*, Derge Kanjur, Dkon brtsegs, Ca, Toh. No. 73.

*Vairocanābhisaṃbodhi*. See *Mahāvairocana-sūtra*.

Vajragarbha. *Hevajratantra* commentary called *Piṇḍārtha-ṭikā*, Toh. No. 1180.

Vajrahāsa. *Tantrarāja-śrīguhyasamāja-ṭikā*, PTT, Vol. 66.

*Vajramālā*, an Explanatory Tantra of the *Guhyasamāja*, PTT, Vol.3.

*Vajraśekhara-mahāguhyayogatantra*, Toh. No. 480.

*Vajravidāraṇā-nāma-dhāraṇī*, Toh. No. 750.

*Vajroṣṇiṣatantra*. As quoted in the *Pradīpoddyotana*.

*Varāhopaniṣad*, in *Yoga Upaniṣads, The*, q.v.

Vasubandhu. *Abhidharmakośa*, with auto-commentary, tr. under title, *L'Abhidharmakośa de Vasubandhu*, by Louis de La Vallée Poussin, Paris, 1923-1931.

*Vimalaprabhā*, PTT, Vol. 46, See *Kālacakra-tantra*.

Vīra, Raghu, and Chandra, Lokesh. *A New Tibeto-Mongol Pantheon*, Part 12, New Delhi, 1967.

Vitapāda. *Mukhāgama-vṛtti*, PTT, Vol. 65.

,, *Muktitilaka-nāma-vyākhyāna*, PTT, Vol. 65.

,, *Yogasapta-nāma-caturabhiṣekaprakaraṇa* Toh. No. 1875.

Wayman, Alex. *Analysis of the Śrāvakabhūmi Manuscript*, Barkeley, Calif., 1961.

,, "Analysis of the Tantric Section of the Kanjur Correlated to Tanjur Exegesis," *Indo-Asian Stuaies*, Part 1, New Delhi, 1962.

,, "Buddhist Genesis and the Tantric Tradition," *Oriens Extremus* 9:1, Feb. 1962.

,, "Female Energy and Symbolism in the Buddhist Tantras," *History of Religions* 2:1, Summer 1962.

,, "The Five-fold Ritual Symbolism of Passion," *Studies of Esoteric Buddhism and Tantrism*, Koyasan, Japan, 1965.

,, "Notes on the Sanskrit Term Jñāna," *Journal of the American Oriental Society* 75:4, 1955.

,, "Contributions regarding the thirty-two characteristics of the Great Person," Liebenthal Festschrift, Visvabharati, 1957.

,, "The rules of debate according to Asaṅga," *Journal of the American Oriental Society*, 78:1, 1958.

,, "Concerning saṃdhā-bhāṣa / saṃdhi--bhāṣā/ saṃdhyā bhāṣā," *Mélanges d'indianisme à la mémoire du Louis Renou*, Paris, 1968.

,, "Totemic Beliefs in the Buddhist Tantras," *History of Religions* 1:1, 1961.

*The Buddhist Tantras*; *Light on Indo-Tibetan Esotericism*, New York, 1973.

,, See Mkhas-grub-rje.

Whitney, William Dwight. *Sanskrit Grammar, Cambridge*, Mass., 1941.

Woodroffe, John. *Introduction to Tantra Shastra*, Madras, 1952.

*Yoga Upaniṣads, The*, tr. by T.R. Srinivasa Ayyangar and ed. by G. Srinivasa Murti; Advar, 1952.

# INDEX

[GS: Guhyasamājatantra, nk: nidāna-kārikā].

A

E



F



G

K



L

M

R

T

U

## W



## Y